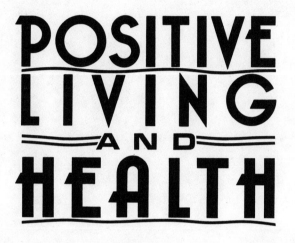

POSITIVE LIVING AND HEALTH

The Complete Guide to Brain/Body Healing & Mental Empowerment

By Mark Bricklin, Mark Golin, Deborah Grandinetti, and Alexis Lieberman of **PREVENTION** Magazine and the Center for Positive Living

FROM AN IDEA OF ROBERT RODALE

Rodale Press, Emmaus, Pennsylvania

The Center for Positive Living is a group within Rodale Press that researches and disseminates information on the nature and achievement of full human potential. This book is its charter publication.

～～～～～～～～～～～～～～～～～～～～～～～～～～～～～～

Cover and book design by Anita G. Patterson
Cover illustration by Greg Imhoff
Book layout by Darlene Schneck and Greg Imhoff
Illustrations by Willyum Rowe

If you have any questions or comments concerning this book, please write:
Rodale Press
Book Reader Service
33 East Minor Street
Emmaus, PA 18098

Library of Congress Cataloging-in-Publication Data

Positive living and health : the complete guide to brain/body healing and mental
    empowerment / by Mark Bricklin —[et al.] ; from an idea of Robert Rodale.
        p.   cm.
    Includes index.
    ISBN 0-87857-854-4   hardcover
    1. Health.   2. Mind and body.   3. Self-actualization (Psychology).
    I. Bricklin, Mark.   II. Rodale, Robert.   III. Rodale Press.
    RA776.5.P67 1990
    613–dc20
                                                                      89-10401
                                                                          CIP

Distributed in the book trade by St. Martin's Press

2 4 6 8 10 9 7 5 3 1   hardcover

To Rita, Julie, Myron, Barbara,
Judy, Sabrina, and Ardie

CONTENTS

~~~~~~

~~~~~~~~~~

CONTENTS

CONTENTS

CONTENTS

CONTENTS

The empires of the future are the empires of the mind.
—Winston Churchill

INTRODUCTION

THE POWER AND PHILOSOPHY OF POSITIVE LIVING

Have *you* ever had this experience?

You're going to bed and it's quite late. But tomorrow morning, you *have* to wake up early to catch the first flight to Chicago or attend a very special A.M. meeting.

So you set your alarm clock. And you tell yourself—*I've got to get up at 6:00. Absolutely.*

The next morning, you awake with a jolt. You fumble for the light, blink, and grab your clock. It says 5:58.

We asked ten people, and every one of them said *yes!* they'd had that very experience—often repeatedly.

But none of us had stopped and thought: *How did this happen?* What faculty in my brain kept accurate time all night long—and then did something to wake me up?

Do I have . . . *an alarm clock* in my brain?

It won't show up on an x-ray, but we say, *yes*—we do have alarm clocks in our brains.

And that's not all.

We have many mechanisms, powers, and talents that don't show up on our x-rays and blood tests, our report cards and résumés.

We have chemical factories that can boost our immune systems in an instant, to help defeat bacteria, viruses, and cancer. We have cameras that can record a scene in full detail and play it back flawlessly 30 years later. Mental theaters where we can rehearse and perfect upcoming scenes in our lives. Superchargers that can pour incredible amounts of energy into our muscles. A record player that will entertain us with any one of a thousand tunes on command. And a computer that will work out the solution to a personal prob-

1

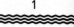

lem while we're working on a tan.

These hidden or unappreciated powers of mind are a major theme of this book. But they are more than a theme—they are a credo to us at the Center for Positive Living. For we believe we can learn to utilize these marvelous powers in our everyday lives—and make life seem not quite so "everyday" in the process.

The trick to doing that is not terribly complex. Remember when we wound the alarm clock, looked at the little alarm hand, and told ourselves we *had* to get up at 6:00 A.M.? In that one simple act, we (*a*) told ourselves that something important was about to happen, (*b*) went through a little ritual, and (*c*) branded into our minds an image of the successful outcome. Our brain listened, because we were "talking its language."

In this book, we will attempt to show you how to elicit the full powers of your brain by talking its language. (One of the things you'll learn, by the way, is that giving yourself a *visual* image—like staring at the "6" on an alarm clock—is probably the best way to communicate with these powers.)

Another credo and central belief of this book is that the mind and body are a unity.

That will strike some of you as obvious. But consider for a moment the word "body." What do you think of? Your heart and pancreas, things like that? And now consider the word "mind." What does that suggest? Your thoughts, probably. And often we use these words as if they referred to distinct entities. My body, we may tell someone, is perfectly healthy. But my mind is a mess.

In fact, there is no commonly used word that quickly gives us a picture of our whole selves—thoughts, brain, heart, and pancreas all as one. We are forced to use terms like *brain/body interactions,* or *the mind/body connection.*

The notion that thoughts are a product of a physical organ (the brain), just as much as estrogen is a product of the ovaries, and that both these products then interact with all other parts of our selves, is . . . well, a tad strange. Almost counterintuitive. How can our *thoughts* exist in the same dimension as estrogen, testosterone, bones, and gristle?

We'll try to answer with a picture. You already know why. Imagine this scene—which you have probably experienced.

You're at a large public gathering. A party, let's say. Suddenly you see someone you haven't laid eyes on in years. You haven't even thought about them for ages. But there they are, across the room. *It's the person you once loved and yearned for with the deepest of passions.* Instantly, you feel your eyes widen. An electric kind of chill goes through you. Your heart races. Your skin goes goose bump, your throat dry, your knees weak, and your ears deaf to the person talking to you.

All in one second.

Ever experience something like that? Let's play it back in slow mo.

First, your eyes (which we think of as purely physical) lighted upon a face. Now, it so happens—though you may not know this—that the brain has a positively phenomenal power to remember faces, far more powerful than our ability to remember almost anything else. In an instant, we picked that face out of a crowd and in another instant dived into deep memory (where legions of faces are stored) to give it a positive identity. In another instant, a powerful emotional memory was accessed, which combined almost explosively with your visual perception. And the shock waves raced throughout the body, causing half a dozen or more distinct physical changes from your eyes to your knees.

And all in one second.

If that is not one perfectly unified system, what is?

Today's new science tells us that these instantaneous communications between brain, nerves, muscles, blood — the works — are not just occasional lightning bolts. The active connection goes on every minute. Every second. With every thought, feeling, and attitude.

We are, literally, what we think.

Research tells us more. It tells us that to the extent our thoughts and attitudes are *negative,* we may be sending messages to every part of our body that encourage fatigue and illness. To the extent they are *positive,* we are sending messages that encourage energy and health.

Thoughts, it turns out, are very much like electrical hormones.

The details are in this book. But we want to emphasize here that you shouldn't think of this as something terribly mystical. The brain, after all, is the king of the body and all its organs. So it is just as natural for the electrical impulses (or thoughts) from our brain to influence our total health as it is for the heartbeat to affect respiration and blood pressure. Maybe more natural. Because the heart is a prince; the brain, king.

Our Ten Positive Instincts

The third theme of this book is that our brains are haunted . . . enchanted . . . choose the word you like best . . . by impulses and desires of which we understand but little.

"Instincts" is not quite the right word, technically. "Instinctual needs" better suggests what we're talking about. But let's call them instincts anyway.

We believe people have at least ten positive instincts that need to be satisfied if we are to approach our greatest potential for health, happiness, and productivity.

Some years ago, Swedish scientists conducted a most unusual study. In an effort to discover the underlying causes of health and illness, they entered the homes of hundreds of people and studied them in their "natural surroundings." Studying people only in medical clinics, they felt, failed to take into account much of their daily lives.

First, they recorded how often each person in each living unit had been ill. Then they measured the precise size of each room in every home or apartment. They noted how many people lived there. They tossed income levels into the calculation, and a lot more. They had a hunch, it seemed, that people living in the most crowded quarters, with the least privacy, would have the highest stress levels and therefore the greatest incidence of illness.

But that hunch didn't pan out. In fact, almost nothing did. No matter how many times they pushed the data through their computer, they couldn't correlate the number of days of illness with any factors the sociologists on the team thought were important.

They hit the answer on one last computer run. The one and only thing that could statistically predict illness was how each person answered a question about whether or not they had a certain . . . *feel-*

4

ing. That feeling was *trivsel.*

Unfortunately, there is no word in the English language which exactly translates *trivsel.* The closest we can come is the phrase "a sense of thriving." "Happy" doesn't quite say it, and neither does "content." Put all three together and what you get is a purely subjective sense of well-being, of, well . . . *thriving,* like a plant that's in just the right place, getting everything it needs to grow, bloom, and express its full potential.

That *trivsel* feeling, we think, is the product of many satisfied instincts.

Here are ten we think are important. Though we all vary somewhat in our need to have them satisfied, each of them deserves attention. They enrich our lives at least as much as, and probably more than, many of the materialistic things we strive for. And more perhaps, even than wonderful accomplishments.

1. The Instinct for Love and Friendship

The human brain is wired for a party line. We've already mentioned our unusual capacity to store and retrieve huge numbers of facial images from memory at a speed that is so fast it can scarcely be measured. But that is only one clue to our intensely social nature.

Researchers tell us that warm, supportive human relationships are perhaps the strongest single psychological predictors of resistance to illness and premature death. A loving relationship to a spouse is the most important of all. But every good friend is like a dose of good medicine.

In *Positive Living and Health,* we'll suggest some ways of deepening and widening your social life, without getting too preachy about it. For most of us, the roadblock is nothing more substantial than not taking the time or making the effort to connect with other people. We get caught up in our little routines, our jobs, and before you know it, we're spending only a few minutes a day communicating with our spouses, and even less with people who could be great friends.

To all you super-busy people, we say: plan on love. Plan on friendship. Plan *time,* even a *place* for them. It won't steal any of your energy, or your productive time. Rather, it will enhance both.

"Human relationships," says Mister Rogers, "are the most important thing in life." That's good enough authority for us.

2. The Instinct to Group Together

Very much related to love and friendship, this instinct finds expression in the amazing profusion of our clubs. Consider for a moment the Optimists, Rotarians, Masons, Knights of Columbus, Owls, Lions, and Moose, not to mention Ralph Cramden's famous Raccoon Lodge. Throw in a couple million fraternities, sororities, softball teams, bowling leagues, rod and gun clubs, scout troops, and churches and you begin to get an idea of the insatiable human instinct to join together with other like-minded folks.

This is no trivial instinct, either. It's easy to imagine that in the earliest days of human existence, individuals who felt no special urge to band together with others often simply perished. Their I'll-go-my-own-way genes were never added to mankind's heritage.

Even today, though, there is a practical aspect to joining up. Sometimes, as with athletic or charitable clubs, there is a meaningful product of the joint effort. But in every case, there is that extra opportunity to make friends and extend the circle of familiar faces and warm smiles that does us so much good.

But let's remember one thing. When the group you belong to defines itself by preaching contempt or outright hatred for another group, the positive energy turns negative. And there can be hell to pay. Literally. Most of the wars in our history were caused or inflamed by just such feelings. Most of the armed conflict we see *right now* stems from the same cause.

Clearly, this group identity instinct can get out of hand. And not just overseas. Fights at high school football games, racial incidents, even some of the name calling in political contests all remind us that we need to keep this powerful instinct purely positive.

3. The Nurturing Instinct

The mere sight of an infant gives many of us a sudden urge to cuddle it. Seeing a child in real distress may almost automatically mobilize us into swift action. Here we come close to a true instinct, one we share with many animals.

Beyond that, however, many people have a strong instinctual need to nurture other people—people of any age—who are suffering. Maybe they're seriously ill. Maybe they're just sad or confused. Maybe there's nothing wrong with them at all— they just look like they could use some encouragement, or a bowl of chicken soup.

If you feel such urges, express them. Some do it by simply sharing health information with their family and friends. Others volunteer as Big Sisters or Big Brothers,

or companions for the ill or infirm. Some do it by caring for pets.

The expression of the nurturing instinct can bring powerful benefits to the giver, as well as receiver.

4. The Instinct to Touch and Be Touched

Some years ago, an unusual experiment was conducted in a university library. As they left the library, students were stopped and asked how satisfied they were with the service they'd received. What the students didn't know was that the study wasn't of the library—it was of *touch.*

The library clerk had received special instructions that half the people checking out were to have their hands touched as they got back their cards. Touched just lightly, almost imperceptibly. But however casual, even meaningless, this contact may have seemed, the researchers found that the students who had been touched had much higher opinions of library service than those who weren't touched.

Many years ago, a famous experiment in a home for foundling children proved that children who were touched and held by nurses grew better and resisted illness better than children who weren't. Recently, this same principle has been found to apply just as well to very small premature babies kept in hospital nurseries. (In some nurseries today, the preemies also get to hear New Age music—aural touch.)

It's a long way from a casual finger touch or gentle cuddling to a full-force, muscle-mashing massage, but we do love them, don't we? Even if our muscles aren't particularly stiff. From the moment the massage therapist lays hands on us to the final feathery stroke, most of us find it an experience of pure bliss. But why?

Touch, we think—for adults as well as tiny babies—is one of the most powerful channels of human communication open to us. *Communication* is the key word. Try massaging your own arm or neck. Feels pretty good— but *blissful?* Hardly.

Likewise, a massage from an indifferent or distracted masseur is completely unsatisfying. The joy of a massage comes largely from the immediate physical knowledge that another person is totally devoting their energy and thoughts to making you feel wonderful. Even if they *are* being paid, it doesn't change the intent—or the result.

Our suggestions: express yourself with touch. Explore the good that exchanging highly attentive massages can do for your relationship with a spouse, child, or friend. Learn to give and receive hugs and kisses more freely.

There are many ways to communicate, but touch is the one that talks the brain's native language.

5. The Instinct for Art

Dancing, you might think, is a rather strange ritual, like yoga, or the Changing of the Guard. But anthropologists report that virtually every society and tiny tribe in the world dances. Every society makes music, sings, performs dramas. And every society goes to great lengths to adorn their bodies with jewelry, hair styles, and clothing they consider beautiful.

The love of art and beauty is not, as we might suppose, a kind of luxury invented by wealthy, developed nations. It's in the genes, right along with our love of friends, human touch, and other positive instincts.

How it got there is not terribly clear. Might there be some survival value to group singing and dancing—bonding people together? Perhaps. But what is the survival value of making beautiful bracelets, of painting on cave walls or chapel ceilings, of staring in wonderment at a beautiful sunset?

And how can we explain the *immediacy* of our response to something as abstract as a pattern of notes, of lines, colors, or words? And how can a mere pattern of musical tones produce a thrill and pleasure in us as powerful as that from a loving caress?

Perhaps all this is the human equivalent of bird songs and brilliant plumage, of coyote howls and whale songs.

We simply don't know the answer.

But we do know that the impulse to make and appreciate things of beauty is an incredibly strong human instinct. More to the point, participating in either half of the equation brings joy and contentment like few other pursuits.

Speaking of participating, remember this: All of today's schools of art and music, all the creative writing classes, have not increased by one iota the number of great works of art, compared to those produced in earlier ages, when such institutions scarcely existed. Art, in other words, does not come from official training—from rules, professors, or critics. It comes from talent, desire, and personal application. Which means none of us should be discouraged by a lack of formal training.

Art is open to all of us. And, even if you can't get it together to create art yourself, you can develop your talent to enjoy *La Boheme* or *La Bamba* as much as any great artist who ever lived.

6. The Instinct to Play

"Johnny plays well with his peers." That comment on a report card may not sound as impressive as an "A" in math. But when Johnny is 40 years old, his ability to "play" may turn out to be more important than his skill at multiplication.

A well-developed instinct to give way to free-ranging imagination, and interact easily with others engaged in the same process, is today considered a premium talent by management gurus.

Games are a quick way to get us past routine, a harmless way to glimpse possibilities inherent in change.

Beyond its practical value, play can act as a kind of garbage disposal for psychological apple cores. Too often, though, this play is rather passive. Watching TV, playing the slots, cruising the mall, that sort of thing.

Take a lesson from Johnny in the playground of his childhood and adulthood. Playing with others brings more fun, more benefits.

Vacations should be playful, too, not just indolent. You're never too old to enjoy a good hour of beachcombing or snorkeling. More and more resorts are offering the opportunity to go off on a little miniadventure. Go for it. You, too, can get an "A" in play.

7. The Instinctive Love of Nature

Recuperating hospital patients, a study has shown, get better faster and can be discharged sooner, if the room they're in has a window looking out on trees.

Nature is another one of those things that speaks the brain's language.

Ask yourself: Of all the beautiful things I've seen, which do I remember most vividly? Our own answer: Yosemite's Half Dome, the Swiss Alps, the redwoods of California, the turquoise water of the Carribbean and the stunning tropical fish you can see through your mask. And yours?

Yes, Notre Dame is magnificent, and so are many paintings. But they don't do to us what even a simple scene of natural beauty can do.

Given the choice, even the most sophisticated of us would rather have a large window looking out on a snow-peaked mountain than a million-dollar mural hanging on the wall.

A glimpse of nature at its finest is like a glimpse of a wonderful, faraway homeland.

It needn't take a mountain to elicit that response. A few houseplants will do it. Some shrubs and flowers in the backyard. A crescent moon . . . a rainbow . . . a tree draped in snow . . . a cardinal at the feeding station . . . a vast V-squadron of geese flying overhead . . . even a small babbling brook or a bunny.

The love of natural beauty is a cousin of the instincts to seek out friends and group identity. Nature often seems like a friend, and we as living creatures are part of her big family.

Besides enjoying nature, we should protect and even nurture it as well. The instinct is there; let it work.

8. The Instinct for Stimulation

Laboratory mice kept in a clean but dreadfully boring environment will not develop as many neurons in their brains as mice brought up in a pen that invites them to burrow, play, and explore.

Bored mice also eat too much. For kicks, evidently.

Now, as you will read within, scientists say that the brain of a bored human being will cause sleep disturbances, and even create physical problems—apparently because *anything* is better than boredom.

So, if we find ourselves getting a bit fat, dumb, and cranky for no apparent reason, we might ask the inevitable question: Are we bored silly?

Could be. Even when our lives are heaped with big piles of responsibilities, and there doesn't seem to be a minute to spare for something new. Keeping busy is one of life's best tonics. But without *some* novelty, *some* surprises, even Mr. Big Executive can turn into nothing more than a hyperactive sleepwalker.

If nothing else, you will find in this book a host of ideas that can bring that regenerating freshness back into your life. And if you say you haven't had a minute to spare for years, we say you probably need it all the more.

9. The Instinct for Altruism

For many years there was a fashionable notion that human beings are first and last selfish. Survival of the fittest. The law of the jungle. Kill or be killed. From a biological point of view, the purpose of life was seen as a struggle to reproduce and thereby pass on the genetic material you possess to the next generation. And after countless generations of such struggle, we've become a race of tough guys.

Now, some researchers who study human behavior are convinced that's only

part of the story. The other is the instinct for altruism.

Let's imagine for a moment that we're primitive people in a primitive land. Life is harsh, food scarce. Powerful instincts drive us to find food, and keep an eye out for danger.

But now, let's say I decide to share my food with you. Or I alert you to danger. I pull you out of a ravine. When I do that, when I act altruistically, two things happen.

First, you're grateful to me. You think: This guy is helping me. So I should help him, too, to make sure he can keep on helping me.

Second, since we live in the same group or clan, it's likely that we actually share a lot of genes. Maybe you're my aunt, my nephew, my second cousin. So when I protect you, I'm actually protecting a great deal of genetic material that is identical to mine. In both ways, altruism actually helps the biological imperative to keep your genes moving on down the line.

Now imagine a large group of people with scarcely any altruistic traits. How long do you think they could survive? Their purely selfish genes would sink into the mud after they'd killed each other off fighting over the carcass of a water buffalo.

So, altruism is not something alien we have to learn, like table manners. It's a positive instinct, wired into the brain cortex along with everything else.

10. The Instinct for Meaning and Purpose

It is entirely possible that the human brain is constructed in such a way as to demand to know why it even exists.

Perceiving *patterns* of events, rather than sheer masses of data from our sense organs, is something familiar to all of us. We quickly take in a scene that includes thousands of people anywhere from 1 foot to hundreds of feet away from us, all sorts of signs, lights, noises, and smells, and exclaim: *Touchdown!*

Instead of chaos, we see artistry. We see victory in the making. In other words: meaning and purpose.

We do this all through our lives, slicing away extraneous data to quickly find the underlying significance of events as it applies to us.

If we *didn't* treat the details of reality that way, we'd soon become overwhelmed, confused, disoriented, anxious, fatigued— and eventually insane.

But does there come a time when the brain begins to consider all the various *patterns* it's exposed to, all the touchdowns and fumbles of our whole lives, and suddenly ask: *What's the score?* In fact, *What game are we playing?*

We think that it does.

And if it doesn't get an answer, we can slowly become overwhelmed, confused, disoriented, anxious, fatigued, and mentally disturbed.

Interesting fact: Virtually every society in the world has religious or spiritual beliefs. No matter how different they may seem at first glance, they all offer grand explanations of why things are the way they are. And they tell the individual exactly what he or she must do to assume a proper place in the great scheme of things.

Some would say this speaks of an instinctual need for God, or spiritual beliefs.

In any case, social scientists say that people who attend church or synagogue live longer than people who don't. And that people who actively participate in groups devoted to a purpose greater than their own lives enjoy the same benefit.

For a look at the opposite end of the scale, consider the aborigines of Australia. The European settlers and their diseases wreaked havoc on these people. But Australian sociologists say the most devastating blow of all to aboriginal culture was the white man's fencing in of their "dream trails." The ritual walking of these sacred trails was an ancient and crucial part of aboriginal spiritual beliefs. Denied access to them, their lives and their culture literally disintegrated.

All of us, to some extent, have our own "dream trails." And sometimes we find ourselves fenced off from following them. We may even—unknowingly—erect those fences ourselves. Fences of indifference. Of cynicism. Of materialistic minutia.

But you can tear down those fences. You can even blaze new trails.

Meaning, purpose, is something that needs to be regenerated from time to time if it is to regenerate us in turn.

One good way to find—or create—that sense of meaning in life is to give the fullest possible expression to the ten positive instincts we've described here. When there is intimacy and friendship, nurturance, altruism, beauty, and all the rest flowing into your life, that sense of high meaning comes more easily.

Mark Bricklin and Mark Golin

BOOST YOUR BRAINPOWER

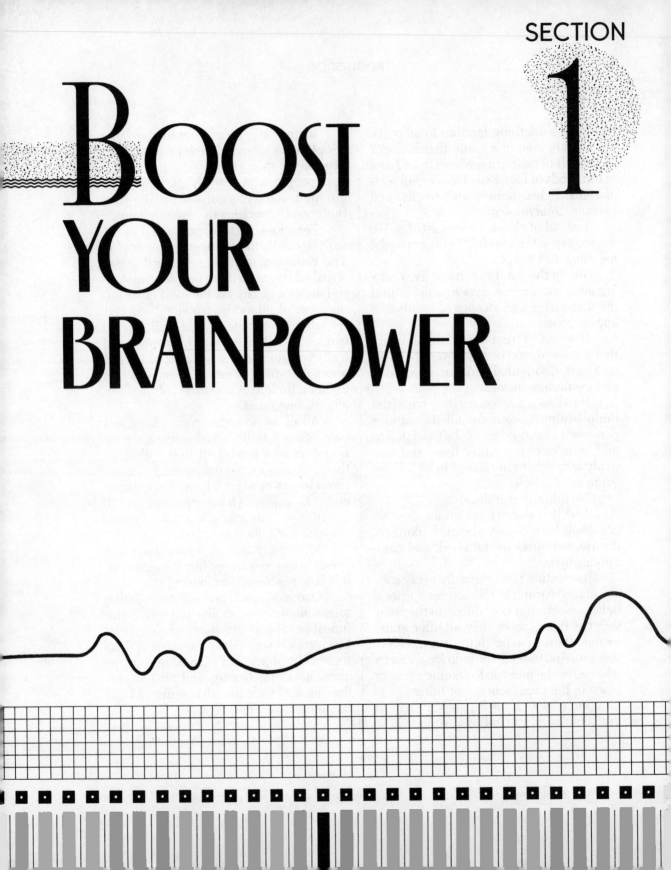

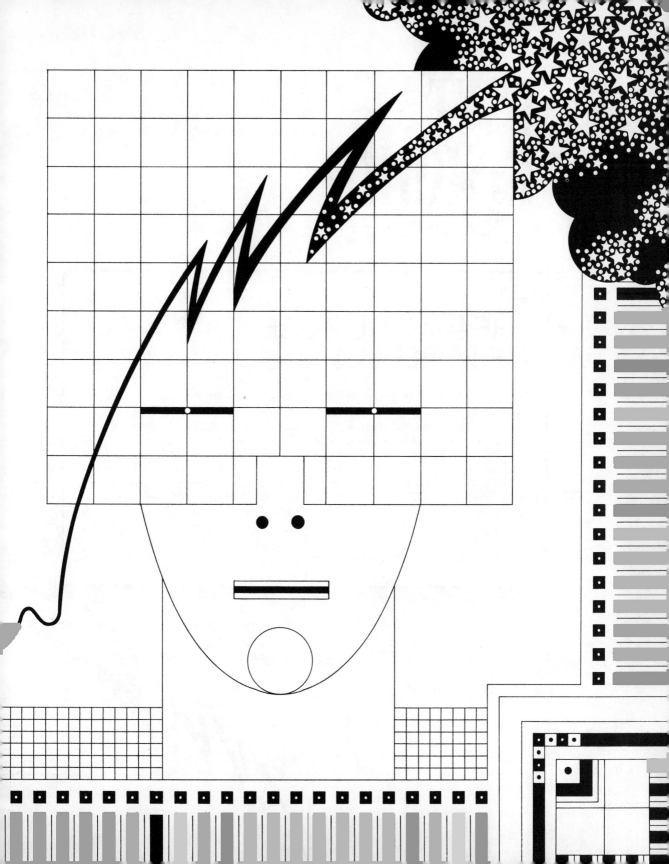

INSTANT INSIGHTS

THE PAINFUL PRICE OF BOREDOM

When it comes to boredom, your own brain can turn into your biggest enemy. The brain hates boredom so much that it will do just about anything to provide itself with the thrill of challenge, says Dr. Augustin de la Pena, professor of psychophysiology at the University of Texas. And that can include inflicting pain on the body.

In its quest for stimulation, the bored brain will first increase the level of REM (rapid eye movement) sleep so that dream capacity is boosted. If that doesn't do the trick, the brain will then increase physical restlessness, which may take the shape of impulsive behavior or workaholism, among other things. Finally, in a last-ditch effort to change the circumstances and provide itself with a new challenge, the brain will even create physical problems such as back pain, high blood pressure, eating disorders, and a host of other ailments.

EXTROVERTS EXCEL WITH COFFEE

Coffee can boost the ability to perform complex mental tasks provided you have the right personality type.

Extroverted, impulsive people are aided by a morning shot of caffeine, according to new research. Thoughtful introverts, on the other hand, are hindered by it. Apparently, coffee "overstimulates" the introverts, who like taking their time making a decision. On simple tasks, however, caffeine boosts the performance of both types. So, if you're faced with simple tasks, go ahead and take that shot of java. If you've got a complex job to perform, think twice.

COLDS AND FLU: DIFFERENT BUT DEBILITATING MENTAL EFFECTS

Whether you've got a cold or the flu seems to make little difference. You still feel rotten. But a team of British and American researchers has found that not only do these fairly minor illnesses reduce mental performance, the way they do it makes a world of difference to your brain.

If your job requires good hand/eye coordination, a cold can make you a klutz. But if what you rely on is a high degree of visual concentration, forget it when the flu hits.

The differences don't stop there. Colds only seem to affect performance while the illness displays all its physical symptoms. With the flu, mental impairment can begin in the subclinical stage, before most of the major symptoms even surface.

One thing colds and the flu do share is this: While they both show the most overt physical symptoms in the morning, the greatest mental impairment occurs in the afternoon. So the tip is, if you've got a cold or the flu, take care of any mental tasks in the morning, even though you may physically feel at your worst.

SLEEPLESS NIGHTS, MINDLESS DAZE

If you find yourself counting sheep all night and welcoming in the dawn without a bit of shut-eye, you can also count on having only half of your mental powers to carry you through the next day, according to recent research from Great Britain. Tests conducted by Dr. James A. Horne, psychophysiologist, seem to show that spontaneity, flexibility, and originality in our thought processes can be seriously undermined by as little as one sleepless night.

Why? Because, Dr. Horne believes, one of the primary functions of sleep is to repair the cerebral cortex from the wear and tear of conciousness.

But while these creative abilities, defined as divergent thinking by psychologists, are out the door, we can still count on our powers of convergent thinking. Convergent thinking is the opposite of creativity and spontaneity and is used in rote situations such as drawing up balance sheets, dealing with well-known, well-defined situations, or taking a true or false test. But even these abilities start to decline if we happen to go two sleepless nights in a row.

The tip? If tomorrow calls for some fast thinking, brainstorming, or unique decision making, get your z's if you want to be in A+ form.

SMART BRAINS ARE FUEL EFFICIENT

Just like any good car, an intelligent brain can go further with less fuel.

The brains of high scorers expend less energy than the brains of low scorers in a test of abstract intelligence, reports psychiatrist Richard Haier of the University of California at Irvine. Haier studied subjects' brains during the test and monitored the rates of glucose metabolization. His scans showed that intelligent brains shift into cruise control while less-smart thinkers need to keep their feet firmly planted on the gas pedal.

Haier speculates that the lower metabolic rate of high scorers could be the result of more efficient neural circuitry. "Although one might assume that a good performer's brain would 'work harder' than that of a subject who did poorly," Haier says, "the opposite is true." He believes that less-intelligent brains may have a higher metabolic rate due to greater anxiety.

Smoke on the Brain

Despite a widely held belief that the nicotine in cigarettes improves your ability to think, recent research conducted by Dr. George Spilich, chairman of the psychology department at Washington College in Chestertown, Maryland, suggests otherwise. While smokers do fine on very simple tasks after smoking a cigarette, in tasks requiring understanding and problem solving they bomb, doing consistently worse than nonsmokers and abstaining smokers. One more reason to stop.

Stay Sharp with Aerobics

Long-term aerobic excercise may help seniors keep mentally sharp, according to the Medical College of Pennsylvania.

A preliminary study there found that men age 60 and older who've exercised regularly for five or more years scored significantly higher than nonexercisers of the same age and intelligence on tests measuring mental quickness and recall.

Going to the Race Track? Leave Your IQ at Home

Intelligence may earn you high IQ scores, but when it comes to the race track and placing bets, you may be better letting your horse sense take over.

IQ may be as irrelevant in picking a winning horse as is the color of the jockey's silks, according to a study by psychologist Stephen Ceci of Cornell University and sociologist Jeffrey K. Liker of the University of Michigan. The two believe that traditional IQ tests may be incapable of measuring some kinds of intelligence.

The two studied a group of 30 bettors at a track in Delaware. The IQ of the group ranged from 80 to 130. But these numbers meant little in relation to the race track intelligence of the bettors. Low IQ subjects did just as well if not better than the higher IQ subjects. (The bettors chose winning horses between 33 and 93 percent of the time.)

The study also showed the same complex brain calculations used by all the bettors regardless of IQ. All 30 gamblers took as many as seven different variables—like track conditions—into consideration before placing their bets.

POWER STEERING
FOR THE BRAIN

Try pulling 6 feet of molding off a wall with your fingertips and you know why someone invented the crowbar. Try unparking your loaded van from a really tight spot and you appreciate power steering. Try getting someone's attention in a crowded room and you know at least one reason why they invented the smile. Leverage, in one form or another, is used by people every day, in almost every conceivable kind of task. Except one—thinking.

Sure, we live in the age of computers, but we're not talking about mere calculating; we're talking about real honest-to-goodness, 100-percent-natural-fiber *thinking*. The stuff you have to do lots of when your job is beginning to drive you crazy, when your relationship is turning into a nonrelationship, when you can't handle your kids, or find time to relax, when you're in a rut—and out of ideas. When what you need is a brainstorm and all you get is intellectual humidity.

It's a place we've all been before, and one where we'll all be again. As long as there is life, there will be lulls—those times when you get stuck and run out of ideas. The only question is, *How long will it last?*

Go see Liz Forrest, the dynamic 32-year-old owner of Innovation Labs in Stamford, Connecticut, and you may be in gear before the day is over. Forrest uses a new technique called, simply, EPS (effective problem solving) that employs a unique form of leverage to get you going again, not under *her* power, but under *yours*. All she does, in effect, is toss some cinders under your spinning wheels.

Forrest spends most of her time running Idea Labs for leading companies, from the Fortune 500 to philanthropic organizations. But the same techniques that have helped companies develop new products, new marketing strategies, and new ideas for growth can do at least as much for you.

What Do You Want?

Brenda, 29, was a junior sales executive working in the office of a small textile company. She enjoyed her work but worried about her future. Chances for promotion to a senior sales position seemed slim. In fact, the company she worked for wasn't doing well. To complicate things, Brenda very much wanted to get more involved in the design part of the industry, but she had no real background in design. She'd thought of moving to a different company, but that would probably entail moving out of state, and she rejected that because of her husband's job. She even thought of quitting and striking out on her own, but she rejected that possibility too, because without her steady income, the family would not be able to meet its mortgage payments.

"Sounds like a soap opera, I guess," Brenda laughed when she met Forrest. Which is part of the problem, Forrest explained. "Most problems start as one big mess. The first step is to sort out what is happening and come up with a simple statement of the major problem. The key to knowing your real problem is to identify the thing you most want in the situation and to isolate what keeps you from getting it." And that begins with the words *"I want."*

Write those words down on a piece of paper and complete the sentence with exactly what it is you want to happen. Brenda had to stop and ponder for a moment. What was the real payoff she was looking for? The *one* important goal? After a few minutes, she wrote, *"I want* to advance myself by getting involved with the design aspects of the apparel field."

Forrest then instructed Brenda to write another phrase under the first sentence beginning with the words *"But I."* Here's where you express the *one* major stumbling block that seems to be keeping you

from achieving your "I want" statement. Don't write down every last pebble in your path, just one big boulder.

Brenda wrote: *"But I* am currently in a sales position that does not involve me in design." The "But I" statement focuses on *you* (in this particular case, Brenda). Don't write down, "But Harry won't let me," because you have no control over Harry. All you can control are *your* actions. At this point, you have the heart of your problem right in front of you. It's also the point where EPS starts to be fun.

Take your pencil and cross out the phrase *"But I."* Over it, write *"And I."*

Why do that? Because, Forrest explains, to proceed further, you have to temporarily knock out of commission the "but" part of your mind. The part that's forever analyzing and criticizing, smothering new ideas in the cradle. So what you're left with is not so much a problem as a kind of paradox, or odd state of affairs. In Brenda's case, "I want to advance myself by getting involved with the design aspects of the apparel field . . . *and I* am currently in a sales position that does not involve me in design."

Notice how different the problem statement rings in the mind without that big, clunky, "but" in there—even though it's as true as the first statement.

Now, Try Wishful Thinking

Now it's time to go wild—almost literally. The next step in Forrest's technique is called, simply, *wishing*. Glance over your problem statement again. Then begin writing down absolutely outrageous,

18

absurdly impossible solutions in the form of wishes. Don't censor yourself—whatever wish pops into your brain, write it down. "Be playful," Forrest advises. "Use fantasy and free association. Keep the wishes coming!"

Do your wishing for as long as you like, but be sure to come up with at least 5. With any luck, you ought to get 10 or 15 real doozies.

Here are some that Brenda wrote down.

1. "*I wish* I could hypnotize Calvin Klein into giving me a job."

2. "*I wish* I could clone myself, send one of me to my job and the other of me to the Parsons School of Design in New York."

3. "*I wish* my husband would get a new job in a town where there were 500 textile mills."

4. "*I wish* my husband would win the lottery and buy me my own factory."

5. "*I wish* everyone I met thought I was a genius."

Give yourself magical powers, Forrest urges.

6. "*I wish* I could fly anywhere in the world on my lunch, buy all the best fabrics and clothing, and sell them from my garage on Saturday afternoons."

Think big, Forrest urges. Really *big:*

7. "*I wish* my eyes could see all over the world and my arms were so long I could reach out and be the first to grab up the exciting new designs to sell."

Wonderful! Now think *small—really* small.

8. "*I wish* I had 20,000 little designers and weavers working in my attic and I could choose what I wanted, make it big, and sell it."

At that point, Brenda felt she was just about through, but in glancing over her list of wishes, she free associated two more wishes from the first eight.

9. "*I wish* I could fly to New York City on my lunch and get orders for the clothes the elves in my attic were making."

10. "*I wish* my next-door neighbor was a fantastic designer and I could get orders for her on my lunch hours in New York City."

What are you supposed to do with all those crazy wishes? you ask.

Well, begin by reading them, Forrest suggests. Let each one bounce around in your head for a moment. Listen for any interesting reverberations. Then pick the one that appeals to you most, no matter how wild it may be.

Brenda chose her last wish: "I wish my next-door neighbor was a fantastic designer and I could get orders for her on my lunch hours in New York City." It had a kind of cozy feeling to it, and while it was pure dream stuff, it *sounded* like something she'd actually enjoy doing.

"Once you've selected your favorite wish," says Forrest, "ask yourself: *'What's the real point of this wish, and how could I translate it into a reality that I could actually work on?'*"

After a moment or two, Brenda decided that the point of her wish was that she didn't have to be a designer herself to get involved in design; she could use her sales ability in working closely with a designer.

Making Your Dreams Come True

But how? That takes us to the real climax of the EPS technique, transforming wishes into ideas. "An idea," Forrest explains, "is simply a more practical way of doing what the wish implies." Again we invoke a facilitating phrase. In this case, it's *"How about."*

Back to pencil and paper. Here's what Brenda wrote.

1. *"How about* teaming up with a first-rate designer and representing her work with the industry."

2. *"How about* advertising for designers who want representation, and asking my boss to let me work late four nights a week so I can go to New York the fifth day."

3. *"How about* finding new designers and asking my boss to let our regular salespeople try to sell their work."

The next step continues to bring us closer to reality. "In the *idea evaluation* stage," Forrest explains, "you study the action possibilities you've written down and choose your favorite. List the strong points or advantages of that idea. Any possibility that has at least three strong points means you may have found a viable new direction, something worth pursuing."

Brenda liked her second idea best, but modified it somewhat, so that she'd ask her boss to allow her to work only four days a week, with a proportionate cut in salary. As an added incentive, she'd tell him that she would give exclusive manufacturing contracts to the company for any orders she got.

Looking for New Directions

Brenda quickly found four strong points to this approach: It permitted her to become involved in choosing designs without actually creating them (which she felt unqualified to do); New York City was only a 2-hour drive from her New England home; her boss—because business was not good at the company—would probably welcome the chance to cut the payroll a little while creating an opportunity for new business; and finally, she'd be able to earn more money without endangering her present job.

What about negatives? Any real roadblocks left in the path you've charted? Brenda could see only two: It might be difficult to find good designers (but certainly not impossible), and her boss might refuse to cooperate. Neither negative seemed overwhelming.

So you, like Brenda, are now ready to write down your plan of action. That includes a strategy for overcoming what Forrest calls the troublesome parts in the idea.

Brenda's plan fell together quickly. First she would discuss the idea with her husband and get his support. Then she'd "trial balloon" the idea with her boss. If he was agreeable, she'd ask for the plan to go into effect only when and if she were able to line up some good designers and exciting samples.

What happens next is strictly up to Brenda (or you) and fate. EPS does not guarantee success stories—only new directions, new opportunities. And, eventually, new problems. "Each action you carry out will create a new situation, which may, in turn, lead you to want something new," says Forrest. "It's a never-ending process."

For all the muscle in EPS, it has a hidden strength that lies not so much in what it *does*, as in what it *doesn't* do. It does not offer a solution to all your problems all at once. Just one problem at a time.

Second, it must be a problem that you personally have control over. There is nothing you can do, for instance, to lower mortgage rates. All *you* can do—and all EPS can help you do—is create ideas for alternative financing, housing choices, ways to increase your income, and so on.

Finally, the opportunity for action that EPS helps you formulate does not presume to be the absolute *best* possible answer to your problem. All it is, really, is a way to get you moving in the direction you want to go.

Maureen, 33, did not see Liz Forrest professionally. They met socially, and Forrest introduced her to EPS. Maureen decided to use the technique on a personal problem. The problem, she felt, was her boyfriend. "No," said Forrest. "The problem is *you*—how you have to choose to handle your boyfriend's behavior."

"Ah so," said Maureen, who then wrote:

"*I want* to have a good and lasting relationship with my friend . . . *and I* am very concerned about his instability and drinking problem, enough to think of ending this relationship."

After making a number of wishes, Maureen chose this one as the most appealing: "*I wish* I were a great psychologist so I could counsel my boyfriend every day and lead him to overcome his self-defeating behavior."

The underlying point of that wish, she decided, was that her friend needed psychological help and that she should somehow encourage him to seek it.

In the "How about" step, Maureen came up with an idea that needed little further work. She would, she decided, give her friend the name of two good therapists she knew of, and tell him that if he did not see one of them, she didn't think the relationship could go on.

Maureen saw a rather intimidating negative to this approach: What if her boyfriend flatly refused? In that case, she would know that their relationship was not that important to her boyfriend, and certainly not worth pursuing.

How this plan turned out, we don't know . . . but suppose it didn't? Suppose Maureen chickened out?

"No catastrophe," Forrest says. "She could go back to the drawing board—literally—and write '*I want* to give my boyfriend an ultimatum . . . *and I* am afraid of the consequences.' Then she could work on a new approach that wouldn't seem like a dreadful ultimatum, but more like a strong suggestion, leaving an escape route for herself. Even that might not work, but it's probably better than to just go on worrying, feeling that you may be wasting your life, and not doing *anything*."

LEARN FOR YOUR LIFE

It's Wednesday—after work, after dinner, and after the news. Roger Peabody is feeling kind of bored and figures he'll do some reading before he turns in. He eyeballs a never-opened copy of *The Story of Philosophy* by Will Durant that his old school chum gave him for his birthday three years ago. Then he eyeballs the steamy potboiler he picked up at the A & P over the weekend. His eyes go back to the first book, then over to the second. Back and forth between the two books.

What's happening in Rog's brain? It goes something like this: "A book's just a book. I know reading is good for me, so why don't I just dive right into that book from the A & P. It'll do me good. Won't it?"

The answer is yes. Reading is good. But reading a book that will challenge your mind is better.

EQUATION 1:
Reading = Good.
Reading Challenging Books = Better.

Roger gets the point and he picks up ol' Will's hefty tome and starts to enhance his brainpower.

Whoa there, you say. Enhance his *brainpower?* We're talking a spot o' learning here, not a brain tune-up.

We're talking both, friend. "There have been studies suggesting that learning, in the sense of taking in new information and keeping your mind active by reading and learning new vocabulary, keeps you alert and sharpens your general intellectual capacities," says Dr. Arnold A. Lazarus, a distinguished professor in the graduate school of applied and professional psychology at Rutgers University.

This brain tune-up keeps your mind sharp and alert. But a good tune-up should also extend the life of the thing being tuned, don't you think? This one does that, too. "Learning won't necessarily keep you from getting Alzheimer's disease," says Dr. Frank Wilson, a neurologist with the Kaiser Permanente Medical Group in Walnut Creek, California, "but it will keep the brain alive, and it will stave off senility."

Roger looks up from a fascinating read about Plato, notices us talking about him, and gets indignant. "Hey! I'm not some Chevy, you know!"

By the time he gets done with that

A 5,000-YEAR-OLD BRAIN BOOSTER

"Short of getting a brain transplant, I think yogic techniques are the most effective way to boost your brainpower," says Dr. David Shannahoff-Khalsa, the president of the Khalsa Foundation for Medical Science in Del Mar, California.

He says that different patterns of breathing taught in Kundalini yoga "speak" to particular areas of the brain in much the same way computer programs cause computers to function in certain ways. This pattern, he claims, will expand and integrate your mind.

"Sit with your spine straight, your feet on the floor, and focus your eyes on the point where your nose and eyebrows meet. Next, keeping your eyes in that position, close your eyelids," says Dr. Shannahoff-Khalsa.

"Use your right thumb to cover your right nostril, rest your left hand in your lap, and inhale slowly through your left nostril. Then remove your thumb, place your right little finger over the end of your left nostril and exhale slowly through your right nostril. Then inhale through the right and exhale through the left. Repeat this alternating pattern. Do not hold your breath in once you've inhaled; begin to exhale immediately. Also, once you're done exhaling, inhale immediately.

"The more powerful the breath, the more powerful the effect, so start moderately at first. Continue for a maximum of 11 minutes (less if you like)."

book, he'll be more like a Rolls, but if he doesn't like being compared to a car, we can oblige. How about a piano?

When you tune up a piano, the notes get sweeter and the music can sound divine. The whole personality of the piano seems different—better. When you learn, *you* change the same way. "People who exercise their minds are more interesting than the ones who don't," says Dr. Lazarus. "They are the kind of people who, when a lull comes up in conversation, might say, 'Let me tell you what I've been thinking about.' They often think about things, and that not only makes them better dinner guests, but it also encourages people to be friends with them. That gives them self-confidence. And *that* enhances their personalities even more."

Not only does the personality of a tuned piano improve, but it's also easier to play, right? Well, it's easier to learn with a brain that's been learning, says Dr. Howard Lieberman, chief of neurosurgery at John F. Kennedy Memorial Hospital in Edison, New Jersey. "That's because the new knowledge gives you more to work with. More knowledge, and, from an anatomical point of view, more connections between your brain cells."

Those new connections, which add to the billions of connections already in place between millions of interconnected brain cells, represent new learning. Thoughts happen when the branches of brain cells, or neurons, connect up electrically, through chemicals called neurotransmitters. So, the more neural connections you have, the more thoughts, insights, and flashes of genius you can have. In short, you get brain potential, not by the pound, but by the neural connection.

What's happening in Roger's head now, you ask? Well, he's thinking, "Wow, I never knew *that* about Plato." Oh . . . sorry . . . you want to know what's happening in his brain.

As far as researchers know, neurons that were never connected before are getting it together for the first time. "It seems likely that new knowledge is stored in new connections between brain cells," says Dr. Jason Brandt, a neuropsychologist at Johns Hopkins University School of Medicine. "As you learn something, or as you practice something and get better at it, I believe permanent changes are taking place in the structure of the brain."

Some researchers even think that learning increases the actual size and complexity of your brain. They got the idea from a rat. Well, a lot of rats—lab rats. In the 1960s, scientists found that rats' brains actually got heavier if the animals were placed in large cages with other rats to play with and lots of toys to stimulate their minds. More recently, Dr. Marian C. Diamond, a neuroanatomist at the University of California at Berkeley, found that the brain tissue of rats doesn't start dying until the animals are the equivalent of 80 human years old, *if,* and only if, the animals keep their minds sharp and in use through play.

Now, there's no proof that learning affects human brains the way it does the rats' thinking caps, but Dr. Diamond has found some clues that make her suspect it just might. She came upon one of her relatively more amazing hints when she examined long-frozen brain tissue from Albert Einstein's cortex (the thinking, top area of the brain).

She found out that the great physicist had 73 percent more glial cells in a portion of the left hemisphere of his brain than found in other men. The glial cells aren't exactly brain cells themselves, but they exist primarily to nourish brain cells. Were there more glial cells because Einstein used his brain more than most of us, or was he so smart because he started out with more brain to work with? No one knows, but Dr. Diamond tends to lean slightly toward the learning-makes-the-mind side: "Einstein's brain might reflect the enhanced use of this tissue in the expression of his unusual conceptual powers," she says.

Look sharp. Roger's glial cells are pumping up.

"Hmm. Plato says that 'the state is what it is because the citizens are what they are.' I guess that means that a country is really just a bunch of people living together, and the way we act has an effect on the way the country is. Just like my family, here. When we're all in a bad mood, we're a mean family. But when we're nice . . ."

That's a lot of abstract thinking going on there. Roger is thinking about ideas that can't be seen or felt—that's abstract thought. "For the purpose of keeping the mind sharp, any abstract reasoning will help you," says Dr. Lazarus.

EQUATION 2:
Thought = Good.
Abstract Thought = Better.

Not only was it abstract thought, but Roger also just engaged in active learning. He involved himself in what he was reading by asking himself what it meant and by applying it to another situation, in this case, his family. "In general, the more active you are in dealing with material you are trying to learn, the more capable you are going to be of actually absorbing the information," says Dr. Keith Cicerone, clinical director of head trauma rehabilitation at the Johnson Rehabilition Institute in Edison, New Jersey.

Active means asking yourself questions, and coming up with brand new conclusions. If you are reading a newspaper article, for instance, Dr. Cicerone suggests you stop after each paragraph and try to guess what the next one will say. Then, compare your expectations with what is actually there. Or when you are learning to work some computer software, try to guess what the next step is before you check the instructions.

EQUATION 3:
Learning = Good.
Active Learning = Better.

So there's the goal: to learn about abstract ideas actively. Now for some examples.

EQUATION 4:
Learning Simple Math = Good.
Learning Logic = Better.
Learning Logic and Then Using It
** in Real Life = Best.**

EQUATION 5:
Learning English Vocabulary = Good.
Learning Vocabulary and Using It = Better.
Becoming Fluent in Another
** Language = Best.**

EQUATION 6:
Doing Jigsaw Puzzles = Good.
Doing Crossword Puzzles = Better.
Writing a Short Story = Best.

"For the purpose of sharpening your mental faculties, learning vocabulary in any language is better than learning simple mathematics, doing crossword puzzles is better than doing jigsaw puzzles, and building a carburetor is better than fixing one," says Dr. Lazarus.

"Why? The more vocabulary you have, the better you will be able to express abstract thoughts," he explains. "Crossword puzzles require a lot of abstract thought, concentration, and vocabulary, so they stimulate a lot of brain cells. Doing a crossword puzzle is quite a good mental workout, while I would think that a jigsaw puzzle is less of a workout because you are not doing as much abstract thinking. And building something requires visualization of the finished product, which is a type of abstract thought."

Roger puts down his book and looks around the room. He seems distracted. He runs his fingers through his hair and tugs at his shirt collar. He's having trouble concentrating. This is a real problem; it's important to concentrate if you're going to get anything out of learning. "The two key words are abstract thinking and concentration," says Dr. Lazarus. "If you can get one of them, that's good. If you can get both, that's even better."

If you have trouble concentrating, it may be because you are hungry, tired, or nervous. Those are pretty easy problems to cure: Eat something, take a nap, or calm down through exercise, meditation, or whatever else works for you.

Whatever you do, don't underestimate the negative power of stress, warns Dr. Herbert Benson, an associate professor of medicine at Harvard Medical School. "Excessive stress or anxiety can undercut

PARLEZ-VOUS SUGGESTOPEDIA?

Can you imagine effortlessly learning 1,000 foreign language words in a day, and remembering most of them weeks later? How about learning a semester's worth of Spanish in just two intensive weeks, and having fun doing it?

Foreign language students in Bulgaria, at Iowa State University, and at the University of Toronto can. They say they've experienced such rapid learning through an innovative new method of language learning called Suggestopedia.

Invented in Bulgaria in the 1960s, this technique for speeding up language learning is based in part on psychology, yoga, and relaxation methods. Suggestopedia also derives much of its framework from the idea of whole brain learning—the concept that the right and left hemispheres of the brain learn differently, and that to learn most effectively, one must teach to both halves.

Proponents of Suggestopedia say that typical language classes teach only to the left brain, which many researchers say is dominant, analytical, and in charge of our verbal skills. The idea of this technique is to excite both the left hemisphere and the supposedly more intuitive, feeling, and associative right hemisphere.

Part of the trick involves reducing tension and boosting involvement in the class by issuing false identities to the students (so they associate mistakes with the other identities); sitting in soft, padded chairs; and using drawing, acting, and conversation to involve all aspects of the intellect.

But the magic in Suggestopedia comes from its special learning concerts. The instructor leads the class through relaxing exercises and then, accompanied by slow baroque music (which some say has the same tempo as the human heartbeat), reads a dialogue in the foreign language while students either read along, with an English translation, or simply relax and absorb.

Since its phenomenal results have yet to be confirmed by a definitive research study, Suggestopedia isn't widely used in the United States. But the educators at one private high school in Silver Spring, Maryland, the Interlocking Curriculum School, have found the technique so effective that they've converted their entire program to use Suggestopedic methods.

your attempts to establish a new learning discipline or pursue an approach to effective problem solving or creativity," he says.

If you really have trouble concentrating, you can train yourself to associate concentration with one particular situation, says Dr. Lazarus. Whenever you want to concentrate, sit in one particular chair, in one particular room, with the lights set up just so. Then, if you find your concentration breaks, get out of the room. When you go back, try to concentrate again. If it doesn't work, leave. Go do something else. Pretty soon, you'll have an automatic reaction; when you're in the special chair, in the special room, you'll focus automatically.

Once you've got the concentration problem licked, learning can still be difficult, especially if you go about it the same old way you used to in school—as though you hate it and it's a chore. If you enjoy the learning process for itself, and don't worry about how well you're doing, says Dr. Benson, you'll learn quickly and painlessly.

Still need help? Try some super-learning techniques to supplement your efforts. We already discussed learning actively—that's one of them. So is taking a nap after learning. (Scientists have proven that a 1- to 2-hour nap at that point can increase your retention.) Here are a few more:

Put forth a regular effort—but take breaks. "Studies show that massed practice, which means that you go at it continually, is not as effective as distributed practice, which is when you have regular rest breaks," says Dr. Lazarus. "If you keep at the learning without a break, you will get fatigued, which will undermine your efforts. My own personal strategy for learning is to go at it for an hour, take a 20-minute break, and then study for another hour."

Taking much more than a 20-minute break in the middle of learning is probably counterproductive, he says, since studies show that, within 1 hour, as much as 20 percent of what you've learned will be lost. That will just make it harder to get back into the subject when your break is finished.

Recent studies show that the process of forgetting happens as the neural connections for that skill break down in the brain. To keep the brain cells connected

ADD UP TO A BETTER BRAIN

Do you remember telling your algebra or Latin teacher, "Why do I have to learn [insert whatever "useless" skill you were objecting to at the moment]? There isn't a chance in the world that I am ever, ever going to use it after this class is over."

Chances are good you still believe that you were right, too. But some psychologists now think that the abstract rules you learned in school have actually helped you solve everyday problems in your adult life.

This is hardly a new idea: Twenty-four centuries ago, Plato wrote, "Even the dull, if they have had arithmetical training . . . always become much quicker than they would otherwise have been." But formal mental discipline fell out of favor in the twentieth century because educators and philosophers stopped believing it worked.

Now it's coming back in style. Researchers recently proved that, if you teach a statistical rule and its use to people, they will apply it to everyday situations unrelated to the ones used to illustrate the rule. And that they'll solve the everyday problems better than before. This trend held for University of Michigan students and New Jersey homemakers alike, even with less than ½ hour of training, so it's likely that it would work for you, too.

(and also to keep your sanity), your best bet is to spend a short time learning every day or every other day, says Dr. Lazarus.

Talk yourself through rough spots. "We give our clients self-statements to talk themselves through difficult activities," says Dr. Cicerone. "One client was easily distracted and very fidgety. We suggested that whenever he started to get distracted, he say to himself, 'Now I have to stop thinking about other things and really try to think about the thing I want to learn.'

"Another client became frustrated easily. So now, when she gets upset, she says to herself, 'Okay, when I am frustrated, I have to stop and take deep breaths to calm down.' Another person tells himself, 'When I get confused, I will go back and see where I got lost.' "

By telling themselves to do things that will get them out of ruts, these people get their activity under control, says Dr. Cicerone. You may be able to do the same by verbalizing a problem of your own, along with its solution.

Learn something easy and something hard. "A good idea is to switch back and forth between things that call for a terrific amount of effort and things that come naturally to you," says Dr. Lazarus. "If you just do things that involve a big effort, you will get burned out. By succeeding at the easier things, you reinforce your ability to do the harder ones."

Using these tips can really help you learn. So it's only fair to warn you that, once you get good at whatever you're learning, you'll have to move on to bigger and more difficult subjects. "If you prac-

NOURISH YOUR NAPPING NOGGIN THE ARMY WAY

Beetle Bailey will be glad to hear that soldiers may soon learn complex battle maneuvers and operations skills while they sleep.

The National Research Council recently reported to the army that some unconventional learning techniques, like sleep learning, may just be worth a 21-gun salute, or at least a second look.

They found evidence that material presented to people when they are in the lighter stages of sleep seems to bolster their ability to remember the information when they are awake. This doesn't mean that learning happens while you're asleep, but it does suggest that listening to tapes of information as you fall asleep or as you wake up may be a super supplement to more conventional types of studying.

tice something, you will get better at it," says Dr. Lazarus. "But once you can do it in your sleep, the activity will no longer increase your mental capacities, though it can maintain them. To improve, you'll need something new and challenging."

WALKING:
THE SPORT OF GENIUSES

Had any good ideas lately?

Don't ask that question of a walker unless you've got a few spare hours to hear him out. Because it seems there's something about walking that does at least as much for your head as your feet.

That notion first struck me in school, when I read that the great English novelist Charles Dickens regularly walked every afternoon for hours at a clip. How did he have *time,* was my first reaction. But then I began to wonder if the unceasing energy and imagination that created *Pickwick Papers, Oliver Twist, A Christmas Carol, David Copperfield,* and all the rest may have been somehow released, or refined by his unceasing footwork.

Some time later, a well-read European psychologist counseled me to take long walks before sitting down to write. "Flaubert did that, you know," he said. "It relaxed him deeply, which permitted his creativity to flow without being crushed by his meticulous writing style. And don't they say," he added, "that his *Madame Bovary* is the finest realist novel ever written?"

"Oh, yes!" replied I, the English major, never having read the book.

It wasn't until I began walking simply because I *liked* it that I remembered all this. And a little research has led me to believe that these two great novelists are part of . . . well, a kind of club. A walking club of creative geniuses. Not just occasional ramblers, mind you, but passionate walkers.

Who else belongs to the club? Well, Aristotle, for instance, the most famous, perhaps, of all the Greek philosophers. Aristotle was so fond of walking while he reasoned that he is considered to have founded the School of Peripatetic (walking about) Philosophy.

Plato, his teacher, was also a great walker.

The great English romantic poet, William Wordsworth, is said to have walked 180,000 miles in his lifetime!

Thomas Jefferson, Ralph Waldo Emerson, Henry David Thoreau, Robert Louis Stevenson, Jane Austen, Walt Whitman, and Robert Frost are also members in good standing.

Bertrand Russell, the brilliant mathematician and social philosopher, said, "Unhappy businessmen, I am convinced, would increase their happiness more by walking 6 miles every day than by any conceivable change in philosophy." Russell himself was vigorous and creative until his death in 1970 at the age of 98.

I would like to say that Albert Einstein thought of E=mc² while he was walking but . . . well, he *could* have, because he too is a member.

So, you're not convinced that walking will loosen *your* genius muscles? Well, listen to this. There is now scientific research suggesting that walking does, in fact, stoke our brains. The phrase used by Dr. Robert E. Dustman is "increased cerebral metabolic activity." That's what he and his colleagues suspect they produced in a group of people aged 55 to 70 who took part in a four-month-long program of fast walking (and occasional slow jogging) on a treadmill, three times a week, an hour at a time. (The walkers had all been sedentary before beginning the program.)

Before-and-after measurements conducted at the neuropsychology research laboratory of the Veterans Administration Medical Center in Salt Lake City revealed that, compared to similar groups who either worked out for strength and flexibility, or who did no exercise at all, the aerobically trained walkers enjoyed much greater improvement in response time, visual organization, memory, and mental flexibility.

"We know," Dr. Dustman says, "that aerobic exercise makes the body able to carry more oxygen, and to better use the oxygen that it carries. We can assume that some of this extra oxygen goes to the brain, which is highly dependent on oxygen for its function. We can also assume that this additional oxygen is beneficial to brain activity. Certain neurotransmitters, for instance, which are involved in motor activity and thinking, depend on oxygen for their metabolism."

This bit of research—supported by the Veterans Administration—zeroed in on the thinking ability of "older" people. Whether or not people of *any* age who also haven't been getting aerobic exercise would enjoy identical benefits, can only be the subject of speculation.

But there is more to high-energy mental performance than specific abilities like memory. And other research suggests that walking *can* help—probably at any age.

One study put students who were in a state of severe anxiety about taking final exams through one of three different regimens: 20 minutes of moderate walking, 20 minutes of meditation, or a pill that was supposedly a tranquilizer but contained no active ingredient. The winner? Walking!

Another study had people between the ages of 25 and 61 participate in a ten-week program of regular walking and jogging. A battery of tests revealed that, compared to another group that didn't exercise, the walkers showed less anxiety, less tension, and less fatigue—while enjoying a greater sense of vigor.

It seems to me that all these changes are just what you need to get the most out of your native intelligence . . . which is why I'm a walker.

———■———

M. B.

THANKS FOR THE MEMORIES

Have you ever thought that you were going 'round the bend just because you momentarily couldn't remember where you put your car keys . . . or your car? As we get older, we're more prone to view innocent memory lapses such as these as harbingers of doom. Today we forgot where we put the keys, but tomorrow maybe we'll forget where we put the children. And then it's downhill from there as our memory slips away just when we need it most.

While this is a wonderfully tragic scenario, it just ain't true. We tend to gloat with pessimistic glee over our mnemonic bellyflops and scarcely give a nod to the majority of the time when our memory is in fine form. Every time we speak, read a book, or drive to the grocery store, we call upon information stored in our memory. As a matter of fact, there is so much of this everyday information stored in our memory that it would take a computer the size of Texas and 100 feet tall to hold the same amount.

So why is it that with all the mental horsepower we've got at our command, we still can't remember what's-his-name even though we met him yesterday? Is it true that as we put on a few extra years, we shed memory abilities, or does it just seem that way?

"The answer is yes and no," says Dr. Robin West, University of Florida psychologist and author of *Memory Fitness over Forty.* "As we grow older, we do experience a definite decline in our powers of attention and concentration, two very important memory tools. On the other hand, the rate at which we forget things we've already learned does not change with age."

Many of the everyday lapses we experience are more the fault of our poor memory techniques than of any physical problem with the brain, according to Dr. West. "Given the use of good techniques, practice, and daily mental stimulation, there's no reason why you can't improve your memory by 50 percent."

Interested? Then let's identify some of our common mnemonic faux pas and see what can be done about them.

Atten-Shun!

We can start by memorizing a little one-liner penned by English writer Samuel Johnson, "The art of memory is the art of attention." When we can't remember a piece of information, frequently it's because we never really paid enough attention to it in the first place. Since we didn't encode it firmly in our memory, it's no suprise that it's not there when we look for it. You're not going to remember where you set your keys because you were putting down the groceries, humming a tune, and wondering what to make for dinner. The keys never had a chance.

Taking the attention theme one step further, in 1890, psychologist William James wrote, "Habit diminishes the conscious attention with which our acts are performed." To put this ponderous statement into everyday clothes, try to remember the sign above the first gas station that you pass on the way to the grocery store or work. Don't feel bad if you can't. Even though you pass it every day, chances are you never really see it. "People commonly turn off their minds when they are performing habitual actions," says Dr. West. "When you are in an automatic-pilot mode, new information has no way of encoding itself in your mind."

How much time do you spend on automatic pilot? The longer we live, the more prone we are to establish habitual behavior patterns. When we were 15, every

day of the week contained a special feature. But by the time we reach a still youthful 30, we've fallen into such a consistent routine that we sort of sleepwalk through the day.

With this in mind, it's no wonder we can't remember what we did at this time last week. It would be like trying to remember something specific about the 3,981st oak tree you pass in a forest of oak trees. Strolling through the forest, you may look at the first couple trees you pass, but after a while their sameness turns off your interest and attention. But suppose you tied a bright yellow ribbon around that 1 tree?

It's exactly that concept that Dr. Curt Sandman put to good use in the treatment of Alzheimer's disease patients at the University of California. Forsaking the traditional medical approach to faltering memory, which encourages the patient to establish a daily routine, Dr. Sandman had his patients tie a metaphoric yellow ribbon around each day by performing some new and different activity. Dr. Sandman had each patient discuss and execute a significant activity with their spouses on a weekly basis. The events ranged from buying a new set of tires to arranging an exotic fruit-tasting picnic.

The results were striking. Two to five days later, 10 of the 13 patients recalled the day of the event four to five times better than a typical day and absolutely as well as their symptom-free spouses! When you put this phenomenon into a personal perspective, the results are not that suprising. Think back to the day you had a fender bender, were on the receiving end of a suprise party, or took a spur-of-the-moment drive to Atlantic City. That day is probably much more clearly etched in your memory than what you had for dinner the day before yesterday.

When you do something out of the ordinary, your automatic pilot is shut off. You start paying attention to actions, surroundings, and people, and by paying attention, you are encoding that information into your memory. According to Dr. Sandman, much age-related memory loss can be warded off if people seek activites that are different, and ideally, fun. "By throwing an enjoyable little wrench into your daily routines, you are not only getting yourself to pay attention, you are also providing the brain with much needed mental stimulation," he explains.

But let's face it. Schedules can get pretty tight. One adventure a week might be all you can fit in. How do we wean ourselves off the automatic pilot during the rest of the week? "While it's easy to remember the unusual, the challenge is to start paying attention to the everyday," says Dr. West. "To do this, you've got to practice the art of observation. By noticing special properties or features of commonplace items, you will have a better chance of committing them to memory."

Observation Equals Memory Conservation

Quick . . . what's on the back of a $20 bill? No need for shame if you don't know. You've probably *seen* the back of a double sawbuck about 500 times. But there is a difference between *seeing* and *observing*. Seeing something allows for a momentary and featureless experience. Observing something means paying attention to

detail — setting the object apart from other things in your mind and memory.

There are many ways to practice observation. In *Memory Fitness over Forty*, Dr. West suggests starting with a magazine photo of a person. Look at the photo and then close the magazine. List the features in the photo. What color were the eyes? What shape was the nose? What about hairstyle and clothing? Was there anything in the background? Having made a list, go back to the photo and study it for two details you missed. Then start again. Do this until you've managed to list every aspect down to the most minute.

Another way to practice observation during the day is to think of a common item that you see regularly. It could be a fountain pen, a building you walk by, or a tile floor. Before you actually come across the item again, ask yourself some questions about it. What is it made of? How many windows? What color? If you can't answer the questions immediately, take a moment when confronted with the object and look for answers. A good example is the $20 bill. If you've got a curious bone in your body (and didn't know the answer), by now you've hauled out your wallet to see for yourself. Having raised a question and then made an observation to answer it, chances are you will not forget the information too easily.

With practice, observation will become second nature. The way you look at things will change as you focus in on details. And the attention you pay to detail will make each object unique enough that it will stand out in your mind and be easily encoded into your memory.

Now you can apply your newfound powers of observation to your behavior. How many times have you left the house only to wonder 10 minutes later if you locked the front door? "To overcome an automatic-pilot behavior such as this, you need to either change the pattern of your action, or find something concerning this routine action that is new and unusual." says Dr. West.

As you lock the front door, for example, note the sound of the lawn mower coming from your neighbor's yard. Twenty minutes later, as you're driving along wondering whether you locked the door, you'll *remember* the lawn mower and then *remember* that you locked the door while listening to that sound. Or, you could focus yourself by changing your routine. If you're right handed, lock the door with your left hand. If you're ambidexterous, lock the door and then click your heels three times saying, "There's no place like home." Later, if you can't remember locking the door, you'll certainly remember the *Wizard of Oz* flashback and know you did your Dorothy imitation *after the door was locked.*

You're Only as Good as You Think You Are

With memory, as with most things, we are our own worst enemy. If you're saying to yourself with a heavy sigh, "Well, my memory just ain't what it should be," then to tell you the truth . . . it probably ain't.

"Lack of self-confidence in memory abilities can be a self-fulfilling prophecy," says Dr. West. "And I mean this in a very real way. A negative self-concept increases anxiety and depression about memory loss whether that loss is real or imagined."

If you don't think anxiety can be a mnemonic roadblock, then think about a

time when you were seriously anxious. How calm and orderly were your thoughts? Does "like a fox in a henhouse" describe the situation? For effective remembering, a clear mind and concentration are needed. These are two things you won't have if you're worrying about your memory. And if you think youngsters are any different, forget it. Test anxiety has sent many young scholars to the showers wondering what happened to their hard-earned knowledge.

"The first step to alleviating memory anxiety is to use a realistic yardstick when evaluating your own abilities," counsels Dr. West. "Many people tend to compare their current memory abilities with an image they have of themselves as a younger person. This is a no-win situation."

It's easy to fall into this trap. As students, we were veritable memory banks of overflowing bits of knowledge. Now it seems as if any scholarly undertaking is difficult. The obvious conclusion is that our memory is slipping. But if we look a little closer at this situation, some plausible reasons (having nothing to do with a failing memory) come out of hiding.

Lack of motivation is often a factor. It's amazing how fast we learn and commit information to memory when there's reward or punishment involved. As a student, you concentrated and memorized your little heart out because a test at the end of the week could make or break you. Be truthful, is your motivational level still the same? Once school is out, we rarely encounter information that has such an immediate do-or-die importance. So in this case, it's not a lack of memory but a lack of a reason to make your memory sweat a little bit.

Diminished effort is another reason why we often don't seem to measure up to

34

our former image. As a student, you probably spent half your life in the library stacks. When was the last time in recent years that you applied that same amount of dedicated effort toward learning and memorizing new information? Do you try studying a new language while cooking dinner, or scan a night class curriculum on the couch while Johnny Carson chats in the background?

"We tend to forget that it always took a lot of effort to commit information to memory," says Dr. West. "And as we get older we need to make an extra effort, giving ourselves every possible consideration to make up for diminishing powers of concentration and attention. Instead, we often give ourselves even less of a chance than when we were younger."

Anxiety, lack of effort, and unrealistic comparisons with past performance can magnify a poor self-concept to the point where we draw in the boundaries and refuse new challenges. "If you do not seek intellectual stimulation and use your memory abilities regularly, you *will* lose them," warns Dr. West. "The exact thing that worried you will come to pass."

If memory is a use-it-or-lose-it ability and lack of confidence is making you hold back, how do you turn the situation around? "The first thing to do is give credit where credit is due," advises Dr. West. "Congratulate yourself for memory successes and examine your failures for plausible explanations."

When you forget a person's name, for instance, don't suddenly start worrying about Alzheimer's. Instead, try to put the incident in true perspective. Weren't you always bad with names? If so, your memory isn't any worse than it ever was. Ask yourself if you were really paying atten-

tion when the person was introduced. If you were looking at something across the room then you didn't forget the name . . . you never learned it. Studying? If the information isn't sticking, assess your motivation level. How important to you is the information? And what about effort? Were you really cracking the books or just sort of window-shopping your way through the text? By questioning what seem to be memory lapses, you'll be amazed at how many of them have nothing to do with your memory.

Tricks of the Memory Trade

Attention, self-confidence, an intellectually stimulating environment, and motivation will get you far in the memory game. But there's nothing wrong with using a few proven memory-boosting techniques to give you more of an edge.

Memory and learning are not far apart, notes Dr. West in her book. When we learn, we take random information and arrange it in a manner that has meaning to us. As we concentrate, and note specific details, it becomes encoded in our memory. But many things we wish to remember, such as lists of items, phone numbers, dates, and random facts are difficult to organize into a cohesive whole because they have no order or inherent meaning. Rather than remembering one thing, which naturally flows into another, we try to remember many different pieces of information that have no connection. A better way — and the secret of most memory techniques — involves organizing small pieces of material into larger groups, giving the items a context we can understand,

and making the information unique in our own minds.

Rote Memory

While rote memorizing is the most commonly practiced of techniques, it is the least useful for committing information to long-term memory. Rote technique is simply repeating information over and over again. You do it when you look up a phone number in the yellow pages and then repeat it until you actually dial the number. "Rote repetition is effective for short-term tasks," says Dr. West. "But you'll find it very ineffective for long-term memory because it does not reorganize the information into a more convenient form. As soon as the repetition is interrupted, the information will be forgotten."

Giving Meaning to Nonmeaningful Material

Rice farmers from the African country of Liberia were given 20 words, divided into familiar categories, to memorize. Not only did they remember a rather poor 9-11 words the first time through, they improved very little with successive tests. However, when the words were incorporated into folk stories, the farmers showed amazing improvement.

Two factors were responsible. First, since the Liberian farmers' culture has a tradition of oral storytelling, the folk story was a more familiar and meaningful form of information to them than a random list of words could ever be. Familiarity and meaning increase memorability. Second, rather than memorizing 20 words, they only had to remember one story. By connecting the words to each other by way of

a plot, the first word provided clues to the second word, and so forth. That gave the farmers an edge in remembering the next word without any hints.

The same technique can be applied to many everyday items you might want to remember, starting with new words for your vocabulary. "Many times, it's hard to draw a line of understanding between a word and its meaning," says Dr. West. "You might be hard put to remember that the medical prefix 'blepharo' refers to the eyelids, because it provides no clues. But you can take the sound of the word and incorporate it into this sentence: I'd blink if I saw a *pharoah*. The sentence reminds you of the word and blink suggests eyelid."

To remember an address such as 1225 Turner Street, you might say to yourself, "I *turned* my life around on Christmas (12/25)." Say you want to remember the name "Sheider." Think of "shy deer." Can't seem to remember that there are 5,280 feet in a mile? Think of "5 tomatoes (5,2[to]8[ate]0[oe])."

While these may seem like make-work exercises that leave you with more to remember than before, they illustrate many of the necessary components of good memory. First, by thinking up a clever framework for the information, you are paying attention and concentrating. Second, you are making the information more familiar. One-two-two-five Turner Street means nothing whereas "I turned my life around on Christmas" does. Third, you are providing yourself with some mental stimulation.

Mental Imagery

Keeping in mind that attention and concentration are the first steps to memory enhancement, the next step is to find interesting ways to practice them. Creating a picture in your mind of what needs to be memorized is one way to make the process fun.

"Think of your mind as a camera," suggests University of Miami memory techniques instructor Elisabetta Ferrero. "If you're not concentrating, then the lens is out of focus. When your memory 'develops' the picture you took, it will be fuzzy and unreadable."

Ferrero suggests that you start by taking a clear picture. "If you need to remember to buy milk at the store, don't just picture a small carton for a few seconds. Make the image stick by infusing it with action and even absurdity. Try to clearly picture in your mind a purple cow kicking a big pail of milk all over a farmer. Give the picture a lot of detail so it's very real to you."

Make the picture large. Most of us tend to conceive mental images on a small scale. If we need eggs, we picture a single egg in our mind. "To really make that image stick, try to picture ten dozen eggs all smashed with their gooey yolks oozing across the kitchen floor," says Ferrero.

Interactive imagery takes this whole technique one step further. Suppose you have a grocery list to remember rather than just one item. In this case you want to create a mental picture in which all the items interact with each other. According to Dr. West, it's helpful to form an action sequence rather than just one picture. That way when you're at the store, you can just run the image like a video.

Let's try bread, milk, celery, pepper, apples, and cucumbers. Keep in mind, the more flamboyant the image, the better you'll remember it.

Walking through the woods you come to the bank of a white river of milk. To make your journey easier you decide to sail down the river and do so on a raft, which is a large slice of bread. The long, green steering oar you're using is actually an enormous celery stalk. The weather starts to turn bad and soon dense flakes of black snow (pepper) and huge red hailstones (apples) begin to fall. Things go from bad to worse as your bread raft sails out to a milk sea where an enemy submarine is waiting. It fires and you see a cucumber torpedo heading straight for you.

Let's leave the story hanging right there. You've read it, now close your eyes and try very hard to actually see yourself in it. Once you have, test yourself five days from now and see if you remember all six items by playing your mental video.

This technique can also be applied to other tasks such as remembering names. "When I want people to remember my name," says Dr. Robin West, "I have them picture a robin flying west. To connect the name to my person, I ask then to include my most memorable feature, long hair, into the image. The end result is a mental image of a robin flying west with long hair streaming behind it in the wind. When they see my long hair, it triggers the image that contains my name."

Association

When you connect a new piece of information to something you already know, you are using association. Say you are walking through midtown Manhattan. You turn onto Broadway, stop in the Winter Garden Theater, see "Cats," and on the way out meet a friend of a friend whose name is Clyde. Each piece of information is naturally associated with the one before it. Clyde, a new piece of information is attached to "Cats," which is attached to Winter Garden to Broadway to Manhattan. A year later, if you couldn't access Clyde's name directly from your memory, you could search under Broadway or "Cats" where the information might still be connected.

The following memory device utilizes the process of association with a second technique.

Peg system. With this technique we can memorize a list of ten or more items or chores by coupling the process of association with mental imagery. The peg system matches the numbers one through ten with objects that rhyme. Before you can use this system you must make and memorize a list. Let's make one up right now: 1 is the sun, 2 is a shoe, 3 is a tree, 4 is the floor, 5 is a hive, 6 is sticks, 7 is heaven, 8 is a gate, 9 is a vine, 10 is a hen.

Once you have committed this list to memory, you can tack onto it new lists of items that you need to remember. Just make a mental picture of each item interacting with one of the numbers. If you need to buy candles, put that under one. Think of the sun melting wax candles on a hot summer day. Also need to make a salad for dinner? Remember it under number two. Picture yourself tossing a salad in a huge shoe. Remember, the more ridiculous the image, the easier it will stick.

That's the imagery part of this technique. Association comes in when you go back into your memory for the list. Rather than trying to remember a stray image having to do with candles, you'll know that number one is the sun. This is the old information you memorized way back. An image of the sun then gives you an asso-ciative trigger for remembering the candles you wanted to buy.

Organization

While it is hardly a trick, organization is a priceless commodity when it comes to memory. Picture a fine meal including an appetizer, a large salad, and an entrée of filet mignon. The filet is the main point of the meal, but if you fill up on the appetizer and salad, you'll have no room for it. When memorizing information, the same thing can happen. You can fill up on unimportant details and end up forgetting key points. That's why you need to organize. What are the important points? Separate them from the fluff and apply yourself to them.

Dr. West suggests organizing and memorizing written material through a method she calls PQRST. The letters stand for preview, question, read, state, and test. "First you should preview the material by reading briefly and identifying the main points. Then, develop questions specifically targeted toward what you want to retain from the reading. Read the material carefully. State or repeat the central ideas and try to test yourself by answering your own questions. Follow all of these steps and you will remain focused on the information that is important for you to remember."

Retention

Okay. You've got a few memory techniques under your belt, but your status as a master of mnemonics is still one crucial step away. The techniques you've learned are a fine way to put information into a

38

storable form. Now you need to make sure you are able to truly retain that information and find it again when you need it.

As unglamorous as it sounds, rehearsal is a mainstay of retention. "But do not confuse rehearsal with rote repetition," cautions Dr. West. "Instead of just reading the information or repeating a list over and over again, make sure you include these steps: Review the strategy you applied. Rehearse your mnemonic. And rehearse your mnemonic with the information you learned."

This basically means repeating the whole process by which you developed your special mnemonic. Using the peg system we discussed, for example, 1 is the sun. Do candles still come to mind? If not, go back over the image, recreate it in your mind as if it were the first time. Rehearse recalling the image with 1 as the starting point. If it isn't working, come up with another image.

How you schedule your rehearsal can be very important. Tests conducted by Dr. Harry P. Bahrick of Ohio Wesleyan University seem to show that information is retained longer and better if practice sessions are distributed over a period of time rather than jammed into one long session or with only short intervals in between.

"There could be many reasons why this occurs," says Dr. West. "First, when you distribute practice over several days, you consciously or unconsciously rehearse in between. Overlearning can also be a factor. Each time you approach a new study session, you have some material retained from the last session. In the second session you overlearn the material retained from the first session and so on. This overlearning increases the likelihood that the information will be remembered."

Recall Strategies

You've utilized good memory technique. You've rehearsed the material. Now that your mind has a viselike grip on the information, how do you get it back out?

"If you've formed good mnemonics, then using the cues you developed should access the information with no problem," says Dr. West. "But there are some additional little advantage makers you can use to ensure good recall."

Pay attention to your mood and physical state, for example. It is often easier to recall information when you are in the same condition as when you learned it. When you're sad, other sad memories seem to come to the surface. Likewise, pain dredges up painful memories from the past. Obviously, it would be difficult to turn your body and mind on and off just to retrieve data you learned when you were in a particular mood. But there is a way around this. "Before sitting down to a learning task, try a few relaxation exercises," says Dr. West. "Later, before calling up the information for a test or speech, do those same exercises again so that your mental and physical state will be the same as when you learned it."

Tip-of-the-Tongue Syndrome

You've probably experienced it. That frustrating feeling that you know something but can't quite put your finger on it. What to do? Rather than hammering away at the question until you're half mad, work around it. If you can't remember the name of that great deli you went to in Philadelphia, try to remember other details about it. With whom did you eat the last time you were there? What did you order? This is the association process in reverse. As you go over other details of the deli you may find that the name is filed in connection with Irv, the guy you ate with. Think of Irv and then the name of the deli might just pop out.

After all is said and done, you may well be thinking to yourself, "This is an awful lot of trouble just to remember a few things here and there. Why bother?" Two good reasons. "Storing information in a rich, elaborate form is the secret of sharp recall," says psychologist Endel Tulving. The process of making information rich and elaborate is one of the finest ways to intellectually stimulate yourself.

Your mind needs this stimulation to stay sharp just as your heart needs aerobic exercise to stay strong. And you may find that tailoring information into sayings and images can be quite an entertaining way to stay in mental shape.

Second, if you don't exercise your memory, you will begin to lose it. There is little doubt on this count. Most of the time, the process can be reversed, but if you don't start now, it won't get any better.

Oh. There is a third reason. If you don't *remember* to lock your front door in the morning, you'll have no one to blame but yourself when your living room furniture is missing.

PASSIVE THINKING: THE POWERFUL ART OF INCUBATION

A couple months ago I was sitting in my office staring at a blank sheet of paper that should have had a story written on it. I knew what I wanted to write about, but it just refused to come out. After tugging at my stubborn brain for a couple of hours, I gave up, ate lunch, read the comics, and found an excuse to wander around the building. Late in the afternoon I came back to that same blank sheet of paper and within an hour there was a finished story smiling up at me. What happened?

Magic was my first hypothesis. Then I thought maybe aliens were secretly beaming ideas into my head from the moon. Faintly suspicious that I might be somewhat off the track, I called Eugene Raudsepp for some inside information.

"It sounds like you were experiencing a form of incubation," said Raudsepp, who is president of Princeton Creative Research and author of *How Creative Are You?* Incubation? Visions of hatching eggs were coming to mind. "Hatching ideas is more like it," replied Raudsepp. "Incuba-

tion is a process in which you cease activity on one process of thought and do something else for a while so that the solution to the first problem has time to take shape and reach maturity."

While incubation is something we've probably all used unconsciously, in recent years everyone, from musicians to corporate vice presidents, has been taking an interest in it. After all, taking a break to solve your problems is a nice way of getting things done. The question is, how does it work, and what exactly can we get from it?

"Currently there are several theories to explain what's happening," says Raudsepp. "On one side, there are the behavioral psychologists who feel that nothing is really occurring at all. By abandoning current trains of thought and starting fresh, you are only getting rid of unproductive ideas that are leading you nowhere."

But there are specialists in the field of creativity who believe that when you take a break from something you're working on, your mind continues to consider the problem even while you're doing something totally different.

"It's a subconscious process, one we are totally unaware of while it's happening," says Raudsepp. "All we see of it is that one day we have an unsolvable problem that just keeps getting worse, and the next day it's solved."

Why should our subconscious triumph over a problem with which we consciously struck out? "Memory is part of the answer," says Raudsepp. "When you are totally concentrating on a piece of work, it's possible that you are blocking off access to certain bits of information stored in your memory that might be useful and pertinent to your work. But subconsciously, these bits of information are easily accessed, then used to solve the problem."

Your Library of Memory

Raudsepp also spoke of something called creative memory. Our conscious mind takes pieces of information and stores them in the memory by subject, much like a library. If you were writing a paper on chemistry, you would go to the science section of the library. Likewise your mind serves up information from a particular part of your memory depending on what you're thinking about. But occasionally information from one section of the memory could be useful on an unrelated problem. A line from Shakespeare might help a company president make a personnel decision. But consciously he doesn't remember that line because his memory

is only releasing information from the business, not the literature section.

A person with a creative memory would have hooked the literature and business information together. He would solve the problem because he knew how to cast a line over boundaries and fish for unrelated knowledge that could help.

For those of us who aren't great at mental fishing, Raudsepp feels that the incubation process does the same thing. "Consciously we rely on the left-hand side of our brain to solve problems and meet social demands. Language and logic are on this side and this is where information is compartmentalized. But subconsciously we work on problems with the right-hand side. This side provides creativity and the ability to see things as a cohesive whole. Creative memory becomes available on this level."

When you incubate, your subconscious creatively accesses all sorts of information and assembles it in a colorful, interesting package—while you're poolside playing volleyball.

How do you incubate? "First you have to assemble data," answers Raudsepp. "Get all the facts and information available concerning your project or problem. Then sit down and give it a good going over. At this point you're priming the pump, so to speak."

Familiarize yourself with the information but make no attempt to solve it yet. This part of the process could take anywhere from 20 minutes to several days, depending on the amount of information you need to look at.

"Then put it away," says Raudsepp. "Go do something else. It could be anything from taking a walk to spending a weekend in New York. But make it unrelated to the project you're concerned with. When you come back, there's a good chance some things have fallen into place, and you're well on your way to finishing your project or solving your problem."

Of course, there are major incubations and minor ones. Some musical composers work on a piece for months and then put it away for two weeks before coming back to it. On the other hand, I've found that a ½-hour break can give me some new perspectives.

"A good way to start incubating is while you're asleep," says Raudsepp. "Think about your problem for 20 minutes before you go to bed. The next morning you may wake up with some good ideas. One engineer used to do this while standing on his head in a yogic position. He said that invariably he'd wake up the next day with new ideas."

While you may not solve the world's problems by standing on your head, incubation is just another example of the many hidden resources we all possess. The process of regeneration is one of discovery — uncovering these resources and putting them into daily practice. The end result is a clearer-thinking, more creative you.

Practice incubating your ideas. Experiment with different break times and see how quickly your subconscious serves up ideas. Find out what activity works best for you — be it a walk in the woods or the roller coaster at Disney World.

M. G.

DO YOU HAVE ONE BRAIN...OR TWO?

"I recently heard two little girls arguing in the New York subway," relates Dr. Julian Jaynes, psychologist and Princeton University professor. "They must have been about 12 years old. The argument heated up as I listened. One finally screamed at the other, 'The trouble with you is you're too left-brained.'"

Anyone who seems too purely logical, methodical, or analytical is likely to be accused of that same brain imbalance these days. Those are the skills and abilities housed in the left division of the front, most intelligent part of the brain, the cerebrum.

On the other hand, if you want to make someone feel really great these days, it's not too hard to fashion the perfect compliment: "You're ever so right-brained." *Too* right-brained doesn't seem to exist. Being too creative or too intuitive—the skills attributed to the right hemisphere of the brain—doesn't seem to be perceived as negative. But it could be, if all your creativity winds up on scattered pieces of paper that you can never find.

Possessing a balanced brain is important these days. Big businesses are spending big money on consulting firms to teach their employees how to balance their hemispheres and bring their brains into the twenty-first century with a more useful, more complete set of skills.

One of these consulting firms, called the Whole Brain Corporation, grosses around $2 million a year, says its founder Ned Herrmann. Whole Brain's customers include Fortune 500 corporations such as Shell, IBM, AT&T, and Du Pont. In his seminars, Herrmann teaches people how to determine their brain dominance profiles using a model that groups skills and abilities into four quadrants—two of which are right-brain oriented and two of which are associated with the left brain. One of his goals: "To help corporations develop a more creative climate and a way to access the creative potential of their employees," says Herrmann.

Corporate creativity moguls aren't the only ones interested in balancing the right and left hemispheres of the brain. Regu-

44

lar folks, just like us, have shelled out from $10 to $1,900 to use light-flashing, electric field-producing, "brain-tuning" machines. Others listen to different "brain-enhancing" tapes in each ear, or take creativity-boosting, hemisphere-balancing seminars.

What's behind this sudden focus on right brain, left brain? Is it warranted, or are we being taken for a ride? "When I think about those girls fighting, and calling each other 'too left-brained,' I have to laugh," says Dr. Jaynes. "The human brain just isn't that simple." Yet a discovery made by Nobel prize-winning Dr. Roger Sperry, psychobiologist, in the 1960s did show differences between the right and left hemispheres and the way they are used. Since that time, scientists have added to that initial insight with a number of intriguing studies. Already several misconceptions about the brain's dual nature have been challenged. Let's take a long, hard look at this research, which points toward a whole new understanding of what Hippocrates called the most powerful organ of the human body, the brain.

Myth: There are two separate brains in our heads, each with its own knowledge, wants, and desires.

Fact: The most straightforward answer to this question is, there's one and only one brain in your head. It is, however, made up of a number of sections: The front, most sophisticated section, the cerebrum, is divided into two portions, the right and left hemispheres. They are connected by the corpus callosum, a thick bundle of nerves that serves both as a communication bridge between the two hemispheres and as an inhibitor, to keep excess electrical stimulation from passing between the hemispheres. As long as your

> # KIPLING'S BRAIN PREFERENCE
>
> Ever wish you had a stronger right brain or a less overbearing left hemisphere? Take a hint from the poet Rudyard Kipling: Both sides are mighty good to have. Here's a portion of his poem, "Kim."
>
> I would go without shirts or shoes
> Friends, tobacco, or bread
> Sooner than for an instant lose
> Either side of my head.

corpus callosum is intact, says Dr. Jaynes, the right and left hemispheres work together, and are in constant communication.

The hemispheres do have different skills, though, and tend to carry out different functions of the brain. The motor or action skills of one side of your body are controlled by the opposite side of the brain, for instance. But there is more to the right/left brain idea than that.

Studies done on epilepsy patients whose corpus callosa have been cut to control the disease are especially intriguing. These patients are often called split-brain patients; Dr. Sperry's Nobel-prize winning work centered on their unique differences.

Dr. Michael Gazzaniga, of Cornell University Medical Center, one of the researchers who worked with Dr. Sperry on his ground-breaking split-brain studies, tested such a patient, called P. S. Dr. Gazzaniga asked P. S.'s right and left hemispheres questions in such a way that only

SEX ON THE BRAIN

Boys are better than girls at math, right? And girls can beat the pants off boys when it comes to English. Or at least that's what we used to think. These days, psychologists are realizing that the intellectual differences between males and females are shrinking.

Reporting in *Psychological Bulletin*, Dr. Janet Shibley Hyde and Dr. Marcia C. Linn noted that verbal test scores of men and women just weren't that different. Out of a group of more than one million people over the age of 5, 48 percent of the men scored above average while 52 percent of the women also did that well.

Other researchers have found that there are decreasing sex differences when it comes to math and spatial skills, too. "Decreased sex differences are partly due to a greater flexibility in gender roles," say the researchers. More girls are taking advanced math classes, for example.

Nevertheless, brain researchers have found that there are physical differences between the brains of women and men. The area of the brain that produces speech, for instance, is located in the front of the left hemisphere in women. In men, it's spread out more, over the front and back of the left hemisphere. That explains why, when people suffer brain injuries, women are less likely to lose their speech than men. There's less of a chance that the area that controls speech will happen to be hurt.

See the accompanying table compiled by University of Western Ontario psychologist Dr. Doreen Kimura for a summary of other brain differences.

| Function | Location | | Summary | |
	Men	Women	Same	Different
Producing speech	Left hemisphere, front and back	Left hemisphere mostly front		Smaller area in women
Hand movements for motor skill	Left hemisphere, front and back	Left hemisphere, mostly front		Smaller area in women
Vocabulary: defining words	Left hemisphere, front and back	Both hemispheres, front and back		Smaller area in men
Other verbal tests: naming words that begin with certain letters; appropriate social behavior	Left hemisphere, front	Left hemisphere front	Same	

one hemisphere at a time would be able to hear the questions and answer them. Because P. S. is one of the relatively rare people whose right hemisphere can produce speech (in most people, only the left hemisphere can speak), the answers were astounding and illuminating. Here's how the exchange went with the left hemisphere:

"Who are you?"

"P. S."

"Where are you?"

"Vermont."

"What do you want to be?"

"A draftsman."

Dr. Gazzaniga also asked P. S.'s right hemisphere the same questions. This time, the exchange went like this:

"Who are you?"

"P. S."

"Where are you?"

"Vermont."

"What do you want to be?"

"An automobile racer."

Which one is the real P. S.? Or are there really two personalities, a daring race-car driver and a sensible draftsman, cohabiting inside P. S. — and maybe inside all of us?

No one really knows, but Dr. Gazzaniga believes that we may have many "personalities" inside our brains. He says that we are only aware of the one that is verbal, and can explain itself in language. We may have many nonverbal modules in our brains that feel emotions and prompt us to take actions that the verbal, conscious self can't control. Then, a part of our brain that Dr. Gazzaniga calls the interpreter comes up with a reason for why we did what we did. The reason, he

says, is just a rationalization, and often has nothing to do with the real motive.

In one of the studies that led to this conclusion, researchers showed the word "walk" to the nonverbal, right hemisphere of a split-brain patient's brain, but kept the information from his verbal left hemisphere. When the patient got up to take a walk, the researchers asked him, out loud, why he was leaving. His verbal left hemisphere was the one that could normally answer most easily, but in this case it didn't know. Nevertheless, it didn't take even a second for the "interpeter" to come up with a reason: "I'm going to get a soda," he said.

"We humans resist the interpretation that things we do are capricious," says Dr. Gazzaniga, "because we seem to be endowed with an endless capacity to generate hypotheses about why we are doing things."

Unfortunately, he adds, this capacity can sometimes backfire, as when we wake up in a bad mood for some inexplicable reason (probably stemming from a nonverbal portion of our brain) but soon rationalize that the mood must be a reaction to the maddening ways of the person in bed next to us.

Myth: The right hemisphere of the brain controls creativity.

Fact: "It's impossible to say that something as high level as creativity could be controlled by one or the other hemisphere," says Dr. Jaynes. The truth is, high-level skills like having a conversation or coming up with a creative idea are really a group of subskills. To be creative, after all, you must be able to identify a problem, remember words used to describe it, know what the words mean, be able to analyze the situation, think up ways to solve it, forecast the future sufficiently to evaluate your solution . . . the list goes on and on. And all these skills are controlled by different areas of your brain—and are housed in both hemispheres, as well as other sections of the brain.

It is true, however, that some people are more creative than others. And that difference may be related to the organization of their brains. You already know that some people—about 90 percent of the population—are right-handed while others are left-handed. And if you're right-handed, probably all your motor skills, like jumping, throwing a ball, or cutting with a knife, are also stronger on your right side. Right-handedness is related to a strength in the left hemisphere of your brain, which controls your right side.

So what does which hand you use have to do with creativity? Well, left-handedness is not, as you might guess, necessarily caused by a strength in your right hemisphere. While no one knows yet why it occurs, many left-handers, explains Dr. Jaynes, actually have what he calls "mixed laterality." This means that both sides of the body, and correspondingly, both sides of the brain, can perform many skills. These people are often called ambidextrous—they can use both hands to cut food, write, and do other things. According to Dr. Jaynes, people with mixed laterality tend to be uncommonly creative. They are also often dyslexic. (Dyslexia is a learning disorder that can cause people to switch letters around, writing the word "said" as "dais," for example.) Some scientists hypothesize that the brain organi-

THE ASYMMETRICAL BRAIN

Mike has 33 allergies—sensitivities to items ranging from pollen to horses. Steve is dyslexic, allergic, and ambidextrous. Both have fraternal twins. And both are unusually creative and skilled at mathematics.

If you subscribe to the theories of the late Dr. Norman Geschwind, a prominent neurologist known for his forays into the frontiers of brain organization analysis, you won't be surprised by these coincidences.

Indeed, Dr. Geschwind's unorthodox theories focused on the linking of these traits. That is, there is a high rate of left-handedness in twins, a high rate of dyslexia, stuttering, and allergies in males and left-handers, and a high rate of creativity among left-handers.

The former neurologist in chief of Boston's Beth Israel Hospital, Dr. Geschwind believed that extra amounts of the male hormone, testosterone, in the uterus can cause the fetus's right hemisphere to grow larger than the left one. The result of the larger right hemisphere and the correspondingly smaller left hemisphere is less emphasis on verbal skills, which are centered in the left side of the brain, and more emphasis on mathematics and creativity.

Where does the testosterone come from? While stress can cause levels of the hormone to increase in a pregnant mother's uterus, the effect is seen more in males. This is because the male fetus's own testosterone augments the mother's levels of the hormone, suggested Dr. Geschwind.

48

zation that causes a person to become left-handed may also cause dyslexia and a high level of creativity.

Myth: The more you use your left brain, the better you'll be able to speak and express yourself verbally.

Fact: Obviously, if you practice anything, you'll get better at it, says Dr. Jaynes. So if you tell a lot of jokes, make speeches, and have debates with your friends, you'll become more proficient verbally.

And, when you tell those jokes, or speak in any other way, it's likely you'll be using your left hemisphere. We know that because scientists today agree that the speech of 95 percent of right-handers and 70 percent of left-handers is controlled by the left hemisphere. Of the rest, about half show right-hemisphere control of speech, and half have control shared by both hemispheres.

But is speech controlled exclusively by the left hemisphere even in right-handers? That would be too simple. After all, what is speech? It's recognizing words, remembering words, understanding tones of voice, putting emotion into your own voice, and even simply shaping your mouth and tongue to produce words. New studies show that each of these tasks is proba-

Half-brained but not half-witted

What would happen if you somehow lost half your brain? Not much, if you are age 7 or under.

Attempting to treat children with such severe epilepsy that a functional life is impossible, doctors have resurrected an old-time surgical practice called hemispherectomy. This procedure, which involves removing the entire epileptic hemisphere of the brain, was tried and abandoned in the 1930s and 1940s because it was so dangerous and unsuccessful then.

Recent advances in medicine have made the procedure workable. And now, doctors are learning that, when you remove half of a child's brain, the other side is able to compensate.

"People think all intelligence resides in the brain, and therefore, if you take out half the brain, the patient ought to be half as intelligent," says Dr. John Freeman, chief of pediatric neurology at Johns Hopkins Hospital. But that's not the case.

Actually, the young brain is remarkably adaptable. After a hemispherectomy, children's humor, personality, imagination, intelligence, and spirit all remain. The brain is able to "rewire"—new areas of the brain take over the jobs of the lost parts.

The remaining half of the brain can't do absolutely everything though. The patients will always be blind in one half of each eye and will have a slight paralysis on one side of their bodies—the side opposite the removed hemisphere.

bly controlled by a different area of the brain. And not all those areas are in the left hemisphere.

Understanding the emotions carried in language, for instance, is a skill carried primarily by the right hemisphere, scientists have found. After adults suffer injuries to the left hemisphere, they often have difficulty conveying or understanding the actual meaning of words. But when the right hemisphere is injured, something entirely different happens. They lose their ability to understand the tone of voice used by a speaker, and stop being able to put meaning into their own tone of voice. It's hard, for example, for them to tell if a statement like, "You're the best," is meant sarcastically or seriously, blandly or passionately, as a statement of fact or as a question.

People with intact brains probably don't think much about how they interpret the tone of someone's voice—they just know. But according to Dr. Jaynes, it is possible that left-handed people, with their emphasis on the skills of the right hemisphere, might be better at decoding the emotions in someone's voice. "These generalizations are easy to come by once you understand basic things, but we just don't know enough yet," he cautions. "It does seem feasible, though. Emotions probably are controlled by a deeper area of the brain than the right or left hemisphere —the limbic system. And it does seem that the right hemisphere has more links to the limbic system than the left hemisphere."

Myth: Right-brained people are more artistic than left-brained ones.

Fact: It is true that the right hemisphere of the brain seems to control many activities we call artistic. "We use the right hemisphere to recognize faces and listen to music, among other activities," says Dr. Jaynes.

As a result, the right hemisphere can be thought of as more visual than the left—and therefore perhaps more artistic. Studies show that the right hemisphere probably understands facial expressions better than the left half of the cerebrum, for instance. And damage to the right hemisphere often results in people being unable to recognize familiar faces.

Some research even shows that people are more aware of what they see in their left field of vision, which sends information to the visual right hemisphere. In one study, Dr. Darlene Kennedy, of Beaver College in Glenside, Pennsylvania, showed 99 college students six line drawings of male faces. A week later, Dr. Kennedy asked the students to pick the faces they had seen out of a larger group of 12 faces. But this time, one group was shown only the left sides of the drawings (the *right* sides of the subjects' faces), another group saw only the right sides of the drawings, and the last group looked at the full-face drawings.

The result: Those who saw the right halves of the drawings did twice as badly in remembering the faces they had seen as those who saw the left halves. Dr. Kennedy concluded that the students actually must have noticed less about the right halves of the drawings when they looked at them for the first time. In other words, their right hemispheres, which saw the left halves of the drawings, were better at picking up information in this way than their left hemispheres. That explains why they had more trouble recognizing just

50

the right half drawings. And it explains why you should play up your right side — it's noticed more.

But do the artistic qualities of the right hemisphere mean that right-brained people are more artistic than left-brained folk? First of all, "there is no such thing as a 'left-brained person,' or a 'right-brained person,'" explains Dr. Jaynes. The two sides simply have different strengths and abilities. And you use both sides all the time.

But interestingly, you may not even use your artistic right hemisphere as much as your left hemisphere when you actually carry out artistic activities. A specialized type of brain scan, the PET (positron emission tomography) scan, can measure brain activity in specific areas of the brain. Using the PET scan, scientists have found that when an untrained person listens to music, there is more activity in the right hemisphere than the left. But when a trained musician listens to music, she is likely to listen in a different way, perhaps analyzing the tones and chords, and will show the most activity in the left hemisphere of the brain.

Myth: You can teach the two sides of your brain to work in balance, or "synchrony," and get greater mental power as a result.

Fact: Makers of the new "brain machines" would have you believe that flashing lights, rhythmic sounds, rotating beds, and pulsed electric fields can "entrain" your brain waves and "synchronize" your hemispheres.

While some users of these machines do report greater relaxation and alertness after a session, scientists are not impressed. "There's simply no evidence in the scientific literature" that these machines can im-

prove your mental powers, says Dr. Stephen Peroutka, Stanford University neurologist.

Not only are scientists not sure these machines work, but they fear that a few of them may be dangerous. Why? Some of the machines actually transmit electric currents, in the form of pulsed electric fields, into the brain.

"Pulsed fields can cause discharge of cells in the brain," explains Dr. Robert Munzer, biomedical engineer, of the Food and Drug Administration. "A pulse could make your arm jump off the table. There are nerves firing in your brain telling your heart how fast to beat. If a pulse can make your arm jump, it might also be able to tell those nerves keeping your heart beating to fire faster or slower.

"Most of these tools have such a weak current that we'd be hard put to say they are dangerous," continues Dr. Munzer. "Then again, no research has been done to show that they aren't dangerous. Really, no matter how small the risk, if there is no proven benefit, you shouldn't use the machine."

"If these devices are strong enough to 'drive the brain' to actually alter EEG [electroencephalogram] patterns—and I don't know that they are—then they're potentially dangerous," adds Dr. Peroutka. "They can induce epileptic seizures in susceptible people, even if they never had seizures before."

Seizures occur when large numbers of nerve cells in the brain suddenly synchronize their electrical activity, say researchers at Stanford University Medical Center. The abnormally synchronized rhythm produces the convulsions, fainting, and episodes of confusion associated with epilepsy.

Even one of the whole brain prophets himself, Ned Herrmann, is distressed by the advent of brain machines. "The thing that really bothers me is the claim that you can automatically, effortlessly 'tune up your brain,'" he says. "I think this is highly exploitative and frequently erroneous. Especially since there are legitimate techniques that can help people access their whole brain."

Techniques that may work better than brain machines: Herrmann recommends certain professionally prepared relaxation tapes (such as those by Dr. Emmet Miller or Dr. Charles Strobel), guided meditation, free association, and brainstorming.

Myth: If you learn to use your right hemisphere more, you will be happier.

Fact: Not only is this idea completely untrue, but studies show that if you were able to use just your right hemisphere, you'd probably be terribly unhappy.

Though most scientists believe that our emotional life is primarily controlled by a deep area of the brain, the limbic system, and not the right and left hemispheres, studies do seem to show that the hemispheres have different moods. It's not as simple as a sad side and a happy side, but scientists have found that areas of the left hemisphere generally carry cheerful emotions, while areas of the right hemisphere are often blue.

Scientists first noticed the link between emotion and brain hemispheres when anesthetizing half the brain in an important test necessary before neurological surgery. Putting the left side of the brain to sleep gives the right free rein — and results in depression. If the right side is put to sleep, the emotions of the left hemisphere come to the fore and the patient feels euphoric.

A recent study conducted by Dr. Geoffry Ahearn and Dr. Gary Schwartz, Yale University researchers, used EEG apparatus to measure electrical brain activity in healthy college students. They asked the students questions that were designed to make them feel happy or sad. They found that when people experienced positive emotions, the frontmost area of the left hemisphere was more active than the right. And when their subjects felt blue, the front lobes of the right hemisphere showed more electrical activity than the left.

Studies of people who have suffered brain damage also support the idea that the hemispheres have different emotions. Neurologists have found that people with severe damage to the left hemisphere often become very depressed. Now it may seem natural to be unhappy about a brain injury, but people with damage to the right hemisphere tend to be oddly indifferent to their disabilities. They've been known to deny that limbs paralyzed as a result of the injury are really theirs and to try to walk on nonfunctioning legs.

Myth: If you're organized and analytical, you are probably left-brained.

Fact: Actually, many organizational tasks are carried out by the right hemisphere. Studies show that the left hemisphere tends to process information in a step-by-step sequential way. It's concerned with details, and deals with information in the order it is presented. The right hemisphere, on the other hand, tends to process information all together, all at once. This skill makes the right hemisphere better than the left at understanding spatial relationships, like how far away a car is, or if a present is going to be too big for a particular box.

The right hemisphere is also able to look at parts of something and see how

TEST YOUR HEMISPHERES

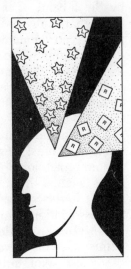

You don't have to go far to find out if you're right- or left-brained. There are tests galore—all in spite of the fact that scientists tell us there is no such thing as a "right-brained" or "left-brained person." We all use *both* our hemispheres.

The problem with the tests: They do measure something, but scientists would be hard pressed to prove that what's being tested is hemispheric dominance, says Dr. Julian Jaynes of Princeton. Here's a small sampling of the sort of questions you'd find on brain-side preference tests. Just for fun, see how you score—right, left, or balanced. (For best results, don't analyze the questions. Just mark the first answer that feels right.)

1. Daydreaming is (*a*) a waste of time, (*b*) amusing and relaxing, (*c*) useful for creative thinking and solving problems, (*d*) a way to plan for the future.

2. How do you feel about hunches? (*a*) You have strong hunches and follow them. (*b*) You have hunches but aren't aware of following them. (*c*) You occasionally have hunches but don't trust them. (*d*) You would never make an important decision based on a hunch.

3. When you have to solve a problem, do you (*a*) take a walk and mull over possible solutions, then talk them over with friends; (*b*) write down all the alternatives, arrange them in order according to priorities, and then pick the top one; (*c*) try to remember how you successfully solved a similar problem in the past, and then do the same; (*d*) wait and hope the problem will go away?

4. Sit in a relaxed position and clasp your hands in your lap. Which thumb is on top? (*a*) Left (*b*) Right (*c*) Parallel

they come together to form a whole. Someone with a functioning right hemisphere, for instance, would be able to see the mixed-up parts of an elephant and rearrange them to look like a whole elephant. Studies done on people who have lost all or part of their right hemispheres show that they can't figure out that the trunk attaches just below the tusks to make a whole elephant head, or that tacking the tail on to the back end would make more sense than just leaving all the elephant parts separate.

5. You are goal oriented. (*a*) True (*b*) False

6. In school, you preferred algebra over geometry. (*a*) True (*b*) False

7. You are very organized, with a place for everything and a system for accomplishing things. (*a*) True (*b*) False

8. You express yourself well verbally. (*a*) True (*b*) False

9. At a party, you are more comfortable listening, instead of being the talker. (*a*) True (*b*) False

10. You can usually tell how much time has passed without looking at your watch. (*a*) True (*b*) False

11. In sports, you often perform better than your training and abilities warrant. (*a*) True (*b*) False

12. You prefer working alone to working in a group. (*a*) True (*b*) False

13. You remember faces easily. (*a*) True (*b*) False

14. You like to redecorate your home often, take trips, and vary your environment as much as possible. (*a*) True (*b*) False

15. You enjoy taking risks. (*a*) True (*b*) False

Scores

Give yourself the indicated number of points for each answer you chose.

1. (*a*) 1; (*b*) 5; (*c*) 7; (*d*) 9.	**6.** (*a*) 1; (*b*) 9.	**11.** (*a*) 9; (*b*) 1.
2. (*a*) 9; (*b*) 7; (*c*) 3; (*d*) 1.	**7.** (*a*) 1; (*b*) 9.	**12.** (*a*) 3; (*b*) 7.
3. (*a*) 7; (*b*) 1; (*c*) 3; (*d*) 9.	**8.** (*a*) 1; (*b*) 7	**13.** (*a*) 7; (*b*) 1.
4. (*a*) 1; (*b*) 9; (*c*) 5;	**9.** (*a*) 6; (*b*) 3.	**14.** (*a*) 9; (*b*) 1.
5. (*a*) 1; (*b*) 9.	**10.** (*a*) 1; (*b*) 9.	**15.** (*a*) 7; (*b*) 3.

Now, add up all the points you scored, and divide the number by 15 to find your average score. The lower your number is, the more left-brained you are. The higher your number is, the more right-brained you are. In other words, if you score an average of 1 point, you are (supposedly) very, very left-brained. If you score 8, you are very, very right-brained. A score of 5 would mean you have a basically balanced brain, with some leaning toward right-hemispheric dominance.

FOOD
FOR THOUGHT

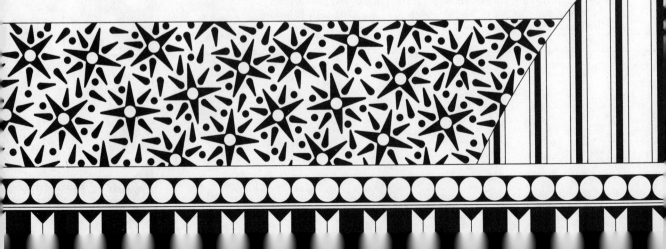

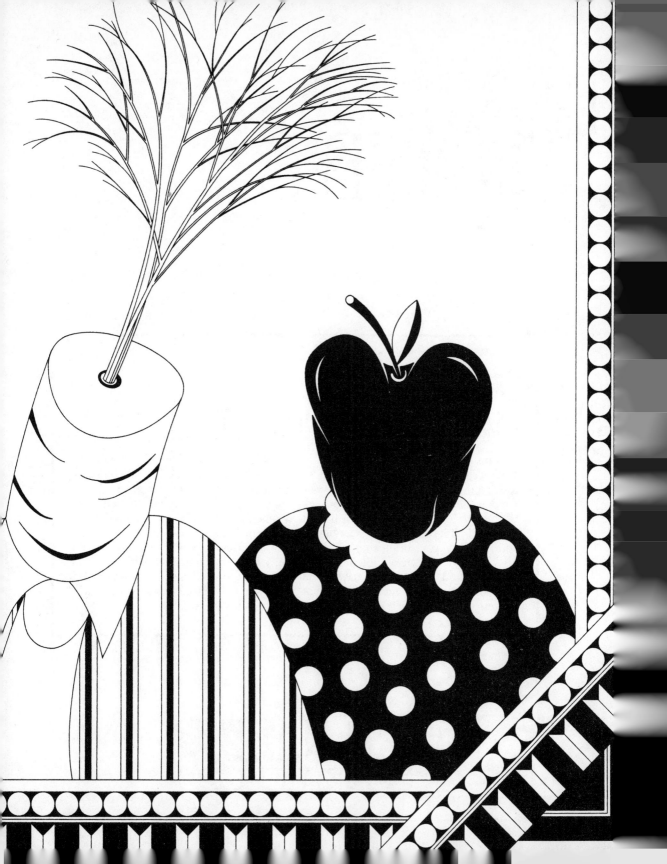

INSTANT INSIGHTS

Depressed? MAYBE IT'S YOUR DIET

It's week three of your new diet. You're climbing the walls and hitting the depths of despair. You curse your weak will and can't believe that for lack of a candy bar you've become a basket case. Well, if it helps any, you can blame your mood on your brain chemistry.

Dr. Guy Goodwin of Littlemore Hospital in Oxford, England, may have found a reason for the nasty mood swings that plague the dieting set: a drop in the production of the mood-affecting neurotransmitter, dopamine. The drop in dopamine production was dramatic in the 20 men and women dieters tested. But women also seem to undergo a drop in another important neurotransmitter, serotonin. Since low levels of serotonin have been linked to mood disorders and depression, it seems that women are twice as vulnerable to eating disorders and black moods.

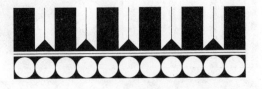

Sorry, Women, This Diet Aid Is For Men

Caffeine does a better job suppressing a man's appetite than a woman's, according to a team of Canadian researchers.

Researchers at Quebec's Laval University gave a group of ten men and women either a placebo or 300 milligrams of caffeine, the amount you'd find in two cups of fresh-brewed coffee. They had the subjects fast for 12 hours. At the end of the fast, the researchers set out an assortment of foods. Pairs of men and women had an hour to eat whatever they wanted. The men ate 21.7 percent less food than the women, according to researchers.

Dr. Angelo Tremblay, professor of physiology and nutrition at Laval, thinks the results confirm what researchers have long suspected: Men are more sensitive to stress. The caffeine acted as a stress inducer, causing the men to reduce their energy intake.

The long-term use of caffeine as a diet aid is another question. Diet pills that contain caffeine and other substances are believed not to work very long; the body simply adjusts to them.

A Relaxing Dessert

How do you spell relaxation? It could be C-H-O-C-O-L-A-T-E C-A-K-E, according to Yale University psychologists. Studies show that smelling — or even imagining — food can induce brain wave changes that are very similar to those that occur during relaxation therapy. An especially soothing mantra, say the psychologists, is imagining your favorite dessert.

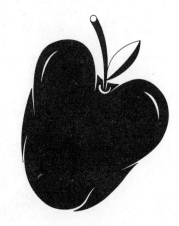

Beer: The Drink That Launched A Civilization

The Romans thought it was barbaric; the French wouldn't even taste the stuff. But if it weren't for the proletarian taste buds of their Neanderthal forefathers and foremothers, neither group would have had the opportunity to sip classic wines made from grapes grown in their own vineyards.

Beer, according to anthropologist Soloman Katz of the University of Pennsylvania, is the real reason hunters and gatherers stopped wandering and settled down on permanent farming establishments. Katz believes that prehistoric gatherers stumbled upon the first beer recipe accidentally. He says wild barley and wheat were collected and stewed in water to make a cereal-type, main-course dish. When this mixture was left out in the sun too long, natural yeast in the air fermented the cereal. Neolithic humans liked the good feelings they experienced from consuming the stuff and decided to grow their own barley and wheat to make more fermented mixtures.

They realized they could no longer wander around and still harvest enough grain for their prehistoric beer, so settling down became the best solution.

"Almost invariably," Katz says, "individuals and societies appear to invest enormous amounts of effort and even risk" to secure mind-altering foods and drinks.

Katz admits there is no direct archaeological evidence to support his theory, but points out that narrow-necked, Neolithic-aged fermentation bottles have been found. Also, he says the world's oldest beer recipe was found inscribed on a Sumerian tablet.

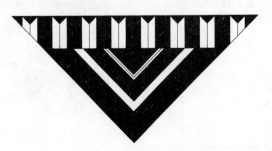

DOIN' THE MEMORY MUNCH

It could be that a better memory is as close as your refrigerator door, according to Veterans Administration researchers in Sepulveda, California. When mice were fed immediately after learning a new task, they remembered the task much better than mice who were fed at other times. CCK, a hormone released from the intestinal tract during eating, seems to be the reason for this mealtime memory stimulation. Even when injected into the stomachs of unfed mice, CCK was able to stimulate memory.

HELLO JAVA, GOOD-BYE JET LAG

Caffeine taken at the right time may help you combat jet lag. So says Charles F. Ehret, an expert in circadian (or daily) rhythms and former biologist with Argonne National Laboratory.

He believes that caffeine acts as a regulator of body clocks.

How can travelers use that to their advantage? This is his advice:

On departure day, if you're eastbound, refrain from drinking coffee until evening. If you're westbound, drink three cups of black coffee in the morning. Ehret says the effects will be even more beneficial if you abstain from caffeine for three days before your flight.

FOODS THAT PLEASE
THE SPIRIT

Every June, the wild blackberries in the field hedges behind our house start to ripen. As early as mid-May, I begin looking at them hungrily each evening as I take our dog Bandit for a walk. First, the little berries are whitish, then yellow. Finally they become dark, ripe, and delicious.

Eating the first blackberries of the year is a special kind of pleasure. I taste in those tiny fruit more than the usual blackberry flavor. They gratify my mind as well as my mouth, and are as well a healing experience for my spirit. That special taste turns a page of my inner calendar. The berry plants, cold and frozen over the winter, have revived. An old friend has come back, and memories of other years return.

Why am I telling you this story? Because it brings home in one simple event the way we, plants and Earth itself, regenerate in unison.

There is a rhythm that unites us with the natural world. The more we learn to feel that rhythm and get it into the mainstream of our lives, the stronger our spirit can be. And the healthier we can become.

Do you need a field and a hedgerow in your backyard to feel that regeneration of the spirit each year?

Contact with the soil itself definitely helps. Best of all is the taste of each season's new crop from your own garden. The idea of regeneration through food then comes home to your spirit in an intensely powerful way. But even away from the land itself you can find food that nourishes and regenerates your spirit.

Knowing the basic principles of the regeneration idea is essential to learning to recognize that special feeling. I will review those principles for you quickly.

First and most important, be aware that the earth has a healing nature. Life may be hard at times. We can be sickened. But all around us—and within us as well—is the spirit of healing and regeneration. Every form of life shares that benign force.

How powerful is that healing nature of the earth? To me, the answer is simple. The power of healing is much stronger than we have yet begun to understand. Just "getting better" after an illness is something quite familiar. But there are more ways to "get better" that we haven't either discovered or put to full use. Those ways are potentially so useful that we actually need different words to talk about and appreciate them.

That's why I stress so strongly the word regeneration. It means more than just to be healed. To regenerate is to become formed again, often in a way better than we were before. There is a positive quality to regeneration. When we understand regeneration, disturbance in our lives becomes an invitation to heal so powerfully that we can actually improve on our lives before. A new momentum of improvement comes into our lives.

What is the best and quickest way to feel regeneration? By eating special food, naturally. For food is not just a collection of protein, carbohydrates, minerals, and vitamins. It is those things and more. And the "more" has to do greatly with the spirit.

Think about the taste of food for a moment. From one year to the next, I remember those blackberries that grow in our field. They are unlike any other berry I eat. But the specialness I taste is more about the place and time they grow than about the berries themselves.

You must have had a similar experience. Did you ever buy apples from an orchard stand along a country road and relish a special taste in that fruit? Or eat an orange from your own tree or a nearby grove? Probably you have, and have tasted the place the fruit grew as well as the fruit itself.

Describing that precise "flavor of place" in the words we use to talk about the common flavors is impossible. Experiences of the spirit take us beyond ordi-nary language. They speak to us in mysterious ways that we know and feel, but which we can't express easily. Actually, we don't need words to describe those spirit flavors. To experience and remember them from year to year is enough.

You can easily share the spirit flavors, though, as well as the feeling of regeneration they generate. Think about how your family gathers for a Thanksgiving meal and how you share a special flavor of turkey on that day. Eaten at another time, turkey doesn't taste the same. Nor is it, in a sense, the same food. Any other time, turkey is just meat. On Thanksgiving, it's also a symbol of gratitude for blessings received.

Practical Uses for the Spirit of Food

Most Americans still eat too much of the wrong kinds of food. Our diet is overly rich in calories and fat, and tends to lack fiber and some vitamins and minerals.

Many people have the facts about food and nutrition in their minds. They know which are the more healthful foods and which to eat sparingly. But taste gets in the way of their good intentions. Their way of eating lets them taste food in the mouth only, and not enough in the mind. So they go on year after year failing to put good nutritional knowledge to practical use in their lives.

You can begin to deal with that problem by getting yourself closer to knowing and "tasting" the spirit of food. Now is a perfect time to do that. And I have some practical suggestions about how you can get started.

Start with a resolution to eat more fresh fruits and vegetables. Almost any diet can be improved by eating more of them. That's one reason why they are important. But another is that these fine foods connect us very directly to the earth itself. One minute they are plants with roots nestled in the soil. And the next they can be part of us, tasting good in the mouth but also reaffirming the support we get from a healthy soil.

Think about that again for a moment. Fruits and vegetables are unique kinds of food. The gap between their lives and ours can be measured in inches and seconds. They are packaged by nature, cooled by the air of evening, and warmed by the noontime sun. And the idea of regeneration is embodied in their very nature.

Yes, you can buy them in almost any store and get all their benefits of taste and good nutrition. But when you come close to where they grow, see the beauty of the entire plant of which they are a part, and touch the soil from which they come, some-thing can happen in your mind. A new dimension of taste is offered to you, and you are free to try to sense it or to let it pass.

My hope is that, this summer, when fruits and vegetables are growing almost all over this country, you will go looking for the spirit of these wonderful foods. Start by walking around where you live, in search of gardens and yard trees bearing fruit. You can just look or also talk to the people who culture them.

Later, go into the country around the place you live and find the fruit and vegetable farms that let you "pick and pay." Most people pick and pay to save money. But in the process of saving you get so close to these plants that you can see and feel their whole nature. You and the plant stand together on the common ground of the earth. Your eyes take in a more complete picture of what you are eating. And that is a profound benefit, if you can open your mind to the possibility that food has a spirit taste as well as the regular flavors.

Robert Rodale

NUTRA-BRAIN

A healthy mind in a healthy body—that ancient Greek ideal is probably familiar to you. And you know that you need vitamins to protect your body's well-being. But did you know that you need a healthy diet, supplied with all the necessary nutrients, to have a healthy mind, too? Scientists have shown that many vitamins and minerals not only nourish the body but also have important and far-reaching effects on your mood, your mental functioning, and even your general outlook.

"A deficiency of any nutrient that is used by the brain can cause irritability, depression, and mental malfunctioning—and just about every nutrient is used by the brain in some way," says Dr. Brian L. G. Morgan, a research scientist with the Institute of Human Nutrition at Columbia University College of Physicians and Surgeons. Some nutrients are especially important to the brain, but, cautions Dr. Morgan, "there's no good evidence showing that vitamins in large doses can cure mental disorders unless the disorder is caused by a deficiency."

Are you getting enough of the right nutrients to keep your head hale and hearty? To be sure, protect your mind from deficiencies of the following nutrients.

Vitamins

Thiamine

Thiamine, or vitamin B_1, is central to carbohydrate digestion. Since carbohydrates break down into simple sugars, like glucose, which fuel the brain, this vitamin is crucial to your intelligence. "A deficiency of vitamin B_1 is responsible for the bizarre behavior sometimes seen in alcoholics," says Dr. Morgan. "Many alcoholics can't metabolize carbohydrates, so their brains don't get enough energy to function properly. If an alcoholic has the DT's (delirium tremens), they can be treated with B_1 and magnesium."

In fact, Dr. Morgan says that people who drink a lot of alcohol need to protect themselves from a deficiency of B_1. "Since the alcohol impairs absorption of this vitamin, those who drink large quantities should take a once-a-day vitamin that will supply them with the Recommended Dietary Allowance (RDA) of vitamin B₁," he says.

Recommended intake: The recommended intake of thiamine is 0.5 milligram per 1,000 calories consumed. That means about 1.0 milligram daily for most women and between 1.2 and 1.4 milligrams for most men. Older people, people who consume a lot of alcohol, those who overcook their food, dieters, and those who don't eat many foods high in thiamine (like vitamin-enriched cereals and breads) need to be the most careful of deficiency.

BEST FOOD SOURCES OF THIAMINE

Food	Portion	Thiamine (mg)
Brewer's yeast	1 tbsp.	1.25
Sunflower seeds, dried	¼ cup	0.82
Rolled oats, dry	1 cup	0.48
Wheat germ, toasted	¼ cup	0.48
Rye flour	¼ cup	0.20
Navy beans, boiled	½ cup	0.18
Salmon steak, broiled	3 oz.	0.18
Soy flour, low-fat	¼ cup	0.18
Beef liver, braised	3 oz.	0.17
Brown rice, raw	¼ cup	0.17
Whole wheat flour	¼ cup	0.17
Beef kidney, simmered	3 oz.	0.16
Kidney beans, boiled	½ cup	0.14
Soybeans, boiled	½ cup	0.13
Chick-peas, boiled	½ cup	0.09

Niacin

A severe deficiency of niacin causes a disease called pellagra, says Dr. Morgan. One of the symptoms of this disease is mental deterioration. Other symptoms of pellagra common only in underdeveloped countries are severe sensitivity to the sun and violent diarrhea.

Those living in developed countries like the United States are very unlikely to have pellagra today, but it is proof that a serious deficiency of niacin can cause poor mental functioning.

BEST FOOD SOURCES OF NIACIN

Food	Portion	Niacin (mg)
Chicken, light meat, cooked	3 oz.	10.6
Swordfish, broiled	3 oz.	10.0
Beef liver, braised	3 oz.	9.1
Halibut, baked	3 oz.	6.1
Salmon steak, broiled	3 oz.	5.7
Beef kidney, simmered	3 oz.	5.1
Peanuts, dry-roasted	¼ cup	4.9
Tuna, white, canned in water, drained	3 oz.	4.9
Peanut butter	2 tbsp.	4.3
Chicken liver, cooked	3 oz.	3.8
Beef, lean, cooked	3 oz.	3.5
Brewer's yeast	1 tbsp.	3.0
Brown rice, raw	¼ cup	2.4
Avocado	½ med.	2.1
Cod, baked	3 oz.	2.1
Sunflower seeds, dried	¼ cup	1.6
Almonds, shelled	¼ cup	1.0

Recommended intake: According to the National Academy of Sciences, the RDA for niacin is 18 milligrams a day for men aged 23 to 50, 16 milligrams a day for men aged 51 and over, and 13 milligrams a day for women over the age of 23. If you take large amounts of niacin, you may have a harmless but unusual side effect: flushing. Your skin will tingle and turn red, as if you had an instant sunburn. The flush will usually fade within an hour or two, and, if you take niacin regularly, the reactions will diminish.

Vitamin B₆ (Pyridoxine)

This vitamin is used in the brain to help produce an important brain chemical called serotonin. "If you have a deficiency of B_6, then you may not produce serotonin at a normal rate," says Dr. Morgan. "A low level of serotonin could lead to depression."

Those using oral contraceptives must be especially careful to get enough B_6, says Dr. Morgan. "Oral contraceptives make the body use B_6 less efficiently. Some doctors feel that if you are depressed and if you are taking oral contraceptives, you could lift your mood by taking B_6," he says. He adds that, while this treatment is controversial in the United States, manufacturers in Spain add vitamin B_6 to oral contraceptive pills.

"Keep in mind that the vitamin will be doing its chemical thing to the brain within a few days of taking it," says Dr. Morgan. "So if it's going to work, it should work within just a few days." He recommends giving B_6 a month to work, however, in case there are other events in your life that are confusing the effects of the vitamin.

Recommended intake: The RDA for vitamin B_6 is about 2 milligrams a day. Excessive amounts could cause irreversible degeneration of the nerves, Dr. Morgan warns.

BEST FOOD SOURCES OF VITAMIN B₆

Food	Portion	Vitamin B₆ (mg)
Beef liver, braised	3 oz.	0.77
Banana	1 med.	0.66
Chicken, light meat, cooked	3 oz.	0.51
Sunflower seeds, dried	¼ cup	0.45
Atlantic mackerel, baked	3 oz.	0.40
Lentils, cooked	1 cup	0.35
Halibut, baked	3 oz.	0.34
Tuna, light, canned in water, drained	3 oz.	0.32
Brown rice, raw	¼ cup	0.28
Salmon steak, broiled	3 oz.	0.19
Broccoli, raw, chopped	½ cup	0.14

Vitamin B₁₂

This vitamin is crucial for the proper functioning of your nervous system. If you have a deficiency, you could experience mood changes, forgetfulness, mental confusion, and depression. Sounds like senility, doesn't it? You won't be surprised to learn that vitamin B_{12} deficiencies are often misdiagnosed as senility.

"There are a lot of people in mental hospitals who are getting less than optimal amounts of B_{12}," says Dr. Morgan. "And if you have a severe deficiency of B_6

you will appear to be senile." That's because vitamin B_6 is needed to produce myelin, the material that insulates your nerves and helps electrical messages sent through the nerves to get to their destinations. Vitamin B_6 is also needed to form blood cells. Since blood cells carry energy all over the body, including the brain, a deficiency of them may affect your mental abilities.

Vitamin B_{12} deficiencies are uncommon in young people, says Dr. Morgan. "Those who eat meat, chicken, fish, or soy products even just once a week have a five- or six-year supply of B_{12} stored in their livers," he says.

But between 3 and 10 percent of elderly patients have vitamin B_{12} deficiencies, reports Dr. Michael Carethers, formerly of the Geriatric Research, Education and Clinical Center at Seattle's Veterans Administration Medical Center.

BEST FOOD SOURCES OF VITAMIN B_{12}

Food	Portion	Vitamin B_{12} (mcg)
Beef liver, braised	3 oz.	60.4
Oysters, raw	2 med.	5.4
Beef, lean, cooked	3 oz.	2.5
Lamb chop, broiled	3 oz.	1.7
Yogurt, nonfat	1 cup	1.4
Haddock, baked	3 oz.	1.2
Swiss cheese	2 oz.	1.0
Milk, whole	1 cup	0.9
Cottage cheese, low-fat	½ cup	0.7
Egg, hard-boiled	1 large	0.7
Cheddar cheese	2 oz.	0.5
Chicken, light meat, cooked	3 oz.	0.3

Given the frequency of this deficiency in older people, Dr. Morgan suggests a thorough B_{12} check for patients diagnosed as senile. If they do have a deficiency, they will either have to improve their diets or receive a series of injections of the vitamin to treat their senility-like symptoms, says Dr. Carethers.

Recommended intake: The body only needs the tiniest amounts of vitamin B_{12} to function properly. The RDA is 3 *micro*grams a day, or three-millionths of a gram. Vegetarians, however, have to be especially careful. Since B_{12} is found mainly in animal food sources, they may be missing out.

Folate

Folate, or folic acid, is a member of the B-complex family of vitamins. And, like many of the other B vitamins, a shortage of it can mimic the symptoms of senility. Dr. M. I. Botez and co-workers at Montreal's Clinical Research Institute report a number of cases of central nervous system abnormalities linked to folate deficiency. Folate is especially concentrated in the fluid of the spinal column—the switchboard of the central nervous system that relays messages between your brain and body. Dr. Botez has found that many of the signs of approaching senility may actually be caused by a folate deficiency "short-circuiting" the nervous system.

Not only does folate preserve the nervous system, but it can also protect against depression. A study conducted by the Department of Psychiatry at McGill University, Montreal, revealed that "serum folic acid [folate] levels were significantly lower in . . . depressed patients. . . . On the basis of our results, we believe that folic acid deficiency depression may exist."

How to cure it? "Based on my clinical observations, it seems that people whose depressions are purely due to folate deficiency do get better with folate therapy," says Dr. A. Missagh Ghadirian, the head researcher in the study.

Recommended intake: The normal adult RDA for folate is 400 micrograms.

BEST FOOD SOURCES OF FOLATE

Food	Portion	Folate (mcg)
Brewer's yeast	1 tbsp.	313
Spinach, boiled	1 cup	262
Beef liver, braised	3 oz.	185
Black-eyed peas, boiled	½ cup	178
Orange juice	1 cup	136
Wheat germ, toasted	1 oz.	100
Romaine lettuce leaves	1 cup	76
Broccoli, boiled	½ cup	54
Brussels sprouts, boiled	½ cup	47
Beets, sliced, boiled	½ cup	45
Cantaloupe, cubed	1 cup	27
Whole wheat flour	1 cup	16

Choline

Can you recall the first words you said today? What did you eat for dinner *yesterday?* If you think your memory could use a boost, you may want to try a dietary approach. Some researchers have found that choline, a nutrient thought of as a vitamin by some nutritionists (it's included in many of the more complete B vitamin supplements), has an effect on memory.

"Our studies show that choline has a weak to moderate memory enhancement effect," says Dr. N. Sitaram, psychiatrist, director of affective disorders at Lafayette Clinic in Detroit.

On two separate days, Dr. Sitaram and his colleagues gave ten healthy volunteers, ranging in age from 21 to 29, either a supplement of choline chloride or an identical-appearing but worthless substitute. Then, after 1½ hours, the people were given two different kinds of memory tests.

In the first, a serial learning test, subjects had to memorize in proper order a sequence of unrelated words. "Choline significantly enhanced serial recall of unrelated words," the researchers reported. "Furthermore, the enhancement was more pronounced in 'slower' subjects . . . than in subjects who performed well."

In other words, the people most in need of help had their memories prodded the most when they took choline.

In the second test, the volunteers read lists of 12 common words. Half of the words were concrete words like table and chair, which can be easily visualized. The rest were more abstract words like truth and hate, which are hard to visualize and more difficult to memorize. In these trials, the subjects didn't have to learn the lists in any particular order.

The results showed that people didn't fare any better overall when they took choline. But they did register much better scores in the more difficult, low-imagery words category. Choline, in other words, seems to selectively enhance memory to meet the challenge of tougher learning tasks.

Should you take choline? Maybe. Dr. Ronald Mervis, researcher, Ohio State University, thinks that supplemental choline may even prevent memory loss from occurring later in life.

Recommended intake: Choline is a natural food substance that is usually safe even in large amounts. Doses used in memory studies have ranged from 1 gram (1,000 milligrams) to 10 grams. Amounts like these, however, should only be taken under the supervision of a doctor. For healthy people, an average diet should supply between 400 and 900 milligrams of choline a day.

BEST FOOD SOURCES OF CHOLINE

Food	Portion	Choline (mg)
Beef liver, braised	3 oz.	578
Soybeans, raw	3½ oz.	340
Egg	1 large	253
Brown rice, cooked	1 cup	218

Minerals

Calcium

A small increase in dietary calcium intake appears to be able to lift your mood, say researchers.

Dr. Kaymar Arasteh, now an assistant professor of psychology at Nebraska Wesleyan University, and his colleagues conducted two studies with calcium. In

one, they gave 47 women and men daily doses of either 1,000 milligrams of calcium or an identical-appearing but inert substitute. At the end of four weeks, Dr. Arasteh found that the test subjects who had felt depressed at the start of the study felt better after taking calcium. The test subjects who had felt fine before the calcium experienced no effect.

Those who took the substitute also felt their moods were slightly better. But they had much less improvement than those who took the real calcium, said Dr. Arasteh.

Some doctors suggest that calcium may also protect people from doses of lead absorbed from the environment. "In high amounts, lead that is absorbed by your body can cause brain damage," says Dr. Morgan. "And calcium, to some degree,

BEST FOOD SOURCES OF CALCIUM

Food	Portion	Calcium (mg)
Swiss cheese	2 oz.	544
Provolone cheese	2 oz.	428
Monterey Jack cheese	2 oz.	424
Yogurt, low-fat	1 cup	415
Cheddar cheese	2 oz.	408
Muenster cheese	2 oz.	406
Colby cheese	2 oz.	388
American cheese	2 oz.	348
Atlantic sardines, drained	3 oz.	322
Milk, skim	1 cup	302
Mozzarella cheese	2 oz.	294
Tofu	3 oz.	174
Pizza, cheese	1 med. slice	144
Broccoli, cooked	½ cup	89

prevents the absorption of lead. But if you are getting enough lead to have an effect on your brain, calcium isn't enough to make a difference. There are powerful drugs being developed that will remove toxic levels of lead.

"There's no evidence to show that the small amounts of lead most of us get from the environment really deteriorate our brains," adds Dr. Morgan, "but if it is a concern, calcium will reduce your absorption of lead."

Recommended intake: Men who exercise can get by with 800 milligrams of calcium a day while those who don't may need more. Some experts suggest women should ingest from 1,000 milligrams a day up to about 1,200 milligrams.

Iron

You already know that your body needs iron to avoid the fatigue, apathy, and weakness of anemia. Did you know that your brain needs iron, too?

Iron deficiency can lead to impaired memory. One study has shown that children with even mild iron shortages have poorer memory and learn less quickly than kids with adequate iron.

"One of the behavioral consequences of iron deficiency is an impairment of mental function," says Dr. Thomas F. Massaro of Pennsylvania State University. "This has been demonstrated both in laboratory animals and in children. Children with a subclinical [not as bad as anemia] iron deficiency can learn—they won't be retarded—but the deficiency will interfere with what they learn."

If you send children with plenty of iron coursing through their veins into a

room and later ask them to report what they saw there, they will remember and name clocks and lamps and rugs and books and many other things, Dr. Massaro says. But an iron-deficient child might remember far fewer objects in the room. Iron deficiency creates a kind of intellectual tunnel vision.

Not only can an iron deficiency sap your learning power, it may also drain away happiness. "There is now substantial evidence that iron deficiency has an adverse effect on brain function," writes a pediatrician in *The British Medical Journal.* "The most noticeable behavioral characteristic" the doctor noted among a group

BEST FOOD SOURCES OF IRON

Food	Portion	Iron (mg)
Spinach, boiled	1 cup	6.4
Beef liver, fried	3 oz.	5.3
Soybeans, boiled	½ cup	4.4
Blackstrap molasses	1 tbsp.	3.2
Roast beef, lean, cooked	3 oz.	3.1
Sunflower seeds, dried	¼ cup	2.4
Lima beans, boiled	½ cup	2.3
Ground beef, lean, broiled	3 oz.	2.0
Turkey, dark meat, cooked	3 oz.	2.0
Broccoli, raw	1 spear	1.3
Peas, frozen, boiled, drained	½ cup	1.3
Prunes, dried, cooked	½ cup	1.2
Almonds, shelled	¼ cup	1.1
Apricots, dried, cooked	¼ cup	1.0

70

of iron-deficient babies studied "was that they were more unhappy than nonanemic babies."

Dr. Morgan assures us that when anemia is corrected, so are the bad mental effects of the iron deficiency.

Recommended intake: Healthy, energetic men and post-menopausal women only need about 10 milligrams of iron a day. The typical younger female needs more; the RDA is set at 18 milligrams for pre-menopausal women.

Supplemental doses of iron should not exceed 30 milligrams daily unless prescribed by a doctor, since iron can be toxic in large amounts.

From Table or Tablet?

You know you need vitamins and minerals to keep your brain running as it should. But where are you going to get them—from the food on your plate or from a vitamin tablet out of a bottle? Some doctors think you should stick strictly to food sources for your nutrients. Others say you may need some help getting all the nutrients you need. "You can't always get all the vitamins and minerals you need through food," says Dr. Eli Seifter, a nutritional biochemist at Albert Einstein College of Medicine in New York. "Especially if you are sick, or live in an area where the soil is mineral deficient, you may need supplements."

A good daily multivitamin is all the dietary protection most people need, Dr. Seifter says. "Your food is the main source, and the multivitamin is just to supplement the food and make sure you get all the nutrients you need."

Obviously, the best source is one you enjoy. So try some of these delicious recipes—each one contains substantial quantities of at least three crucial brain vitamins. But remember, if you overcook your food, you may burn the vitamins right out.

Vitamin Vitae

Ever wonder who takes vitamins? The National Health and Nutrition Examination Survey, analyzed by researchers at the National Institutes of Health and other centers for health statistics, provides some answers.

Twenty-six percent of women take some sort of vitamin supplement, while only 19.4 percent of men do.

People between the ages of 35 and 44 are the least likely of all to take vitamins—only 19.5 percent of them do, as compared to 28.8 percent of those aged 65 to 74, and 20.9 percent of those aged 25 to 34.

Higher-educated folks with 13 or more years of school are the most likely to take some sort of supplement: 28.7 percent of them do. That compares to the 23.7 percent of those who only finished high school and 16.5 percent of people with 8 or less years of school.

The most interesting statistic of all: Nearly 60 percent of surveyed registered dieticians in the state of Washington use some nutritional supplement, according to the *Journal of the American Dietetic Association.*

Brain-Food Recipes

Super Chili

(for folate, vitamin B$_{12}$, and niacin)

2	cups dried kidney beans
1	pound lean ground beef
½	pound calves' liver
1	large onion, quartered
1	green or sweet red pepper, chopped
3	cloves garlic, crushed
3 to 4	tablespoons chili powder
2	teaspoons ground cumin
2	teaspoons dried oregano
⅔	cup tomato paste
1	cup corn kernels
4	teaspoons low-sodium soy sauce
1	tablespoon blackstrap molasses
	dash of cayenne pepper (optional)

Soak beans in water overnight. Place them in a large saucepan with enough water to cover, bring to a boil and simmer gently until soft, about 1½ hours. Drain, reserving 1½ cups of cooking liquid.

Brown beef in a large, hot, lightly oiled skillet. Place liver in a blender with a quarter of the onion, and process on low to medium speed until smooth. Stir liver into browned beef. Chop remaining onion. When meat is cooked through, add chopped onions, peppers, garlic, chili powder, cumin, and oregano. Cook until onions become translucent.

Stir in tomato paste, cooked beans, reserved cooking liquid, corn, soy sauce, molasses, and cayenne. Simmer chili 20 to 30 minutes, or until peppers are tender. Serve hot.

Serves 8

Double-Barreled Oatmeal Bread

(for thiamine, niacin, and folate)

1	tablespoon dry yeast
½	cup warm water
¾	cup buttermilk or milk
¼	cup honey
2	tablespoons butter
¾	cup rolled oats
2½ to 2¾	cups whole wheat flour
1	egg, beaten
¼	cup plus 2 tablespoons brewer's yeast

Sprinkle dry yeast over water. Set aside until yeast bubbles.

In a small saucepan, combine buttermilk or milk, honey, and butter. Heat until butter melts. Cool mixture to lukewarm, then stir in yeast.

Combine oats and 1½ cups of the flour in a large bowl. Stir in dry yeast mixture and egg. Beat vigorously to combine them. Stir in brewer's yeast and enough additional flour to make a stiff dough (go easy, too much flour will make the bread heavy). Work dough well, but do not knead it (it will be too sticky to knead).

Transfer dough to a well-oiled bowl. Brush top with oil. Cover the bowl and let dough rise in a warm place until doubled in size, about 1 hour. Punch it down, then transfer to a well-greased 9 × 5-inch loaf pan. Let it rise until doubled again, about 45 minutes. Bake at 375°F for about 35 minutes. If the top browns too fast, cover it with foil.

Makes 1 loaf

Romanian Onion Stew with Beef and Peppers (*Tocana*)

(for vitamin B$_6$, thiamine, and vitamin B$_{12}$)

¾ pound beef chuck, cut into 1-inch cubes
1 tablespoon whole wheat flour
2 tablespoons butter
2 tablespoons olive oil
2 pounds onions, sliced
1 tablespoon cider vinegar
2 tomatoes, pureed
¼ teaspoon cayenne pepper
3 large green peppers, seeded, cut into chunks
1 cup boiling water

Dredge beef in flour. Heat butter and oil in a heavy, 4-quart stew pot. Add beef and brown on all sides. Lift out beef with a slotted spoon and set aside. Add onions to pot, stir and cover. Cook for 1 to 2 minutes, or until onions are tender. Uncover and cook over medium heat, stirring occasionally, until onions are dark brown. Add vinegar, stir, and return beef to the pot. Add tomatoes, cayenne, peppers, and water. Cover and bring to a boil, then lower the heat to simmer, stir, and cook for 45 minutes, or until beef is tender. Check occasionally, adding more water if necessary (the stew should be fairly thick).

Serves 4

ABSORBING POWER

Don't let the vitamins and minerals you take go to waste. Use this table to maximize your absorption.

Nutrient	Blockers	Boosters	Tips
B-complex vitamins	Cholesterol-lowering drugs and anticonvulsants may interfere with B$_{12}$ absorption.	Take a B-complex supplement so the B vitamins can work together.	Take with meals during day.
Iron	Vegetable and fruit fiber, whole grain fiber, tannic acid (in tea), caffeine, and preservatives decrease absorption.	Viamin C boosts iron absorption from fruits and grains.	Take between meals; buy iron supplements labeled "ferrous" not "ferric."
Calcium	Food fiber, protein, and antibiotics interfere with absorption.	Lactose (milk sugars) and vitamins C and D enhance absorption.	Take before bed; exercise improves utilization.

BREAKING BREAD, BUILDING BONDS

Barbecued-to-perfection chicken, corn on the cob, coleslaw, strawberry shortcake. Cappuccino laced with amaretto, hazelnut cannoli. Lox and bagels, kippered salmon, gefilte fish.

Quick, pick your fare. Got your choice in mind? Good.

Now were you among those who stopped to tally the probable calories, and the protein, vitamin, mineral, and fat content before you made your selection? Didn't think so.

Just how did you choose?

If you're like most of us, you based your selection on preferences that involve taste, texture, degree of familiarity, and even the setting and image you associate with these foods. Maybe you're not consciously aware of it, but you do assign values to food that have nothing to do with their nutritional content. And you're right—food does have a psychological component. By learning to understand it, and master it, you'll be happier and healthier.

You've heard the old saw "you are what you eat." That's only half the story.

How we eat, and with whom, can help us nourish our sense of well-being. Our approach to food can express our individuality or deepen our sense of belonging. It can even enhance romance. The trick is in knowing how.

Social Animals

We human beings are social animals and our food habits reflect that. In cultures both simple and complex, eating is the primary way in which we initiate and maintain relationships. In fact, that's part of what makes us human. As Peter Farb and George Armelagos note in *Consuming Passions: The Anthropology of Eating*, we are the only primate group to observe rules about what is eaten, how it is prepared, and with whom it is to be eaten.

The idea of food as something that connects us to another is as old as our memory. In the womb, sustenance flowed from our mother to us through the umbilical cord. As infants, we fed at the breast or bottle, lovingly cradled in our caretaker's

73

arms. Is it any wonder that some of us never stop looking to food to soothe us, to make us feel connected and secure? Even our language betrays the social and emotional qualities we give to food. The English word "companion," for instance, comes from French and Latin roots that mean "one who eats bread with another."

But lately, our eating habits seem to be getting less and less chummy. For one thing, more of us are living alone. The number of single person households has doubled in the last decade. And even those of us living with family are often too busy ricocheting about—to classes, to work, to the gym—to sit down and enjoy leisurely meals together. According to one survey, fully one quarter of American households share a sit-down dinner less than five days out of the week.

Breakfast is another story entirely. How'd you have yours this morning? Were you among the bright faces gathered around the Wheaties box and the low-fat milk, or were you the one spooning the oatmeal with one hand, and working the curling

THE TOFU PERSONALITY

It's said you can tell a lot about people by meeting their friends. But did you ever consider how much you could infer just by looking at their plates?

Two psychologists did just that, and confirmed what we intuitively know to be true: The foods we choose reflect our self-image. Our choices also affect how others see us.

The study was done by Edward Sadalla, director of the doctoral program in environmental psychology at Arizona State University, and Jeffrey Burroughs, assistant professor of psychology at Juniata College, Huntingdon, Pennsylvania. They found that the stereotypes Americans have of vegetarians, gourmets, and health-food enthusiasts matched closely with the self-descriptions of people who prefer those types of foods.

Gourmets, for instance, are seen—and see themselves—as cultured, liberal, sophisticated people who tend to be interested in glamour sports like sailing. Health-food fans are the ones who—by self-definition and popular agreement—oppose nuclear power, vote Democrat, and drive foreign cars.

Sadalla and Burroughs found less correlation between the stereotypes and self-descriptions of fast-food fanatics and those with a yen for foods like Cheez Whiz and Carnation Instant Breakfast. Why less correlation? Sadalla thinks that's because more people fall into those categories, so it's hard to generalize about specific character traits.

He and Burroughs suggest that the symbolic importance modern man gives to certain foods may be a natural outgrowth of beliefs primitive tribes held about the magical qualities of food.

iron with the other? Or wolfing down a Mc-something, at every red light on the drive to work?

"If the word 'meal' means people sitting down to eat together," says Lawrence Gibson, food consultant and former marketing director for General Mills, "then breakfast hasn't been a meal for a long time."

Think about how far we've come. Just a few millenia ago, an ancestor's résumé might have read like this: "Hunter-gatherer. Expert in foraging and communal meal preparation." Now, we tend to be so busy accomplishing other things, we bring home the bacon but we don't often make time to eat it. And when we do, we don't take much care with how we eat it.

Common sense tells us that skipping meals when we're hungry, or rushing through that bite to eat will take its toll physically. But here's something else to consider: Every time you forgo a leisurely meal with companions or kin, you're also giving up an opportunity for fellowship and emotional nurturing.

How strongly are these values connected to eating? Well, think for a minute about the reason why people living alone tend to take their meals in front of the television, or with a good magazine. What's going on other than an attempt to substitute the appearance of company for real dinner companions? And think about the elderly woman living alone, who loved to cook when she had family at home, but who now routinely staves off hunger pangs with a couple of cookies or some fruit.

"If you talk to the elderly, the malnutrition problem is not just a matter of money," Gibson says. "One of the signifi-

ANOTHER DAY, ANOTHER RESTAURANT

Is the home-cooked meal becoming an endangered species?

More than one in three American adults will eat at least one meal away from home on any given day, according to the people at the Louis Harris polling organization. That's not surprising, considering that many of us are at work or at school during the lunch hour. In fact, half those meals out are lunch.

What is surprising is this: The 37 percent of Americans who are eating out on a single day add up to just under 66 million people, which is more than the entire population of France, Italy, West Germany, or the United Kingdom.

More than 40 percent of us prefer family-style restaurants, while another 32 percent go for fast food. And despite warnings about cutting back on red meat, four of us order meat for every two people who order fish. Steak is at the top of the list for the meat eaters.

Even when we're not sitting in a restaurant, 11 percent of us are buying take-out food and bringing it home on any given day. Fast food restaurants get 58 percent of that business.

cant problems is, it's just no fun to fix foods for yourself. Even meals at a senior citizen center are not a perfect solution because residents don't get the values they associate with food, namely family nurturing and companionship."

Celebrate Your Togetherness

Let's face it. Our lives are busy. But while we may not have the time or the desire to share every meal with kin or companions, we can manage to set aside a regular amount of time for celebratory eating—that is, eating in a way that celebrates our togetherness and renews us. All it takes is a little planning. The fare doesn't have to be complicated.

Singles who are living alone have plenty of options. If you like to cook, join a gourmet circle or organize an exchange where you and a group of friends get together on a regular basis to create a meal, or trade your favorite entrées. If boiling water is just about your speed, interest some friends in joining you in a weekly or bi-weekly exploration of ethnic and other unusual restaurants in your region.

Families can set aside specific times for "big deal" meals, where the menu is worked out by the members, who are also obligated to help with the preparations. If you've got young children in tow, try simple recipes so you can get them involved too. Making veal cutlets, for instance, can occupy three children. One child pounds the cutlets flat, another dips them in milk or egg, a third breads them.

And if you're an older couple living in a nest that's just emptied out, don't get into the habit of skimping for yourselves because you don't have to feed the kids any more. Indulge each other. Recreate the romantic meals of your newlywed years. This is prime time to rediscover dinner by candlelight with linen napkins. After all, look at what you survived as a team. Aren't you worth it?

Declare the Dinner Table a Demilitarized Zone

Eating together sounds great in theory. But whether it is great depends upon how you get along with the people at your table.

"It's important to have time when we get together to bond and interact," says Jane Hirschmann, coauthor of *Are You Hungry?* "With a lot of families, when both parents are working and the kids are being dropped off at day care in the morning, dinner hour is premium time for coming together and sharing experiences. The unfortunate thing about the dinner hour in many homes is that instead of sharing time together, people are arguing and yelling at each other about the food they're eating. It really detracts from the experience."

If that sounds familiar, why not declare your dining area a demilitarized zone, and adopt rules consistent with that attitude? You can even create a sign to serve as a reminder until the idea takes hold.

How do you keep the truce in effect? Begin with a meeting in which you talk to each member about how you want the meal together to strengthen the family rather than divide it. Tell them that constructive suggestions are okay, but personal blasts, from now on, are forbidden. Ask what you can do as a family to make mealtime more enjoyable. Maybe you'll want to decide in advance that certain topics are best reserved for family pow-wows when you're not eating. To enforce this, you can even strike a pact. Anyone who breaks the rules—and this includes Mom, Dad, Grandma, and Grandpa—has to eat the rest of the meal alone, some-place inappropriate, like the basement.

Try to keep the peace after dinner, too. "I'd suggest a quiet period surround-ing digestion," says Dr. Mark Tager, who practices wellness-oriented medicine in Oregon. "It does little good to consume good food and then damage digestion by stress."

Acknowledge Your Common Past, Present Ties

Those were the good old days, weren't they, those holiday meals at Grandma's that used to last for hours and hours? Those feasts where the table kept filling up with course after course of your tradi-tional favorites? Years later, the aroma of even one of those foods can probably still bring back a highly charged memory. Certain dishes seem to serve almost as a gastronomical family photo album.

How does that happen? It happens because those meals filled you up with something more than calories. What else? A feeling of belonging to a cultural tradition, of being part of a larger whole.

"I associate family ritual eating with euphoria, a sense of well-being, a feeling that all is right with the world," says Gibson. "Serving good, traditional food, whether it's pasta or lox and bagels or whatever, is

RED, WHITE, AND ETHNIC

Joey LaBriola drives a Ford Bronco, likes his Levi jeans, and is avid about baseball. You'd be inclined to think that as a third-generation Italian American, most traces of his ethnic background have faded away.

But sit down to eat with him and you may see something else. It's probable that Joey is still eating Italian and loving it. Maybe not as often as his parents and grand-parents did, but often enough to call it a regular part of his diet.

Old food habits, food anthropologists find, linger as the last vestige of an ethnic culture.

"Clearly, ethnic background still affects food tastes," says Lawrence Gibson, for-merly of General Mills. "For some people, the preferences are tremendously tenacious." Even something as simple as a favorite des-sert can be a function of habit. Pastry, for example, is an English custom, while cakes are an eastern European one. Which does your family prefer? What foods are your "comfort" or "special celebration" foods?

Regional food preferences in America correspond with the settlement patterns of its immigrants. What we loosely term American-style cooking is a favorite with 55 percent of the people in this country. Yet, on the East Coast, Italian food is a favorite, while on the West Coast, Mexican and Chinese foods are considered tops. Peo-ple in the Midwest and South tend to like American-style best, according to the Louis Harris polling organization.

78

demonstrating caring, giving love. It's also demonstrating expertise and skill."

And while newlyweds might disagree, the authors of *Consuming Passions* maintain that "eating can bind a pair together more effectively than sex, because people eat more often and predictably than they have sexual relations."

You can easily strengthen your mealtime bonds with family or friends by asking them to help you share in the making and eating of traditional foods. If you can learn enough about the customs of the region where you were raised to explain why the foods became a tradition, so much the better.

Or, if you've moved, perhaps you can start some new traditions, based on foods common to where you live now. Why not explore the farmers market in your area and talk to the local historical society about what the colonists, pioneers, or Indians who settled your area ate? What a great theme for a dinner or block party! Let the foods you eat give you a deeper sense of the place you've chosen to live.

A Word about Balance

Foods do affect us emotionally. But we do a disservice to ourselves and our bodies when we look to food exclusively to make us feel soothed, connected, and secure. How do you know when you get that craving for a serving of hot apple pie, chocolate mousse, or rice pudding, that the emotional boost you need wouldn't be better accomplished by taking a hot, scented bath or a bicycle ride through the country?

THE EDIBLE SOCIAL REGISTER

How tight are you with your social circle?

One way to answer the question is to look back over your date book and think about ways in which you've shared food and drink with the people you consider friends.

George Armelagos and the late Peter Farb, authors of *Consuming Passions,* say that "any invitation to share a meal or snack conveys its own nuance of social information."

According to the hierarchy they devised, you know you're at least not being sneered at when someone asks you to join them for a cold lunch or morning coffee. When you gain a few more points, maybe you'll be asked to a barbecue or buffet.

Cocktails alone are for acquaintances the hosts don't care to spend much time socializing with. If your hosts really like you, they'll ask you to stay past the cocktails and join them for a sit-down dinner. That's about as intimate as it gets, with the possible exception of an invitation to dinner and then breakfast the following morning.

Hopefully, you know by being attuned enough to your body to stop eating when you're physiologically full. That, in itself, is enough to give a sense of mastery.

"Most of the food problems in this country are what we call calming problems," says Hirschmann. Overeaters take a feeling—maybe loneliness, emptiness, or anger they're unable to express—and translate the language of feeling into the language of food.

"They're reaching out for supplies," she says. "Unfortunately, it's the wrong kind of supply. At this point in their lives, food is only symbolic of the care they're really seeking."

When you learn to reconnect eating with "stomach hunger rather than mouth hunger," says Hirschmann, you are "reparenting yourself and showing yourself you can meet your own needs. Then you can really be with the people with whom you dine. And you can experience the real joy of eating and connection with a physical need."

BEVERAGES AND THE BRAIN

Coffee and tea. Wine, beer, liquor. These libations have been around for ages, accumulating meaning and lore. No wonder it's sometimes tricky to be sane around them.

Maybe you're the type who feels you just can't conquer the day without your morning java. That's not exactly a modern view.

Madison Avenue can say what it likes, but the first Coffee Generation lived more than a thousand years ago in Ethiopia. Nomadic warriors there used to harvest the ripe cherries from the wild coffee tree to produce a "courage cocktail," a mixture of crushed cherry and animal fat that they'd serve at the little "pep rallies" they held before warring with other tribes. It wasn't until after A.D. 1000, that the Arabs figured out how to boil the seeds inside the cherries to make a hot drink.

And so an industry was born—as well as a new vehicle for social interaction.

If you think coffee's got history, tea predates the wheel. And alcohol, historians suspect, has been around since before recorded history. Could be that the hangover is as timeworn as the Stone Age.

All three beverages certainly have staying power. Maybe that owes partly to the weight of the myths and ritual uses that developed around them. The myths speak to the fascination these psychotropic—or mind altering—drinks held for early man.

Tea was so highly regarded by Tao alchemists of Asia that they considered it an essential ingredient in the elixir of immortality. The folks who christened "whiskey" must have had the same concerns. The word evolved from a Gaelic phrase meaning "water of life." There's even a Christian folk legend that coffee was brought to earth by the angel Gabriel.

Times have changed. Where the earliest consumers of caffeine and alcohol saw magic, we see biochemistry.

But it's not hard to understand how those notions about magic got started. Caffeine and alcohol go right to work on the central nervous system, producing quick and evident changes in mood, behavior, and capabilities. That bottle of brandy or that fragrant pouch of freshly ground Colombian blend might not carry warning labels that identify them as drugs, but they are classified as such.

That's right—caffeine is medically classified as a habit-forming drug. Considered the mildest drug in its category, it takes its place alongside barbiturates, amphetamines, and alcohol—other examples of psychotropic agents. There's even a term for caffeine addiction—caffeinism.

The Caffeine Blockade

You know that coffee, tea, or cola can perk you up when your alertness is on the wane, but have you ever stopped to wonder just how they work?

Researchers at Johns Hopkins University School of Medicine have shown that caffeine has a molecular structure similiar to adenosine, a chemical your body makes to do a variety of jobs. (Adenosine is a known vasodilator or blood vessel widener, and can also function as a sedative.) Receptor molecules for adenosine are distributed in various tissues throughout the body.

When adenosine locks onto special receptor molecules in the brain, it reduces the spontaneous firing of neurons in the cerebral cortex, cerebellum, and locus cerules. Put caffeine in your system and you effectively lock adenosine out. The caffeine attaches itself to the receptors instead, allowing the neurons to keep firing. It also blocks the vasodilator effect, causing blood vessels in the brain to constrict.

In fact, that's why you'll find caffeine in many headache-relief preparations. The substance is believed to reverse the dilation of blood vessels that create a vascular headache.

It doesn't take caffeine long to effect these changes. Within minutes after you ingest it, caffeine passes into your central nervous system, saturating body tissues in approximate proportion to their water content. In 15 to 45 minutes, the caffeine reaches its maximum level in your bloodstream. And then it begins to dissipate, metabolizing at the rate of about 15 percent an hour. So if you're drinking coffee to help you wake up for the drive home, be sure to allow enough time for it to kick in.

How long it takes you to clear all the caffeine from your system depends on your individual chemistry. The half-life of caffeine—the time it takes your body to eliminate half the amount consumed—is said to be about 5 to 6 hours for the typical adult, but about twice that for users of oral contraceptives. In other words, if you're on the pill, and you drink a cup of strong black coffee at 9:00 A.M., dosing your body with 120 milligrams of caffeine, you'll still have 60 milligrams in your system at 9:00 P.M. Maybe tea with dinner isn't such a hot idea after all.

What happens to your alertness, your manual dexterity, and your coordination while the caffeine is in your system are questions science still can't answer with any real authority. New studies have contradicted old ones, or turned up flaws in them.

What is known is this: If you're tired, or bored, low doses of caffeine can improve

81

CAFFEINE COUNTDOWN

Not all coffees are created equal. The same holds true for tea and chocolate. Brazilian coffee blends typically give you more of that caffeine jolt than Colombian blends. And the American and English teas usually have more of the stuff than the oriental varieties.

If you're curious about your average daily intake, consult the table below. Remember that a number of factors affect the caffeine content, including how—and how long—the beverage was brewed, and how large the serving is.

Product	Caffeine (mg)
Coffee (5 oz.)	
Brewed, drip method	60-180
Brewed, percolator	40-170
Instant	30-120
Decaffeinated, brewed	2-5
Decaffeinated, instant	1-5
Tea (per bag)	
Twinings English Breakfast	80
Twinings Darjeeling	74
Red Rose	69
Lipton	68
Tetley	65
Lipton decaffeinated	10
Chocolate	
Baker's chocolate (1 oz.)	26
Dark chocolate (1 oz.)	5-35
Hot cocoa (5 oz.)	2-20
Chocolate milk (8 oz.)	2-7
Milk chocolate (1 oz.)	1-15

Product	Caffeine (mg)
Soft Drinks (12 oz.)	
Mountain Dew	54
Tab	46.8
Coca-Cola	45.6
Shasta cherry cola	44.4
Pepsi-Cola	38.4
RC cola	36.0
Drugs	
Dexatrim	200
Vivarin	200
No Doz	100
Excedrin	65
Darvon	32.4
Triaminicin tablets	30

your concentration and accuracy on simple tasks like typing or math computation. Other studies show that a low dose, about what you'd find in a single cup of coffee, can immediately improve your reaction time.

And because caffeine causes marked increases in the levels of fatty acids in the bloodstream, it can boost your endurance. (Fatty acids are able to convert to energy, if needed.) Olympic athletes know this; use of "high levels" of caffeine is specifically banned by the International Olympic Commitee.

On the negative side, caffeine may impair short-term memory. One study at the University of North Dakota showed that caffeine impaired recall ability by about 20 percent. Students were asked to recite word lists immediately after they'd heard them. Those in the caffeine-free group did significantly better than their counterparts. You might keep this in mind next time you're meeting a group of new people whose names you want to remember. You'll also want to keep your caffeine intake below 150 milligrams if you're crafting or repairing something that requires manual precision. Studies show that more caffeine than that can cause your hands to be unsteady.

Keeping an accurate count of your caffeine intake is not easy. There is much variation from brand to brand and brewing method to brewing method. See the box "Caffeine Countdown" on page 82 for more information.

Ounce for ounce, coffee packs more of a caffeine punch than most other beverages. But tea, chocolate products, and soft drinks also contain caffeine.

Certain nonprescription drugs may have even greater concentrations of it than coffee. When adding up your milligrams, be sure to include all the sources.

You can probably get away with a cup or two of coffee a day, or its equivalent, without really deleterious effects, provided you aren't pregnant, or suffering from ulcers, heart-rhythm abnormalities, premenstrual syndrome, or panic disorders. But be sure to keep your intake well under 500 milligrams daily.

More than 500 milligrams a day will speed you on your way to caffeinism, a

83

GETTING THE CAFFEINE OUT OF THE BEAN

Have you ever wondered just how they remove the caffeine from the coffee bean?

According to *The Book of Coffee and Tea,* the raw green beans are softened with steam and water. Once soft, they're flushed with a solvent, usually one containing chlorine. The mixture is agitated, just like clothes are in a washing machine, and the solvent soaks into the beans, helping to draw the caffeine out. After about an hour soak, the solvent is drained off. The beans are heated and blown with steam, to dissolve any remaining solvent. Coffee manufacturers may repeat the process up to 20 times to arrive at a product 97 percent caffeine free.

The extracted caffeine is purified and used in soft drinks and pharmaceuticals.

84

chronic low-level poisoning with symptoms that include sensory disturbances, nervousness, insomnia, and digestive distress.

Know that no matter what the dose, caffeine can increase the effects of thyroid preparations and amphetamines, and decrease the effectiveness of sedatives, sleeping pills, pain relievers, and narcotics.

Liquor's Systematic Approach

The difference between caffeine's effect on your system and alcohol's is much like the difference between turning a light switch on and flicking it off.

Caffeine is a stimulant. Alcohol is a depressant. If someone were to hook you up to an EEG (electroencephalogram) machine, you'd find that your brain waves slow down after alcohol is introduced to your system.

That's the reason why you don't want to mix alcohol with other depressants like tranquilizers or medication for high blood pressure. If you slow your system down too much, you risk shutting it off for good.

And be aware that the hotter your body, the drunker it can get. Researchers at the University of Southern California School of Medicine have found the first evidence of a direct relationship between body temperature and brain sensitivity to alcohol. Tests on animals show that a rise in temperature increases alcohol's potency. If the same holds true for humans, a normally safe dose could become progressively more harmful as the mercury rises. Maybe that's why a beer after a long hot summer hike can knock you for a loop.

Alcohol's effect on your brain is very systematic. First it disables the intellect, hampering judgment, memory, and problem-solving abilities. Eventually, it breaks down more fundamental functions, like balance and coordination.

To understand the route alcohol takes through the brain, follow the blood-alcohol level. The higher the concentration of alcohol in the blood, the more regions of the brain affected.

Let's follow what happens to Joe, who, at 150 pounds and eager to drink, is ideal for this discussion. Joe's first drink of the night, a 12-ounce glass of beer, puts about ½ ounce of pure alcohol in his system (5

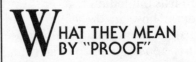

WHAT THEY MEAN BY "PROOF"

You see it on every bottle of alcohol, a numeral followed by the word "proof." As in "Vodka, imported, 100 proof."

You've probably guessed that proof has something to do with potency. Just how did this curious custom start?

It began in the early days of the distilled liquor industry in England. Distillers determined alcoholic content, or proof, by applying a mixture of alcohol and water to gunpowder. The ratio that would just permit the ignition of the powder was considered 100 proof.

In the United States, proof refers to twice the percentage of ethanol (ethyl alcohol) by volume. For instance, a liquor labeled as 90 proof contains 45 percent ethanol.

ounces of wine or one shot of liquor would do the same thing).

He expels about 10 to 20 percent of the alcohol through his lungs. And because he has no food in his stomach to slow the absorption, the rest passes quickly from his small intestine to his bloodstream. This first drink pushes his blood-alcohol level to 0.024 percent. His thirst is quenched, but not much else has changed.

If he knocks back another beer immediately, his blood-alcohol level rises to 0.05 percent. Now his central nervous system takes notice. As the alcohol meddles with his prefrontal lobes, Joe may act on impulses he'd normally restrain. (A study at the University of Washington suggests that the stronger the conflict between his impulse and his inhibition, the more likely he is to engage in uncharacteristic behavior.)

At this point, Joe's memory has lost some of its sharpness. If you engage him in a debate right now, you're likely to find his logic isn't so hot, either.

Two more beers, one right after the other, and Joe's blood alcohol level rises to 0.1 percent. Police would consider him legally drunk. Watch him at the pool table, and you'll see something's off with his coordination. It also takes him longer to react.

Another two—he's up to six—and he's managed to depress the entire motor area of the brain, and affect the limbic system, which mediates emotional behavior. Joe's just broken off with his girl; he starts getting alternately weepy and angry after someone asks about her. His blood alcohol concentration registers at 0.20 percent.

At 0.30 percent, Joe is having a hard time hearing and seeing. The alcohol is causing chaos in more primitive centers of the brain, which regulate wakefulness, among other things. Joe seems to be fighting sleep.

If he manages to remain conscious, he could drink himself into a coma. Once his blood-alcohol level exceeds the 0.4 or 0.5 percent mark, it begins to depress the lower center in the medulla that controls breathing and heart rate. And if he stops breathing, he's dead.

Joe's big mistake through the evening has been to drink nonstop. At his weight, his liver could metabolize about ½ ounce of pure alcohol an hour. If he had a beer or two at 9:00 P.M., when he got to the party, and waited until 10:00 to have his next one, and 11:00 to have the one after that, he could have maintained a pleasant "buzz" while keeping his faculties pretty much intact.

As Dr. Robert Linn points out in his book, *You Can Drink and Stay Healthy,* it isn't how much you drink that's the real key, it's the way you space your drinking. In other words, three shots in an hour will cause more internal disruption than five or six spread out over 5 hours.

Now that you're familiar with how one night of drinking affects the brain, it will probably come as little surprise to learn that chronic drinking inflicts permanent damage. But did you know that too much booze can actually destroy brain cells?

An Australian study of chronic alcoholics and heavy social drinkers found that their brains tended to weigh less than those of nondrinkers who were similiar to them in both age and weight.

The researchers found that the drinkers had smaller and fewer neurons, the

C STANDS FOR CLEARING

If you're planning on doing a little social drinking, you might want to take some vitamin C beforehand. A study at the University of Michigan Medical School shows that vitamin C, taken before you start drinking, may counteract some of the effects of alcohol by speeding up its clearance from the blood.

Researchers had 20 healthy young men take either a placebo (sugar pill) or 1 gram of vitamin C five times a day for two weeks. Then they threw a beer blast for the guys. For 2½ hours, the men drank a carefully monitored amount of alcohol. Blood samples were taken every hour for the next 10 hours.

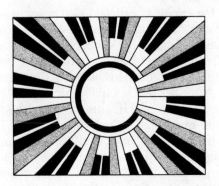

In half the men, pretreatment with vitamin C speeded up alcohol clearance from their blood. It also improved the men's color discrimination and motor coordination. It did not do anything, however, to limit alcohol's impairment of their intellectual function.

cells we think with. The tissue loss was evident in the superior frontal region of the brain, and is believed to be only partly reversible even after years on the wagon.

Other studies have shown that alcoholics suffer from a reduced level of endorphins, the brain's natural opiate. But it's unclear whether this lack causes individuals to drink more or is the effect of too much drinking, or both.

Strategic Use

You've learned how caffeine mimics the body chemical adenosine and how alcohol depresses brain functioning. Obviously, a little of either goes a long way.

One way to limit yourself to occasional use of mind-altering beverages is to stock plenty of substitutes. Nose around in your cabinets. Do you have mineral or seltzer water, fruit juices, natural or low-sodium bouillon, or caffeine-free herbal teas on hand?

Another way is to learn to question your impulse. Are you simply thirsty? A healthier beverage is just as likely to quench your thirst. Do you need to wake up? Try some deep breathing, yoga-style alternate-nostril breathing, or take a walk outdoors.

If you want to soothe jangled nerves, why not treat yourself to 15 minutes of progressive muscle relaxation or a long soak in a scented bath. Or learn to meditate. You'll find that the irritations that used to make your blood boil don't even produce a simmer.

One way to firm up your resolve to cut back is to begin a regular aerobic exercise program, preferably first thing in the morning. The exercise will help you feel you really do have self-discipline, and that will boost your self-esteem. Studies suggest that intense, sustained exercise will boost levels of brain chemicals that help improve your mood. Physical activity also serves as a healthy release for anger and anxiety.

Should you decide to decrease your caffeine consumption, be sure to do it gradually. Abrupt withdrawal can cause mild to severe headaches, depression, and nausea. Reseachers have found that habitual caffeine use increases the density of adenosine receptors in the brain, probably in an effort to let adenosine do its normal job.

When caffeine is withdrawn suddenly, adenosine locks onto these extra receptors, causing the blood vessels in the brain to dilate. Nerve endings in the vessel walls fire in response to the dilation, producing a headache.

Caffeinics Anonymous does not yet exist. But there's lots of outside help for the alcoholic. The newer programs employ a combination of non-narcotic medications, nutritional intervention, counseling, and education in coping skills, like Progressive Relaxation. The Acupuncture Clinic of the Lincoln Medical and Health Center in New York even uses acupuncture treatments to stimulate the renewal of endorphin production, which the addiction has shut down.

If you're struggling with a dependency, take heart. Physician David Hawkins views addiction as the side effect of a natural human drive—the search for more satisfying mental states. "It may be a failed attempt at legitimate goals: The exploration of creative possibilities, a more positive attitude, greater social ease, and self-understanding," he says.

Worthy goals, all of them. But chronic drinking, time has proven again and again, is the wrong route.

UP, DOWN, AND NEUTRAL: GETTING YOUR BRAIN IN GEAR

Take this quiz to see if you eat smart.

1. You've got an important brain-storming meeting at 1:30 P.M. For lunch, you have (*a*) two slices of pizza and a soft drink; (*b*) a baked potato, green beans, and a portion of vegetarian lasagna; (*c*) a lean slice of turkey, green beans, and a glass of milk.

2. It's 10:00 P.M. and you're in the living room watching a disturbing television documentary. You're worried it will keep you awake tonight, so you reach for a sleep-inducing snack. Your choice is (*a*) a handful of dry cereal, (*b*) a bowl of cereal with milk, (*c*) a glass of warm milk.

3. You have 1½ hours before your airplane takes off to get the dog to the neighbors, get yourself and the kids packed, and call the airport limo—and you haven't had anything to eat since breakfast. You grab something to munch in the car. It's (*a*) an apple, (*b*) a plain bagel, (*c*) a chicken leg.

If your answers spell out a word that means the same thing as taxi, you win the Cerebral Gourmet Award for understanding how food affects your mood. If not, read on for an explanation of the answers and some amazing facts about how you can use diet to harness your brain processes and get the mind effects you desire.

ENERGIZING EATS

In a slump? High protein, low-fat foods like these will lift you up in no time, says Dr. Judith Wurtman of Massachusetts Institute of Technology: beans, very lean beef, low-fat cheese, skinless chicken, eggs (but don't have more than two or three a week), fish, lentils, skim milk, peas, shellfish, tofu and other soybean-based foods, low-fat yogurt.

Rule of thumb: Protein foods, like meat, fish, and dairy products, will make you alert, while carbohydrates, such as pasta and bread, will calm you down or make you sleepy.

Corollary number one: Protein mixed with carbohydrates acts like protein alone.

Corollary number two: Fruits and vegetables are neutral, and won't calm or alert you.

A Chemical Tug-of-War

Researchers, including Dr. Judith Wurtman, a nutritional biochemist at Massachusetts Institute of Technology and author of *Managing Your Mind and Mood through Food,* have found that eating carbohydrates or protein activates different brain chemicals, called neurotransmitters, which either relax you or pep you up.

"When I first explain the relation between food, mood, and brain chemicals to my patients," says Dr. Wurtman, "they often begin to look uneasy or doubtful . . . [But] there is absolutely zero risk in the food/mind/mood strategies I've developed. The mood-modifying chemicals involved, including dopamine, norepinephrine, and serotonin, are always present in your brain. You will not be introducing any foreign substances into your body. Nor will you be inducing any unusual changes in the chemical processes that normally take place in your brain. You *will* be harnessing those processes, using them to achieve more of what you want at work and in your personal life."

MEDICINE IN THE COOKIE JAR

What's your snack profile? Is first choice always a starchy or sugary tidbit? Do you find yourself craving carbohydrates much more than usual? Even all day long? If you answered yes to these questions, scientists say you could be going after these foods to relieve a bad mood or even depression.

Research shows that when you eat carbohydrates, a chain reaction begins in the brain that results in the production of a calming brain chemical called serotonin. Based on this fact, some scientists suspect that certain people use cookies, cakes, and other carbohydrates deliberately—but unconsciously—to actually medicate themselves out of a mild depression.

"If you're not seriously depressed, there's nothing wrong with using carbohydrates to make yourself feel better," says Dr. Judith Wurtman of Massachusetts Institute of Technology. "It's just like taking an aspirin when you have a headache."

But if your carbohydrate cravings seem excessive, and are accompanied by other signs of depression like insomnia, oversleeping, or an inability or lack of desire to work or socialize, you could have a more serious problem that warrants the attention of a physician, says Dr. Wurtman.

The best part of Dr. Wurtman's strategies is that they use foods we have in our cupboards and freezers already. Like skinned chicken, lean beef, low-fat cottage cheese, ice milk, crackers, and muffins. One note of caution before we go on: If you have ever been diagnosed as having hypoglycemia (low blood sugar), you should check with your doctor before you follow any of the strategies discussed here. In fact, it's a good idea for just about everyone to consult with a physician before making major changes in eating patterns.

Once that's out of the way, the next question is how to put Dr. Wurtman's research to work for you. To get an idea, let's have another look at that quiz we started with.

What about lunch before the important brainstorming meeting in question number one? The right answer is (c) a lean slice of turkey, green beans, and a glass of milk. That's because the proteins in the turkey and milk contain an amino acid called tyrosine. According to researchers, the tyrosine gets into the brain and is used to develop a group of neurotransmitters called catecholamines, which include norepinephrine and dopamine. These are alertness chemicals that take effect in your mind 20 minutes to 1 hour after eating protein. To get this effect, you should always eat the protein before anything else. How much? Choose from this list: 2 to 5 ounces of lean meat, poultry, seafood, or fish; about a cup of low-fat yogurt or cottage cheese; 2 ounces of low-fat cheese, like skim-milk mozzarella; or two eggs (but limit yourself to a maximum of three eggs a week to cut down on cholesterol, warns Dr. Wurtman).

What was wrong with the other two choices? It's true that the two slices of pizza with a soft drink do have protein in the form of cheese. Since protein mixed with carbohydrates counts as protein, that should do the trick. But all the fat in the cheese plus the grease you often find on even the best slices of pizza will cut way down on the protein effect. Always remember to choose protein meals that are low in fat to avoid that kind of slow-down interference.

As for the baked potato, green beans, and vegetarian lasagna, well, they are pure carbohydrates and neutral vegetables. If that's your midday meal, you may be nodding during the brainstorming meeting, not sparkling.

Calm Cuisine

Foods that are low in fat but high in carbohydrates will trigger the brain chemicals that may soothe you when you're being driven up a wall. Dr. Judith Wurtman of Massachusetts Institute of Technology, suggests you try these foods when you need to calm down: bagels, bread, cereal, low-cal cookies (like gingersnaps and tea biscuits), corn, crackers, muffins, pasta, air-popped popcorn, potatoes, unsalted pretzels, rice, rice cakes, rice pudding, rolls.

The Sandman Strategy

What if you want to sleep easier tonight? Take another look at question two. Probably, your first guess was a glass of warm milk. Well, it might help you nod off if you *think* it will, but that's just a mind over body trick at work, says Dr. Wurtman. Actually, milk has enough pro-

PRAWNS FOR PAWNS

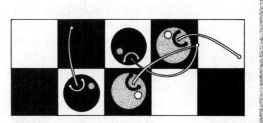

What's the ultimate brain fuel? Experts say protein is just the thing to jump-start your brain when you need it to be really alert. And that carbohydrates—sugar in particular—will focus a jumpy brain. Are they right? We decided to check it out with the people who demand the most from their brains—chess champions. See if you spot the important similarities in their favorite, most effective pre-game meals.

Maxim Dlugy, 1985 World Junior Chess Champion, favors elegant restaurant meals. He says, "I try not to eat right before the game—I allow about 2 hours to digest, and I try not to make it too heavy.

"Before the last game I won, I ate shrimp for an appetizer, some veal for a main course, and then a fruit tart for dessert. Also, if the game takes a long time, I eat chocolate while I play to give me energy."

Sergey Kudrin won the U.S. National Open in March, 1987. "About 2 hours before a game, I try to eat some meat so I will have enough energy to play for 6 or 7 hours," he says. "I also have a starch with it—it doesn't matter what—and a vegetable if it is available.

"I always avoid dessert, but if I am very hungry during the game, I will have some fruit. I especially like to drink tea during the game."

Lev Alburt, 1985 and 1986 U.S. Chess Champion and 1987 U.S. Open Champion, is the most particular of all. "In Russia, my favorite food before the game was black caviar. Since I came here in 1979, it is harder to find caviar in restaurants. But it's still my favorite food before the game, and I have it when it is available," he says. "I like it best with dark rye bread and butter. It is very light and provides a lot of energy for the small volume.

"Also, it is good for the brain to have something sweet. Häägen Daz rum raisin ice cream, I think is good. And during the game, I always eat chocolate."

Caviar, shrimp, veal, meat—the breakfast of chess champions always involves protein for a super-alert performance. During the game, when they are probably tense and need to focus, these winners eat sugar in the form of fruit and chocolate. Our conclusion: Food strategy just may be the best chess strategy of all.

tein in it to keep you staring at the crack in your bedroom ceiling for hours. And milk combined with cereal will have the exact same effect as milk alone. Remember: Protein mixed with carbohydrates acts like protein alone.

The best sleep-inducing strategy is to eat plain carbohydrates, like potatoes, corn, bagels, and muffins, which will trigger the sleep-inducing brain chemical serotonin. Serotonin is made in the brain with the amino acid tryptophan.

But here's a surprise fact: There's *no* tryptophan in carbohydrates. Tryptophan is actually found in very small quantities in protein, says Dr. Wurtman. But there are so many other amino acids trying to pass the blood/brain barrier and get into the brain after you eat protein, that tiny, weak tryptophan often gets stuck outside. When you eat carbohydrates, however, insulin is produced by the brain to break down the sugars in the carbohydrates. That insulin also tells most of the amino acids to leave the brain and go into your body's muscle tissue. This leaves the opening to the brain clear for tryptophan from previous meals to get in. Once in the brain, the tryptophan is used to make serotonin, which helps you slow down and fall asleep.

So the right answer to question two is (*a*)—dry cereal. If that doesn't suit your palate, try some instant hot cereal made with boiling water, or instant hot chocolate made with water, suggests Dr. Wurtman. But remember, you'll get a better effect from a low-calorie bagel than from a rich piece of fudge—the fat in the fudge will get in the way of digestion. Furthermore, the blood/brain barrier is so sophisticated that you'll get the same effect from one bagel as you will from ten, so don't overload on calories needlessly. Your best bet is to eat 1 to 1½ ounces of pure, low-fat carbohydrates 15 to 30 minutes before you hit the sack.

Calm and Capable

Finally, let's look at question number three. You're harried, in a rush, and have loads of things to get done on an almost impossible time schedule. But, none of the activities involved needs a super-alert mind—after all, you won't be driving. All you really need is a calm mind so you can get through the next 90 minutes without bursting a blood vessel. The tension of the day is already keeping you on your toes—if you eat a protein snack like the chicken leg (with the skin off) it might make you so alert that you'll fall right off your toes. The apple, like all nonstarchy fruits and vegetables is neutral; it'll help you avoid hunger, which is useful, but it won't calm you down.

What should you eat? The answer is (*b*) a plain bagel, which will help the amino acid, tryptophan, get beyond the blood/brain barrier and into the brain, where it can spark the production of serotonin. That same brain chemical that helps you fall asleep when you're lying awake in bed will calm you when you're harried. It won't make you fall asleep, though: "If you're hyper, the serotonin will just bring you down to normal levels," says Dr. Wurtman.

In fact, eating carbohydrates to produce serotonin can even be helpful when you want to be completely alert. It will calm you enough to focus your thoughts when you are so excited by an idea that you can't control your racing mind long enough to get the idea down on paper. Unfocused? Try a carbohydrate snack like a sugared soft drink (liquid snacks are digested faster than solids). Within 10 to 15 minutes, you'll find your mind clearing and your ideas taking shape.

Reviewing Your Options

Let's review for a second. To calm down, focus, or fall asleep, eat 1 to 1½ ounces of low-fat carbohydrates 15 to 30 minutes before you want to feel the effects.

(continued on page 96)

THE DRIVING FORCE OF ROAD FOOD

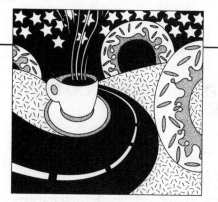

It's 2:15 A.M. on I-80, the radio is blaring, the oncoming headlights are glaring—and you're so tired you're swearing. Driving late at night isn't fun, but it's something we all have to do, at least occasionally. The next time you're stuck behind the wheel in the wee hours, you can make it a safer and slightly more pleasant experience by eating the stay-awake way.

"When you need to drive late at night, you must fight the natural tendency of your body to follow its normal 24-hour sleep/wake cycle," explains Dr. Judith Wurtman of Massachusetts Institute of Technology. "This cycle dictates that as night approaches, body temperature will drop and metabolism will slow."

To fight this tendency to go to sleep while you're driving, have a late lunch that is large enough to let you wait until around 10:00 P.M. for dinner. This will help fool your system into thinking it's still daytime when it's really not. Then, your nighttime meal should be exceptionally light, says Dr. Wurtman. "Hungry is fine. It's hard to fall asleep when you're hungry," she says. "But people get drowsy when they eat a lot."

Both meals should begin with low-fat protein foods. "The best meal choice is one you buy at a supermarket and carry in your car," says Dr. Wurtman. "Bring yogurt or lean slices of chicken," she suggests.

If you must eat in a fast-food restaurant, absolutely stay away from fatty foods. British studies show that eating high-fat foods while on the road lowers the driving ability of professional bus drivers, explains Dr. Wurtman. Best bets in fast-food restaurants?

"Go with the salad bars," she says. But don't touch the coleslaw or potato salad—cottage cheese, which is a good source of protein, is a better side dish. And skip fatty, mayo-loaded salad dressings. Vinegar or lemon juice are good substitutes.

The only other acceptable fast food is a burger, says Dr. Wurtman. "Everything else is loaded with fat. Especially milk shakes, hot apple pies, and french fries. Stay far away from those."

When you head back to the car, bring along something to drink. The restaurant probably offers you a limited choice: a cola drink, which has caffeine and sugar, or coffee. Maybe you lean toward the cola—all those calories will give you energy, right? Wrong. "Go with the coffee rather than the soft drink," says Dr. Wurtman. "The soft drink doesn't contain nearly as much caffeine as the coffee, and it's got a lot of sugar, which will tend to put you to sleep late at night." Caffeine has been proven to dramatically improve performance during a tedious task like late-night driving, she says.

"If you don't like the taste of coffee," adds Dr. Wurtman, "you can buy skim milk and mix the coffee into it. And feel free to put a teaspoon of sugar in your coffee; 1 teaspoon is a far cry from the several tablespoons of sugar in a soft drink."

Other tips: get plenty of fresh air, take exercise breaks, and if you must munch, stick with fruit or nuts rather than candy.

KEEP A FOOD/MOOD DIARY

"Some people are extraordinarily sensitive to the effects of food on mood, while others barely react at all," says Dr. Dan Kaplan of Philadelphia. To find out how the food you eat is affecting your feelings, Dr. Kaplan suggests you keep a food/mood diary.

The first step is to get a small notebook you can carry with you, he says. Before each meal or snack you eat, jot down how you feel. Use the table below as a guide or photocopy it and then just check off your state of mind. (In the table, snacks are listed as meals, and meals are labeled by number. Breakfast, for instance, is meal 1. Lunch may be meal 2, unless you have a midmorning coffee break, in which case that will be meal 2 and lunch will be meal 3.)

Next, write down everything you eat in your notebook, labeling clearly what meal it is, and what day it is. Then, an hour after your meal, write down your state of mind again. When you are evaluating your mood, don't think for a long time about it. Your first reaction is likely to be the most accurate one.

Continue with this regimen for four days, writing down everything you eat, and how you feel before and after. Whenever possible, try to eat the same foods each day. This will help you see which of your emotions are a result of the events of the day and which are caused by your diet.

At the end of the four days, says Dr. Kaplan, analyze your preliminary results. Did certain meals make you feel tired? Did others help you feel alert or energetic?

You may be able to modify your diet with just this information. If certain meals make you tired, reserve them for the evening. If others get you going, have them in the middle of the day. And if some meals seem to consistently make you sad, avoid them completely.

You may notice, however, that you feel sleepy after an afternoon snack of rice cakes and orange juice but wide awake after a snack of rice cakes and cottage cheese. You won't be able to tell if rice cakes make you feel tired or alert. The way to determine which foods cause which specific reactions is to test them individually.

Dr. Kaplan suggests you choose which foods you want to test based on the initial four days worth of data. Then, after fasting half a day, record your state of mind, eat just one of them, wait an hour, and then record your mood again. Test the same food at a few different times of day, and on different days. Then go on to the next food. Soon you'll have a good idea of which foods affect your mood for the better, which for the worse, and which have no effect at all.

FOOD/MOOD DIARY   Day _____

	Meal 1 before/after	Meal 2 before/after	Meal 3 before/after	Meal 4 before/after	Meal 5 before/after
Alert Vigorous Sharp Motivated					
Relaxed Calm Focused Patient					
Irritable Grouchy Tense Agitated					
Sluggish Apathetic Slow Sleepy					
Sad Blue Despairing Unable to cope					

96

Liquid will be absorbed faster. Fat will just get in the way of digestion. (And eating double the recommended amount won't double the relaxation but might end up doubling your weight.)

To pep up, eat 2 to 5 ounces of low-fat protein. Eating more will have no additional effect on your brain chemicals, so it's useless to gorge yourself. You'll feel the effects of the protein almost as quickly as those of carbohydrates, but you should be aware that the digestion process will also get in the way of maximum alertness. You're best off if you eat about 2 hours before an important meeting, interview, presentation or exam, to allow time for digestion. Eat any earlier and you may be hungry again by the time of the meeting. Eat later, and digestion will still be using up energy that could be going to your brain.

Dr. Wurtman offers some other simple rules to keep your performance top notch at crucial moments.

● Eat very low-calorie, low-fat meals — about 400 calories — before you need to perform. Being too full is just as bad as feeling starved. (But be sure that the meal before this meal was sufficient, so you won't be hungry.)

● Don't snack just before you must perform at a high level and definitely try to avoid a carbohydrate snack, like the pastries often served at coffee breaks.

● If you must eat while you perform (for example, during a business lunch), eat a small, low-cal, low-fat, neutral or protein snack an hour before the meeting, such as some low-fat yogurt, a piece of fruit, or a cup of clear soup. Then, pick at protein foods like fish and neutral foods

like salad (without dressing) during the meeting. Make sure the calorie total of the business meal is exceptionally low — around 400 to 500 calories will help you avoid sluggishness.

● Drink no alcohol the day of the important meeting, interview, exam, or other crucial performance.

● Don't pick this moment to kick your caffeine habit, or to start one up. Keep the caffeine level in your body just where it usually is, whether that's very high or less than none. If you'll need to be alert in the late afternoon, however, do drink a small amount of caffeine an hour before, unless you are so sensitive to it that you know it will make you feel ill. Otherwise, the natural rhythms that slow your body down in the late afternoon will dull your sharp wits and could ruin your presentation.

Keep in mind that these ways of eating will have slightly different effects on different people. Most of the differences are purely individual — they simply vary from person to person. Some common tendencies, however, have been found by researchers. Extroverts, for instance, tend to react more strongly to the slow-down effects of carbohydrates than do introverts. And older people tend to be much more sensitive to food than younger ones. In fact, those over 40 often find a protein breakfast causes them to feel anxiety, while folks under 40 may find it sharpens them up for the day. And women often get sleepy from the same amount of carbohydrates that just relaxes men.

The best way to find out if Dr. Wurtman's advice is going to make your life more pleasant and productive is to try it. You might even want to chart your reactions to food by keeping a diary like the one described in the box "Keep a Food/Mood Diary" on page 94. While her theories are not universally accepted by nutritionists, some find them helpful. Here's one success story.

"One of my patients was a big-city radio disc jockey who had a little problem. He kept falling asleep at the mike," relates Dr. Dan Kaplan, a Philadelphia medical nutritionist. "He would put on 5 or 10 minutes of solid music, and then would get groggy and even nod off while it played. After he started missing cues to go back on the air, he came to see me.

"After making sure he didn't have any neurological problems, I asked him about his diet. I found out that all the time he sat at the mike, he was gobbling down crackers and candy. Apparently he was very sensitive to those carbohydrates. Now that he eats nuts and fruit while he's on the air, he stays alert and his life is back in tune."

SELF-ESTEEM: THE PEDESTAL YOU NEED TO BE ON

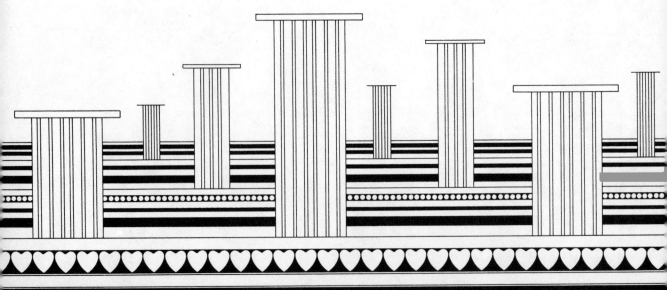

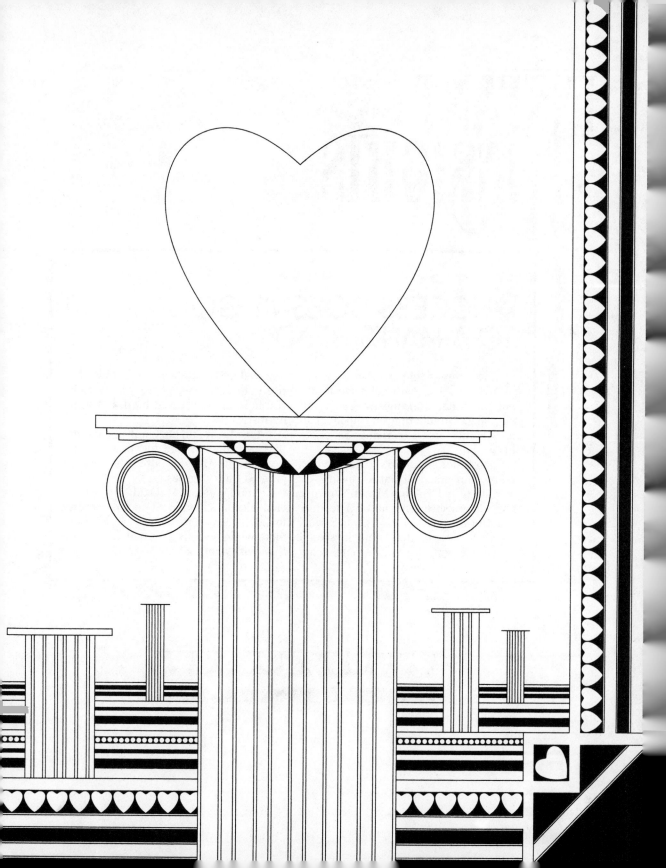

INSTANT INSIGHTS

SUCCESS DOESN'T GO TO A MAN'S HEAD

The things that make a man feel most manly, that really get his testosterone pumping, are things we suspected all along: Humiliating an opponent in an athletic contest. Affixing "M.D." to his name.

Testosterone, man's main sex hormone, appears to be status-driven.

A study by Dr. Allen Mazur, Syracuse University sociologist, and Dr. Theodore Lamb of Wittenberg University in Springfield, Ohio, found that men who scored a decisive win in a tennis match (and received a $100 prize to boot) showed a rise in testosterone. There was no such rise in men who played hard, but won narrowly.

Dr. Mazur and Dr. Lamb also found that new doctors had higher levels of testosterone the day after they were granted their degrees.

And Dr. James M. Dabbs, Jr., a psychologist at Georgia State University, found that a man's testosterone level rises more when he converses with a woman than with another man.

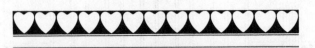

THE IF-AT-FIRST-YOU-DON'T-SUCCEED DEPARTMENT

- Abraham Lincoln lost seven elections for various public offices.

- The royal bengal tiger, considered the premier predator of the Indian subcontinent, only catches its prey once out of every ten attempts. Field observers report that the African lion has much the same record of success. Yet both creatures reign supreme.

- "Superman" was rejected by every major comic book publisher before being accepted by Detective Comics. The character—invented by two boys still in high school—was soon selling over one million copies of every comic book he appeared in.

- A popular songwriter in the late 1920s turned out a song that was not particularly popular. A few years later, a second recording of it proved equally unmemorable. Several more years passed, and yet another band recorded the obscure number. Only this time, the rhythm was slowed way down, giving it an entirely different feel. Quite unexpectedly, the song became a smash hit. And that's how Hoagy Carmichael's "Stardust" began its meteoric rise to being the most recorded song by any American composer.

- Mary Higgins Clark was a widow with five children when she decided to become a writer. With no university education, and having worked only as a secretary and airline attendant, it didn't seem like an easy road. And with all those children, the only time she could write was from 5:00 to 7:00 A.M.—before the family woke up.

Her first manuscript was rejected. So was her second, third, fourth, and fifth. Her tenth, fifteenth, and twentieth. The years rolled by. The rejection slips kept rolling in. Twenty-five. Thirty. Thirty-five. Not until six years and 40 thanks-but-no-thanks form letters accumulated did she make her first sale—for $100.

In 1988, Clark became the first writer in history to sign a publishing contract worth over $10 million in guaranteed royalties. That, on the basis of best-sellers like *Where Are the Children?*, *A Cry in the Night*, *The Cradle Will Fall*, and *Weep No More, My Lady.*

Along the road, she found time to get a college degree at night, graduating summa cum laude, and serve as president of the Mystery Writers of America.

HIGH SELF-ESTEEM INCREASES DRIVE

When faced with a problem to solve, a decision to make, or a riddle to answer, do you persist until you have the correct solution? Or do you think a little bit and then give up? That depends on your level of self-esteem, says Dean McFarlin, psychologist at the State University of New York at Buffalo.

High self-esteem, McFarlin claims, is directly related to perseverance. Individuals with low self-esteem, are more likely to give up.

Thirty-four undergraduate women were given an extremely difficult test, designed to produce failure. Afterwards, they were told of their failures and then given geometric puzzles to complete, three of which could not be solved. Some students were told this, others were told all could be solved, and the rest were told nothing. In studying the results, McFarlin found that those with higher self-esteem, who were told all the puzzles were solvable, persevered longer in trying to solve them than those with less self-esteem. He speculates that after being told of their initial failure, those with high self-esteem felt a need to redeem themselves and try harder.

The group that was told nothing about the tests, McFarlin says, showed no variation between low and high self-esteem individuals. In the group told some of the problems were unsolvable, high self-esteem individuals readily accepted the fact while low self-esteem subjects appeared to work harder to solve them. McFarlin speculates that those with low self-esteem were not sure if the inability to solve the problem was due to a lack of a solution or to their own ineptness.

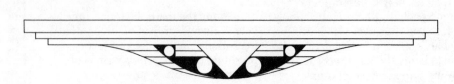

READ THIS WHEN THINGS AREN'T GOING WELL

How badly can you botch things up and still manage to escape with your self-esteem in an upright position?

Consider this true story of an architect and a building.

In the mid-1950s, he received a commission to build a public entertainment center, which was to cost about $5 million and take a few years to construct. Somehow, though, things didn't go well. He was soon months behind schedule. Then . . . *years.* As expenses mounted, people began to suspect there was a fundamental flaw in his design. No matter how he modified his plans, the building just wouldn't go up. A special bond issue had to be floated as the cumulative cost surpassed first $25 million, then $50 million, then $75 million. The press lambasted and mocked him. The whole project became a kind of national joke.

Finally, nearly ten years and $100 million over budget, the building was completed.

How would *you* feel at that point if you were the architect? Like wearing a mask for the rest of your life?

Joern Utzon, who *was* the architect, didn't have that reaction. Not long after the job was finished, his building came to be regarded as one of the most exciting pieces of architecture of the twentieth century. A whole nation took pride in it. It became, in fact, a symbol of the country itself, and helped draw in millions of tourist dollars.

That long, painful, "botched-up" job sits on the shore of Australia's largest city, the stunning international landmark known as the Sydney Opera House.

THE ART OF BOOSTING YOUR CONFIDENCE

How's your self-image? To find out, take a moment to complete the sentences below:

1. I relate to others (well/poorly/easily/with difficulty)

   _____ .

2. At social gatherings, I am _____ .
3. People tend to (like/dislike) me _____ .
4. My personality is _____ .
5. I am a (good/bad/okay) person _____ .
6. At work, I am usually _____ .
7. My co-workers think of me as _____ .
8. My intelligence level is _____ .
9. My appearance is _____ .

Next, rate each answer as positive ("I relate to others well," "My intelligence level is good for accomplishing most of my goals"), negative ("I am a bad person," "People tend to dislike me"), or neutral ("My personality is average").

Now count up your positive answers and your negative answers. "Usually, you will find that in at least one area, whether it is your appearance, your personality, or your mental functioning, there will be one or two things you don't like," says Dr. Fred D. Wright, director of training at the Center of Cognitive Therapy, University of Pennsylvania, who suggested this test. "That's okay. But if you have more negative answers than positive ones, then you are probably experiencing a low self-image."

A low self-image, however, is not a permanent characteristic the way having red hair is. "You are not born to be shy or underconfident," says Dr. Wright. "If you work at it, you can certainly change." All it takes is effort.

The first thing to do is decide where your efforts could be most effective. Some people have an extremely low self-image. "If you're down and you're always down, you have a problem best worked on with a therapist," says Dr. Wright. But most other people can make small, simple changes in their lives that could have an enormous impact on their self-image.

Begin with a very small change, says Dr. Wright, something with guaranteed success. Go to a hairdresser or barber, for instance, and ask for a new style that will really flatter your face. Or ask a friend to go shopping for a new outfit with you.

These small, appearance-oriented changes won't change you inside, but Dr. Wright says they will trigger a semiconscious thought process in you that goes something like this: "Gee, I look really good. Attractive people are smart, capable, responsible, and nice. (Studies show that we believe that the better looking a person is, the better person he or she is). So I guess I must be smart, capable, responsible, and nice."

It all has to do with creating an image, says Dr. Wright. By creating a confident image, you can actually convince yourself and others that the image is a real one — and by doing that, you make it real. "If you behave a certain, positive way and act

PUMPING IRON STRENGTHENS SELF-IMAGE

Well-developed biceps are good for more than just lifting heavy boxes and opening stuck windows. Strong muscles can actually lift your confidence level, too, studies show — and it works for women as well as men.

Researchers have found that strong males were significantly more satisfied with themselves than their muscularly weaker peers. And a recent study reported in the *Journal of Sports Medicine and Physical Fitness* found that women with greater upper body strength had better self-esteem than those who were weaker.

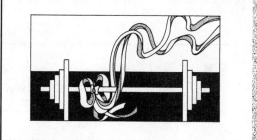

a certain way," he says, "people will begin to treat you differently, better. Your behavior is rewarded by the way others begin to treat you, which tends to reinforce that behavior and enhance your self-image."

Keep looking sharp and carrying yourself confidently, and pretty soon you might notice that you're *feeling* a lot more confident. But don't stop with superficial changes. That's only the beginning; your

106

self-image can get much better. You see, it's not the actual changes you make that matter. The important thing is to trigger the mental pats on the back you can give yourself and the satisfying compliments and smiles you can get from the people around you. Once you have those coming in, they will play off and intensify each other. The more people compliment you, the more you'll like yourself. And the more you like yourself, the better the messages you'll send out to others. Those I-like-myself messages will make others like you even more.

Best of all, the boost in confidence you can get from that first small step will make it possible for you to go on and make longer-lasting changes in your life.

One of those should probably be developing your self-discipline. Discipline may be the most potent force there is for improving your self-esteem. It's what lets you start a regular exercise program and stick with it. It's what helps you learn a foreign language or go back to school at night.

"I think discipline can help improve your self-esteem," says Dr. Wright. "Many people see having the self-discipline to stick with something as very difficult. People think 'Exercising regularly is going to be tough and I don't know if I can do it.' Then, if they succeed, it is very image-enhancing because they thought they wouldn't succeed."

Begin a Spiral of Success

"Really, any activity you try involves taking a risk. You always risk not doing

---

WHAT YOU THINK IS WHAT YOU GET

Think people like you? Then they do. Doubt it? Then they probably don't. Psychologist Rebecca C. Curtis and her associate, Kim Miller, of Adelphi University in Garden City, New York, randomly divided 60 undergraduates into pairs and had each pair chat for 5 minutes. Then, they separated the pairs, and told some that their partners liked them and others that their partners didn't like them. None of this was true, of course.

Later, they had the students meet again for another conversation. This time, the researchers looked for clues. They found that when students were led to believe they weren't liked, they acted in unlikable ways, making less eye contact, sitting further away, and revealing less information. But when students thought their partners liked them, both partners got along better.

In a related test, Curtis found that, regardless of their researcher-provided ratings, the students who felt good about themselves were more likely to believe that the other students liked them.

well, which would lower your self-image," says Dr. Wright. But that kind of risk taking is the road to even greater self-esteem. "It's a numbers game," he explains. "The more times you take a risk, the more chances you have to be successful. The more successes you have, the more confident you feel. The more confident you feel, the more risks you take and the more successes you have. It's a spiraling effect."

Self-discipline, of course, will maximize your chances for success, Dr. Wright says. But he warns against seeing each task or activity you try as a test to be passed or failed. "If you set up a test for yourself to see, for example, if you have the self-discipline to walk a mile every day, then you have the possibility of failing, which can be image-damaging," he says. "But if, instead, you see the activity as an experiment, then you can only collect data. If an activity doesn't work out, you end up saying, 'I guess I'm not that good at walking a mile every day,' or 'Hmm, ballroom dancing is not for me,' instead of things like 'Darn it! I have no self-discipline. I'll never amount to anything.'"

Some people, though, find passing their own tests exhilarating. They prefer to see their activities as pass/fail enterprises rather than as calmer data-collecting experiments, says Dr. Wright.

Once you have discipline and the confidence that comes naturally from it, you'll be capable of moving on to the really big, tough changes that could, if you choose, make your life just the way you want it to be. You might decide to look for a better job, work on your relationship with your spouse, or get involved in a new out-of-work interest. Do you think changes on that scale are beyond you? Maybe they

How Fat You're Not

If you're a woman and you think you're unattractively overweight, you might want to check with a friend. There's a good chance you're not.

Researchers at St. George's Hospital Medical School in London asked 50 female staff members—all of normal weight for their heights—to estimate the widths of their bodies at the bust, waist, and hip levels by moving two points together or apart on a bar. They also had the women estimate the width of a box, just to test their measuring abilities.

Well, the women were all on target with the box, but they consistently overestimated themselves. They were over by 24 percent for their busts, 28 percent for their waists, and 16 percent for their hips.

are—but that's now. See them as a long-term challenge. And remember, the first step toward meeting a big challenge is a very, very small one.

"Whatever it is that you want to accomplish, break it down into steps," says Dr. Wright. "Do something that you can succeed at immediately. Let's say you're thinking about moving to California. The first step is to get some information about California from the library. No matter how low your self-image is, you can do that right away and succeed. Then take a trip out there, and chalk up another sucess. Next talk to someone who lives there."

Look happy and you will be

Forcing a smile will actually force *you* to find life funnier, concludes social psychologist Fritz Strack of Mannheim University in West Germany. He gathered 92 subjects and told them he was testing their physical skills. Then he had them rate on a scale of zero to nine the funniness of a group of cartoons while they held a pen either between their lips or between their teeth.

The results showed that cartoons viewed by those with the pen between their lips rated 4.32, while those viewed by teeth-holders had a higher score of 5.14. The explanation: When held between the lips, a pen causes the mouth to contract, making

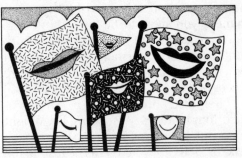

a smile nearly impossible. But when held between the teeth, the pen causes the cheeks and the sides of the mouth to stretch, forcing a laughing expression.

"If you really want to appreciate humor," says Strack, "it's important that you smile —even if you have to fake it a bit."

The trick is to do something small to build up your confidence, and then take another step toward your goal in the wake of that success. And that should be your method of operation whether you want to ask your boss for a raise, strike up a conversation at a party, take a trip to New York, or just improve your self-image.

Striding Down the Road of Confidence

Here are a few more tips from Dr. Wright to help you along your confidence-building way.

Have patience and be gentle with yourself. "Accept yourself the way you are," says Dr. Wright, "and then change what you don't particularly like. We don't have to beat ourselves into change. If I am shy and I don't like it, I can say to myself, 'Okay. I'm shy. Now what am I going to do about it?' rather than 'I hate myself because I'm shy.'"

It's also important to realize that there are some things you can't change. "If you are a short person, you must learn to live with being short," says Dr. Wright. "But you may be surprised to learn that you can also learn to *like* being short. We can change our perceptions much more easily than most of us think—with some effort and self-questioning. After all, how awful is it really to be short?"

Act "as if." "This can be very rewarding," says Dr. Wright. "I do it often with patients." Basically, it involves acting as if you are whatever it is you want to be. If you are shy, act as if you are not. If you are awkward, act as if you are suave. "You pick someone whom you admire. Perhaps he is outgoing and confident. Then imagine how that person would respond to others and behave. When you've got a grip on it, give his behavior a try for a few days and see if it fits. Certain parts will feel all wrong. They will alienate your friends or get you into trouble. But other parts will feel great from the beginning. You can keep those."

Lots of people, he says, object to this exercise because they feel it's phony. Dr. Wright disagrees. "First of all, it's very difficult to take on all the aspects of someone else so a lot of your own personality and style will be there from the start," he says. "But in reality, you are not pretending behavior. How can you pretend to *act*? You are actually *trying* new behavior. You may start out acting like Jane, but if you like the behavior and continue it, you are no longer acting like Jane. You are acting like yourself. It's your behavior pattern now.

"The reason a person might think she is being phony is that we often think that our present behavior is the only type of behavior we can have. But it's not true. Our behavior can be modified," he says. "Is it worth the effort, is the only question."

One word of reassurance: In the beginning, says Dr. Wright, you might act outgoing but still find yourself anxious about it. Generally, he says, the anxiety will go away after a short time.

Begin in a new environment. If the people where you work think of you as only a follower, for instance, take charge for the first time someplace where no one knows you. You could be a volunteer for the local Red Cross or emergency squad perhaps. Present yourself there as a leader —someone they can depend on, and someone who has a lot of good ideas.

"It's easier to make behavioral changes in new environments," says Dr. Wright, "because you don't have to worry about what people who are significant to you will think, and because your old behavior patterns won't be reinforced by people who are used to the old you." And don't worry, when the new you gets comfortable in this alternate environment, it'll start showing up back at work when you least expect it.

Learn a skill. "A sense of accomplishment is one of the best confidence boosters around," says Dr. Wright. Learning Japanese, quilting, or how to fix a tractor could get you thinking, "Hey, that was tough and I did it. I must be pretty great."

Rehearse your new ways of acting. If you know that certain situations make you shudder, practice them at home. Speak in front of a mirror or role-play with a friend. "I think that any type of rehearsal is useful for those with low self-esteem," says Dr. Wright. "Do a mental rehearsal in your head. Or practice striking up low-risk conversations with people like receptionists and cashiers. This kind of practice is important because it enables you to learn that many people will like to talk to you, and that nothing terrible happens even if you get rejected."

Take time to value who you are now. While you're working on the small changes that could add up to a new you, don't forget that you already have lots of great qualities. "I tell my patients, 'Okay. You have a long list of negative things about yourself. Now take a week and write down just as many positive things,'" says Dr. Wright. Try that exercise yourself; you may be surprised how well you do. Or, at the end of every day, make a habit of telling a friend or spouse about your best accomplishment of the day. They'll love to hear it and you'll love telling it.

"This is especially important for people with low self-esteem," says Dr. Wright. "Living with a low self-image is like driving down the expressway with a car that is out of alignment and keeps pulling off to the left. You must spend a lot of energy pulling in the other direction just to drive straight. You have to pull hard in the positive direction and notice all the positive things in your life because your negative thoughts are so automatic."

BEAUTY—AND PERSONALITY— ARE IN THE EYE OF THE BEHOLDER

When you see a very attractive person, do you automatically think she's probably smart? Is your first impulse to like her? If so, then you've already proven to yourself what many researchers have learned— appearance counts for more than just looks.

Dr. Judith Waters, psychologist and a professor at Fairleigh Dickinson University, found in a recent study that better-groomed women may be offered from 8 to 20 percent higher salaries than women who are not groomed as well.

She showed potential employers photos of women before and after having their hair color and makeup routines improved. The after photos got higher ratings and higher salary estimates.

"Attractive individuals are evaluated more positively across a wide range of dimensions," says Dr. Joyce Brothers. "Research on job applicants, potential dating partners, and ill patients shows that improving one's level of attractiveness increases the likelihood that others will evaluate you more positively. We seem to subconsciously believe a stereotype that 'what is attractive is good.'

"One study, on college students applying for a job, demonstrated that subjects who were well groomed and appropriately dressed for interviews were judged to be more confident, more at ease during the interview, and more effective than those who were groomed and attired less attractively.

GIVE WELL, LIVE WELL

"I never thought I could swim distance before. But when I found that I could be effective helping people, I realized that I could do anything I set my mind to. And now I can swim a mile," says Susan Silbert, sociologist, assistant professor of sociology at California State University, Northridge, and founder of One Voice, an emergency aid agency.

"Six years ago, I wouldn't have spoken in front of two people. Today, I'll stand in front of a thousand and speak. That's because the cause is so important to me," says Suzy Perkins Yehl, creator of Rainbows for All God's Children, a support group system for children who have lost a parent through divorce or death.

"I can't feed the whole world or even the whole city, but in my own small way, I can make a tremendous difference. And it's a good feeling. You always get more self-esteem and pleasure from giving than from receiving," says Jack Berlin, owner of a Los Angeles wholesale produce business who gives food to the needy.

What do Susan Silbert, Suzy Perkins Yehl, and Jack Berlin have in common?

Although they lead very different lives, with different concerns and interests, they each have found that they can help others and make a difference in the world. And they each feel more capable, more confident, *better* about themselves as a result.

We all want to solve the problems of the world, but many of us feel that we aren't in a position to *do* anything. "I've never met anybody who didn't care about the world, but they don't do anything because they think they can't," says Silbert, Not only do we think we can't do anything, but we also feel truly terrible about it. "You don't have to rot in guilt and impotency," she says. "You *can* do what you believe in."

And if you do, don't be surprised if you start feeling like a million bucks. That's because mowing your elderly neighbor's lawn, smiling at a stranger, or serving food in a soup kitchen are some of the most effective ways there are to help you feel useful, important, needed, loved, and generally terrific.

"Reaching out to help others brings about a tremendous amount of self-esteem,"

111

(continued on page 114)

Volunteer Yourself for Success

When you think of volunteering, you may picture yourself answering phones at a long table or stuffing endless mounds of envelopes. But actually, the world of volunteerism offers many exciting opportunities. As a matter of fact, many top-level publishing, public relations, and advertising executives cut their teeth through volunteer work. Combine the good feeling you get from helping people with the opportunity to earn yourself some experience, and you've got a package you can't beat.

Have a look at this list of jobs volunteers do for some typical large, medium, and small organizations; see if anything sounds like an exciting way to spend *your* free time.

Sierra Club (large)

- Analyze survey data.
- Combat industries that pollute.
- Communicate with the press.
- Conduct polls.
- Endorse and support environmentally concerned political candidates.
- Lead hikes.
- Lead local Sierra Club groups or state-wide chapters.
- Lead trips.
- Learn about environmental issues through workshops.
- Lobby local, state, and federal governments.
- Monitor acid rain in your backyard to help combat it.
- Organize a letter-writing campaign.
- Organize membership meetings.
- Organize town meetings.
- Present slide shows.
- Participate in public education.
- Form a strategy to influence Congress to support an issue.
- Work on the political action committee.
- Write and produce television videos on environmental issues.
- Write letters to editors of newspapers.
- Participate in youth education.

Mount Sinai Hospital in New York (medium)

- Act in films geared toward health education.
- Assist in cancer research.

- Develop brochures.
- Participate in emergency room procedures.
- Participate in health education.
- Hold and feed babies.
- Participate in occupational therapy.
- Perform music for patients and staff.
- Preview videos for health education.
- Participate in physical therapy.
- Participate in rape crisis intervention.
- Rehabilitate patients with disabilities.
- Participate in social work services.
- Participate in spiritual guidance.
- Participate in therapeutic play with kids.

Lehigh Valley AIDS Services Center in Pennsylvania (small)

- Analyze surveys determining how people with AIDS will be treated in the future.
- Answer a hotline.
- Be a buddy for someone with AIDS.
- Communicate with the press.

- Document information on AIDS and possible cures.
- Participate in hospice work.
- Lead a support group for people on whom AIDS has had an impact.
- Give legal advice.
- Lobby the local, state, and federal governments.
- Join in prison and street outreach.
- Participate in public education about AIDS.
- Organize a food bank.
- Organize demonstrations to increase the availability of experimental drugs.
- Organize social events for people with AIDS.
- Raise money through grants, donations, and events.
- Translate foreign languages.
- Work with employees, co-workers, and relatives of those with AIDS.
- Work with the welfare department.
- Write educational pamphlets.

says Dr. Edward Eismann, a social worker who founded UNITAS, a community counseling and support agency for young people in the Bronx. "I think a lot of people's self-esteem is low because they have never developed a sense of pride in their own abilities. These people need to develop a sense of themselves in some way. It might be through meeting a special friend, falling in love, having a religious experience, or being deeply trusted by someone."

Helping others, says Dr. Eismann, can be a way to simultaneously prove yourself worthy of someone's trust, develop skills, and make a profound connection with both the people you help and the other helpers. "I would say that one of the main reasons people help others is to feel good and useful," he says.

Poverty of the Soul

"One Voice actually developed as an outgrowth of a race relations class I was teaching," says Silbert of her emergency aid agency. "At the end of the class, we decided that poor race relations were the result of poor human relations." The class decided to do something about it, and raised a thousand dollars to make up food baskets for 70 families. The next year, they fed 500 families, and now they're a year-round emergency aid agency with over a thousand members. If people need jobs, food, surgery, funeral, or rent money, One Voice can help.

"At One Voice, we have a two-pronged approach," she says. "First, we try to help those who are in the kind of poverty most of us recognize—generally hungry, poorly educated people. Then there is another kind of poverty that we attack. Poverty of the soul. We go out into the community, asking people to recognize and heal that poverty in their lives by joining us in fighting the more easily recognized poverty."

In doing so, they make a connection with those they help. "I think a lot of insecurity and lack of fulfillment exists because people haven't realized their connection with other people," says Silbert. One of the best ways to forge that connection is to do something you believe in for the good of yourself and others, whether it's registering people to vote, leading a scout group, or volunteering at a hospital.

The Long-Life Connection

You may find that the social contact you get from raising money for a worthy organization, helping your neighbors, or coaching the Little League, is what makes it all worthwhile for you. The bonds that form between you and other members of your organization, and also between you and those you help, are among the deepest and most emotional that exist between human beings. "That bondedness is essential for your well-being," says Dr. Eismann. "When you are alone in the world, no self-esteem is possible."

Not only can social bonds improve your self-esteem, they may also lengthen your life. In a study of 2,700 people in Tecumseh, Michigan, that lasted more than a decade, those with many social contacts tended to live longer than more isolated individuals, according to investigators at the University of Michigan's Survey Research Center.

In another study, Dr. Lisa Berkman of Yale University and Dr. S. Leonard Syme of the University of California at Berkeley, both epidemiologists, followed nearly 5,000 residents of Alameda County, California. Over nine years, they found that those who were unmarried, had few friends or relatives, and shunned community organizations were more than twice as likely to die during that time than people who had these social relationships. That was true regardless of race, income, level of activity, or other lifestyle factors.

Twenty years ago, when Dr. Eismann first set up UNITAS, he was able to form bonds with children from a culture completely unlike his own, the children of the Bronx. He was initially hired to be a clinician at the local mental health center there, but soon found that the children who really needed his help weren't coming to the center. "I wanted to work, so I went outside and began to walk around in the streets," he says. "Pretty soon, I began to make friends with the kids. I chatted with them, listened to them, and when problems came up, I was able to help work them out."

At the end of that first summer, says Dr. Eismann, a woman who lived on the block came up to him and said, "Don't think we mothers weren't watching you every second that you were out there with our kids. But we like you, so you can stay."

Today, UNITAS is a large, government-funded organization, but it still operates on the principle of meeting the kids on their own turfs, bonding with them, and helping them learn to communicate with each other in a more loving, peaceable way.

Eternal Youth

When Louise Montgomery answers the phone at Friendship House, the Portland, Maine, shelter for the homeless she and her husband opened in 1985 with their savings, her voice is full of youthful vigor. So it's a bit of a surprise when she starts to tell her story. "The last thing I thought I would do at the age of 72 was open a shelter for the homeless and live in it," she says. "But I feel so rewarded through this work I am doing. Nothing I have done in the past 30 years has been so gratifying."

How does Mrs. Montgomery handle being on 24-hour call, raising the donations that keep Friendship House running, and planning for future projects like the summer camp she would like to open for disadvantaged children? "One of the beautiful advantages of being my age is that I can get along wonderfully with just 4 or 5 hours of sleep," she says. "And I'm blessed with great energy."

Some preliminary studies indicate that, as much as her great energy and good health are allowing her to do good works, the good works may be just the thing that *gives* her that health and energy in the first place.

A Tecumseh, Michigan, study revealed that doing regular volunteer work, more than any other activity, significantly increased life expectancy. Men who did no volunteer work at all were two and a half times as likely to die during the study as men who volunteered at least once a week. (The results for women were not as dramatic, perhaps because many women spend so much time helping others without formally volunteering.)

In another study, psychologist David

(continued on page 118)

These Groups Want You

Ready to dive into the world of volunteerism? You could start your own organization that addresses your particular vision. But it might make more sense to find a small, local group with goals that speak to your own. Or join the local chapter of a large organization that appeals to you. One way to find local organizations is to check in the blue pages of your phone book under "Volunteer Center" or "Volunteer Bureau." Or, send a self-addressed, stamped envelope to VOLUNTEER—The National Center, 1111 N. 9th St., Suite 500, Arlington, VA 22209 (703) 276-0542. They can give you information about volunteer opportunities in your area. Another possibility is to peruse the partial listing of national organizations below, and get in touch with them to find a local contact.

American Red Cross
17th and D Sts. NW
Washington, DC 20006
(202) 737-8300

Association of Junior Leagues
825 3rd Ave.
New York, NY 10022
(212) 355-4380
(Women's civic service, ages 18-45)

Boys Clubs of America
771 1st Ave.
New York, NY 10017
(212) 557-7755

Girls Clubs of America
205 Lexington Ave.
New York, NY 10016

Gray Panthers
311 S. Juniper St.
Suite 601
Philadelphia, PA 19107
(215) 545-6555
(Older adults)

Interfaith Hunger Appeal
468 Park Ave. S
Suite 904A
New York, NY 10016
(212) 689-8460

Kiwanis International
3636 Woodview Trace
Indianapolis, IN 46268
(317) 875-8755
(Men's civic service club)

National AIDS Network
2033 M St. NW
Suite 800
Washington, DC 20036
(202) 293-2437

National Association of Town Watch
P.O. Box 769
Havertown, PA 19083
(215) 649-7055
(Work against crime through local crime watches, other crime prevention activities)

National Coalition for the Homeless
1439 Rhode Island Ave. NW
Washington, DC 20005

National Committee on Youth Suicide
  Prevention
67 Irving Pl. S
New York, NY 10003
(212) 677-6666

National Community Action Foundation
2100 M St. NW
Suite 604A
Washington, DC 20037
(202) 775-0223
(Head Start, Meals on Wheels, etc.)

National Gay and Lesbian Task Force
1517 U St. NW
Washington, DC 20009
(202) 332-6483

National School Volunteer Program
701 N. Fairfax St.
Alexandria, VA 22314
(703) 836-4880
(Provides leadership for school volunteers)

Older Women's League
1325 G St. NW
Lower Level B
Washington, DC 20005
(202) 783-6686
(Middle-aged and older women's issues)

Oxfam America
115 Broadway
Boston, MA 02116
(617) 574-8800
(International development)

Rotary International
1600 Ridge Ave.
Evanston, IL 60201
(312) 328-0100
(Civic service club)

United States Jaycees
P.O. Box 7
Tulsa, OK 74121
(Civic service, ages 18–35)

Volunteers in Technical Assistance
1815 N. Lynn St.
Suite 200
Arlington, VA 22209
(703) 276-1800
(Places volunteer consultants in foreign countries to
assist technical development)

118

McClelland of Harvard University showed students a film of Mother Teresa, the ultimate altruist, working among Calcutta's sick and poor. Tests on students revealed an increase in immunoglobulin A, an antibody that helps defend the body against certain diseases.

Follow a Vision

Ready to drop out of the human rat race and join up with the cooperative human team? Then the only question left is where to start.

Just plunge in, says Silbert. "You just do something," she says. "Whether you join an organization that exists, start one of your own, smile at people in the supermarket, meet your neighbors, start a recycling group, treat people in a human way . . . whatever you choose, you'll feel more human, and more fulfilled. And you'll be making a difference."

If you're going for large-scale involvement, however, your first step should be to choose your priorities, say the directors of the Giraffe Project, a group dedicated to promoting and honoring people who, as they put it, stick their necks out for the common good. If you set out to save the whole world at once, all you'll end up with is sore feet and no energy, they say. Instead, think about what's really important to you, and choose an area where you have the skills and support to be effective.

Next, picture your goal. Get a grasp on where you're going with your project — that's the vision that will compel you to move onward. "We started by sitting around and dreaming," says Silbert of the start of One Voice. "Then we took very small steps,

slowly, one at a time, and soon we saw the dreams coming true. We realized that the only reason they hadn't before was because we hadn't tried."

After that, to get your project underway, you must learn all you can about the situation in which you are involved, and then find other people who will want to work with you. Motivate them with your vision.

The final step before success is hard work and persistence. "People ask me how I managed to get Rainbows for All God's Children underway," says Yehl of her support group system for kids. "My answer is you work real hard every day."

In 1983, there were 50 children participating in Yehl's pilot program in her neighborhood. Today, there are over 40,000 kids involved in Rainbow projects throughout 33 states and four foreign countries. "Now I can say to others, if you have a dream, follow it," says Yehl. "If you have a belief, stand up for it. Because I know that it can work."

Start with Your Beliefs

"To be really powerful, your vision has to be rooted in a belief system," says Dr. Eismann. To have the staying power to get through the hard times, there has to be a reason for what you do, he says, whether it is religious, political, or philosophical. Without that, when things get difficult, you'll wonder why you bother — and you just might quit. "I have to make sense of my life in order to keep at something that is difficult year after year after year," he says.

"For me, that belief is that life has a

purpose. The purpose is to create a cooperative brother- and sisterhood among all people. The work I do is to help youngsters understand their peers and parents better. That, to me, is living out what I believe. It's a way of making that brother- and sisterhood become incarnated right here and now."

If you are to be truly effective in your efforts, part of your belief system must be that it is worthwhile to help people and to give of your time without much, if any, financial reimbursement. That can be tough to do in today's me-first world, says Silbert.

"A lot of the values that we are taught in society directly counter values that we would like to hold. Many of us were taught, for instance, that we have to look out for only ourselves or we'll get stomped on," she explains. "It's more courageous today to be a loving, humane person than to be a cold, distant person, because loving is not a value that is supported in our society."

Care for Yourself, Too

As you reach out to others, don't forget that you can only be effective as long as you, yourself, are cared for. The trap: You may like how important you feel if you become indispensable, but you will also be pressured by thinking, 'If I don't do it, no one else will.' That kind of pressure may make you feel needed but it will weigh you down. Besides, if you are always so busy doing for others, then you will not meet your own needs. And how will you feel if your needs don't rate even *your* attention? *Un*important.

"It can be very discouraging to help others," says Dr. Eismann. "Those who do usually don't get adequate support in their efforts. When you help somebody, you must have a friend who will listen to you, encourage your project, and support you emotionally. No one can do it alone." So take care of yourself, and keep lots of friends around who will give you a boost when you need it.

The Way the World Should Be

Remember that your goal is to be important and useful, but not indispensable. You want the changes you make to continue after you decide to work on something else. So you can't be the only one supporting them.

One of the best ways to ensure that your goals are shared by others is to work as part of a group of people, *all* of whom are important to the project. That group could be a national organization geared toward large-scale changes; a small task force, like a block association, working on a specific issue in your community; or a human services business, like a hospital. One of the most fulfilling groups to work with is the one you live in—your neighborhood.

Charlie E. Muller, Jr., has lived with his wife in West Lebanon, New York, since he retired from the Air Force in 1972. "I always used to say, 'If I retire, I would like a trout stream in the front and deer in the back,' and that's what we have here," he says. But Muller has done more than simply commune with nature. For the past ten years, he's gotten to be an institution in this small town.

By working through the town's

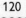

120

churches, Muller has been able to raise money, which he distributes to people with specific emergencies in West Lebanon. "If a person is sick and they need help, I can give them help," he says. "Say their car insurance needs to be paid quickly. I do that. Then I refer them to agencies for continued help. There was one man who lost his job. I worked out a budget for him, and I bought him a car for $200 so he could get around.

"I save the people who have fallen through the cracks. We have assistance available, but it's long term. Most of my assistance is short term," he explains.

The beauty of Muller's project is how personal it is. He wins the confidence of people in trouble, and helps them without judging them. And he gets help from the rest of the town in the form of emotional support and contributions. "I spend on faith," says Muller, who will often put up money on his own. "And I always get it back.

"I was in the Air Force for 25 years, and I've been around the world. But to me, this is the way I would like to see the world be, everyone helping their neighbors."

ALL PAIN, NO GAIN: THE ORDEAL OF PERFECTIONISM

To the class, it seemed like a harmless question. "What about the brain waves of dolphins?" came a student's query from the back of the room.

The teacher, in graduate school after raising three children, seemed shaken. She didn't know the answer. She stared at the floor and wondered, for the third time that week, why she ever thought she deserved to get a master's degree. She was too stupid. And now the whole class knew it.

Two depressing weeks later, with the help of her therapist, she learned one of the most important lessons of her life. She, along with millions of other people, had a nemesis called perfectionism.

You probably know some perfectionists—those self-mandated superpeople who crusade through life with sky-high standards but are usually grounded trying to meet them.

"Perfectionism is the world's greatest con game," says Dr. David Burns, Philadelphia psychiatrist and director of the Institute for Cognitive and Behavioral Therapies at Presbyterian Medical Center of Philadelphia, in his book *Feeling Good*, "It's a concept that doesn't fit reality."

What it does fit is the distorted set of beliefs perfectionists have about themselves.

Somewhere along the line, perfectionist people picked up the message that "love, respect, and reward will be theirs, if only they can be bigger and better and more wonderful than they actually are," Dr. Burns says.

A Breed Falling Apart

When perfectionists connect their self-worth with success, the result can be a loss of happiness and satisfaction with life.

"This is one of the most common themes we see in therapy," explains Dr. Burns. Like Dr. Burns's patient who expected her cerebrum to be brimming with handy little facts on the brain waves of dolphins and other scholarly matters, "these people just can't live up to the unrealistic expectations they have for

122

themselves. And when they fall short, they somehow believe they're a total failure and deserve to suffer."

That suffering often shows up as depression and anxiety, marital and sexual problems, and difficulty forming and maintaining relationships. The pressure of perfectionism may also predispose some people to problems such as alcoholism, the eating disorders anorexia nervosa and bulimia, and obsessive-compulsive behaviors.

Superseekers can be caped in different kinds of perfectionism. "Most perfectionists aren't like Tony Randall's compulsive character, Felix Unger, on 'The Odd Couple,' " says Dr. Scott Pengelly, psychological consultant for Nike and Athletics West. While Felix declared war on all imperfection, whether it was in his slovenly roommate Oscar, his job performance, or his underwear drawer, "most perfectionists are just trapped by the illusion that they can achieve perfection in certain areas if they push hard enough, usually areas they consider extremely important," he explains.

Dr. Burns points out three places where perfectionism can breed.

At work. Dr. Burns once lectured to a group of insurance agents on the pitfalls of perfectionist thinking. The salesmen nodded in agreement and applauded when he was finished. This was followed by a rousing address from the president: "People, we were number two this year. That's not good enough. Being number one is the only thing that counts!"

"Pushing for perfectionism may not be the winning strategy you think it is," Dr. Burns says. "Each perfectionist thinks it can help make for a better performance,

when actually it cripples the person with procrastination, emotional misery, and insecurity."

In a study of more than 700 men and women, Dr. Burns discovered perfectionists experience distress and dissatisfaction with their careers and personal lives.

ARE YOU A PERFECTIONIST?

Just because your house is messy or your checkbook won't balance doesn't mean you don't have a streak of perfectionism somewhere that could be holding you back. Experts point to four behavior patterns that may indicate a deep-down desire to be perfect.

Procrastinating. You put off giving a dinner party until you have perfected a soufflé recipe, installed new carpeting, and repaved the driveway for the big event.

"Finished product" thinking. You overlook the satisfaction from *doing* something, like organizing a fund-raiser, and aren't happy until it's all over and the money's in the bank.

All-or-nothing thinking. You slip up on your diet and eat a sundae; you feel that one indulgence means you're weak, your diet is a total failure, and you don't deserve to ever see your toes again.

Mental filtering. You dwell on the bad reviews of your latest book and discount the success of your previous two that got you an honorary degree from a university and a spot on Johnny Carson's "Tonight" show.

And he found no evidence that they were doing any better or making any more money than their nonperfectionist peers.

"Despite what we've been taught," he says, "perfectionism appears to be all pain and no gain."

In your relationships. Many perfectionists fear criticism and react defensively because they just can't stand the thought of being wrong. This can alienate others, resulting in conflicts in marriage and professional relationships.

In the bedroom. Although occasional impotence is normal, perfectionists may turn this into a castastrophe with the ego- and erection-deflating attitude, "Unless I'm a great lover, I'm less of a man." Perfectionist women may place the same burden on themselves, basing their self-esteem on the girth of their thighs.

Another type of perfectionist is one Dr. Pengelly calls a "hope I" perfectionist. He sees many of these people both in athletics and in business. The tendency here is to get so wrapped up in thinking, "I hope I break this record," or "I hope I can save this project," that all the worry wins out and the goal is lost. "Perhaps no mistake is uglier than the brutal concept, 'I am how I perform,'" says Dr. Pengelly.

When all of society appears to back up their be-the-best attitude, it can be hard for perfectionists to realize that they're only hurting themselves.

"Our whole society puts a premium on perfection," says Jim Quitno, pastor of Grace Lutheran Church in Spirit Lake, Iowa, who's seen a lot of perfectionism in his 15 years of counseling.

"In the workplace, we push our people to work as fast as they can, and when they are working at peak capacity, we may call in an efficiency expert to see how we can squeeze out even more productivity.

"We are a culture in which parents go to Little League games, sit in the bleachers, and criticize their children for only making it to first base. If he had really tried, he could have made it to second. We're never satisfied."

A Quest for Love

While culture may serve as perfectionism's reinforcement, childhood may well be the root of the problem.

"Many of the people whom I have seen have the idea that somehow, if only they were perfect, their parents would love them," says Dr. Asher R. Pacht, clinical professor of psychology and psychiatry at the University of Wisconsin-Madison. The child of a parent who gives either inconsistent, conditional, or absolutely no approval may try harder and harder to "win" the love that's not being given.

One 35-year-old career woman Pastor Quitno saw came from another kind of home that can breed perfectionism—the supersuccessful environment. Her father was a dynamo both in the community and in the state legislature. Her mother headed all the best organizations in town. Growing up in this home, she was often praised for her accomplishments. But she felt that she had to measure up to the level of her parents' success and their high expectations for her.

The fact that she's simply not as talented as her mother nor as aggressive as her father set her up for some guilt-building failures.

123

Patricia DePol knows the pressure of living up to superparents. A recovered anorexic, she is now assistant director of the American Anorexia/Bulimia Association and a firm believer in making children comfortable with success and failure. "I was aware of subtle feedback growing up," she says. "There definitely was pressure to perform. What I know now, and what all parents should let their children know, is that love and assurance shouldn't be connected to being perfect."

A Better Approach

Perfectionists need to learn self-acceptance and let the air out of their overblown standards. The trick is to change the no-win mindset and think in more constructive ways.

In his book *Feeling Good,* Dr. Burns explains some effective ways to overcome perfectionism through cognitive therapy, an innovative form of treatment based on the theory that, "You will feel the way you think."

"You can break out of perfectionism by learning to identify negative thoughts, recognizing the distortions in them from perfectionism, and learning to substitute more realistic and positive thoughts," he explains.

"When I was helping the teacher who felt like a failure for not knowing about the brain waves of dolphins, we looked at what negative thoughts crossed her mind right after that class. She was thinking, 'I should have known that. I must be a lousy teacher.' She saw that those negative thoughts were illogical for several reasons: She had never learned about dolphins,

she knew deep down that no one can be expected to know everything, and she could have easily turned the challenge to her into challenge for the class by saying, 'That's a great question. Let's all research this and find out the significance of it.' Eventually, she learned to think about herself in a more compassionate and realistic way, and her self-confidence improved."

Costs Outweigh the Benefits

Another method Dr. Burns recommends is to write out a "cost/benefit analysis." List all the advantages and disadvantages of thinking about something in a perfectionist way.

Take the compulsive car washer, for instance. Every neighborhood probably has one: A person who insists on washing his car every Saturday, even when it's not dirty. For this behavior's advantages, he might list that, "It feels good to have the spiffiest car in town." And that's probably about it.

His disadvantages might read, "I have no time for softball anymore. I spend a fortune on cleaning products, and I should own stock in Turtle Wax. I get really upset whenever it rains. I wish death to all birds." It won't take long to find out where all the tension's coming from. Once a person realizes that perfectionism isn't helping, it will be that much easier to give it up.

Dr. Burns suggests conducting a mini-experiment, where a person refuses to give in to a perfectionist habit for a certain amount of time. This can be upsetting at first, but riding it out until the worst of the anxiety is over will gradually help the person realize he can tolerate being imperfect.

One perfectionist felt intense guilt if all the windows in her house weren't washed every day. Using Dr. Burns's refusal method, she would pick a day and not go near the windows. Every hour and then every day that she got by without washing them would bring her closer to beating her habit, until she was comfortable with a more reasonable washing schedule.

Pastor Quitno offers a substitute motto for the many perfectionists whose fear of failure keeps them from trying anything new: If anything is worth doing, it is worth doing poorly.

"That motto certainly violates our cultural stress on excellence," Pastor Quitno admits, "but it can help a perfectionist.

"I'll say, 'Can you win an Olympic medal for swimming? No. Then does that mean you shouldn't swim? No.' Gradually, a perfectionist can see that even in the areas where he sets rigid standards, there will always be room for improvement—and inadequacy, too."

"Learn to celebrate smaller goals," suggests Dr. Pengelly. "Jack Nicholson thinks a movie is good if it has two good scenes in it. I think a ten-cut record album is a good buy if it has two really nice songs on it. If you don't go looking for perfection in yourself, you'll probably surprise yourself and find satisfaction."

And remember, adds Dr. Pacht, "True perfection exists only in obituaries and eulogies."

WRITE A RÉSUMÉ
FOR THE REAL YOU

"What do you do?"

It's a big question, but one that many people have whittled down to the size of a toothpick. You'll normally get this inquiry fired at you when someone wants to find out what sort of work you do. And usually, you'll respond in kind: "What do I do? I check the air pressure inside tennis balls at the Spaulding factory." Or maybe you say in sort of a resigned voice, "I'm a housewife."

But Is That *All* You Do?

While the kind of work you do or have done accounts for some of your time and reflects part of your personality, there are still all those activities, feelings, and experiences that occur outside the workplace that are just as important to figure into a total concept of who you are. But we seldom treat these extraprofessional pursuits to the much-needed attention they deserve. The result? Too much of our self-respect or identity depends on something as arbitrary as a job title.

"Actually, there are three ways that people tend to identify or define themselves," says Dr. Emmett E. Miller, a Menlo Park, California, physician who, as a trendsetter in body/mind healing for the past ten years, is known nationally for his series of self-help tapes. "The first and most primitive way is by what they have. Who are you? One man might answer that by saying 'I own three limos.' Number two is by what a person does for a living. The third and healthiest way people identify themselves is by recognizing their internal value system and emotional makeup. In other words, they look at who they are underneath the nice car and great job."

Why is the third way the best way? One reason may be that your eggs aren't all in one basket. By basing self-esteem largely on where your desk is located, you could well be setting yourself up for a fall. What happens if you get a salary reduction? What happens when you retire? If you don't give yourself credit for excellence in other areas of life, you've got nothing to keep your identity afloat in emotionally troubled waters. "People who are in touch with their real identity weather the storm better because they have a more varied and richer sense of themselves due to the importance they attach to their personal lives and activities," notes Dr. Miller. "I guess you could say that for these kinds of people their lives *as a whole* are their profession."

If we do need to make our lives our profession, as Dr. Miller suggests, a great way to start is with a résumé. We've all had to create one somewhere along the line. Only this time we're going to put down the things that have happened or are happening in our private lives. For example, have you ever taken care of someone who was ill? That goes down on your résumé. Perhaps it would look something like this:

1984-1985 CAREGIVER — Nursed my invalid aunt back to health. Duties included dispensing medication, monitoring dietary intake, providing mental comfort and love, administering humor when patient's spirits were low, and more.

Qualifications: Responsibility, caring nature, gentle humor, sympathy, a strong will.

Or maybe you take a long walk in the woods every evening right around sunset. Picture that on a résumé.

1985-Present WALKER — Take long walks in the woods. Duties include the exercising of the body, mind, and spirit through aerobic activity; casual nature studies; and the enhancement of my perception of beauty.

Qualifications: Dedication, a need for self-improvement, the ability to relax, a talent for hearing and seeing, a love of nature, a good rapport with myself.

Now you may very well be saying to yourself, "All this just from a stroll through the underbrush?" Of course. When you realize that you learn from everything you do, then you might surprise yourself with how much you know. But what you *like* to learn and do is as important as how much you've learned. Add another section under each activity (under *Qualifications*) entitled *Comments*. Here you can put down how you felt about what you were doing and the changes you think it made in your life.

To see the complete pattern of the real you, the résumé should be complete. Suspend the critic in you and don't look back at what you've written until it's done, whether it takes you a day or a week. When it's finished, type it up in standard résumé form and head for a quiet place to look things over.

"There are several possibilities that may occur when you meet yourself," suggests Dr. Miller. "First of all, you might look at your résumé and see a completely new you — a person who rarely gets a chance to emerge during the daily rat race. This new person may have different needs than you do. If so, it could mean that you have been focusing your attention on other people's needs at the expense of your own, even though you didn't know you were doing it. Ask yourself, 'Do I like this new person? Do I want to see more of him?' To do so you might start by closing your eyes and picturing this new person operating in your life."

You may look at your résumé and for the first time be very impressed with just how rich in experience you really are. You may also find that throughout your life you've had a strong affinity for a particular activity and have gained so much experience in it that you could capitalize on it in the future. You might also be surprised to find out that you don't really like what you're doing with your life right now and that's why you've been vaguely unhappy for the past year.

Whatever thoughts come to you, you're experiencing something we call regeneration—a new way of looking at your internal resources, encouraging growth in the direction that makes you happiest.

After all of this heavy thinking, take a minute and go back to the last time someone asked you, "So, what do you do?" If your answer was something about the air pressure in tennis balls, or retirement, take another look at your résumé and remember it. The next time someone asks you that question, why not turn to them, smile, and say "I live . . . and I do it quite well."

MAXIMIZING IN THE MIDYEARS

Some people say it starts at 35 and runs up to 59. Others say 40 to 65. But in fact, midlife is something of a mysterious Bermuda triangle; you never seem to know where it starts and ends, you just somehow end up in the middle of it. The trick is to chart a course through these waters that leads to adventure rather than stagnation.

Traditionally, midlife tends to throw the biggest waves at three parts of life: our careers, our marital relationships, and our confidence in our own creative abilities. But as far as the experts are concerned, midlife could be about the best thing to happen to us in relation to all three. It's a matter of applying our experience, showing a willingness to change, and using a little imagination.

Career Changes

Remember when you finished school? The working world was a mysterious and exotic land that lay just beyond the pur-ple horizon. It's been 20 years since you set out on that adventure and suddenly, as you settle down behind your desk one dreary Monday morning, the thrill is gone. Maybe the job has become routine. Perhaps it's been many a moon since your last promotion. Or, it could be that *you* have changed and your current career just isn't fulfilling your needs anymore. Whatever the reason, it is not unusual for this to occur at midlife, and it just might be that you are ready to join the ever growing number of people who are leaving behind the security of their former jobs in search of new and more enjoyable careers. If a change is just what you are looking for, here are a few things to consider.

Be careful that you aren't changing careers for the wrong reasons. "Ask yourself if you're not trying to find a certain excitement and satisfaction in your job that in fact should be provided by your marriage," says Dr. Michael Nichols, author of *Turning Forty in the Eighties*. "If this is the case, a career change won't help."

Are you running away from an unpleasant boss? You may be leaving a career

129

130

you enjoy very much just to avoid one person. Before bailing out, see if there is any way to make a lateral shift in the company.

Give your current position one final all-out effort. "Maybe you've been in a slump and haven't really been giving it your best shot," says Dr. Nichols. "You only get out of a job what you put into it. Work harder. Work smarter. Do this for another month. If the thrill is back, then you have solved your problem. If not, then it's definitely time to move on."

Investigate your past job experience and interests to gain clues for a new direction. Dr. Beverly Potter, author of *Maverick Career Strategies,* has a favorite story concerning a man who switched from a career in engineering to paralegal work. "The man had been a competent engineer and then a competent paralegal assistant, but in all honesty, he was nothing extraordinary. What made him a real star was when he found a prestigious firm that was looking for an engineer familiar with legal terminology. Instantly he went from mere competence to being the only man who could successfully fill a highly specialized position."

Are you harboring some past work experience that, in combination with your present knowledge, could make you uniquely qualified for an unusual job? List all your work experience and see if you can't mix and match. But don't stop there. If you are an avid hobbyist, throw your extraoffice interests into the pot. Your present business knowledge, mixed in with the hours you spent in the basement puttering around with that combination television/microwave oven/blender might

just land you a managerial position with the electronics firm of your dreams.

Decide if you are a team player or a loner. It's the decade of the entrepreneur, and you've probably seen some of your friends make the prospect of starting a new business very attractive. Before taking the plunge yourself, Dr. Nichols suggests you take a look at your past record. "Some people enjoy the security offered with a job in a large firm and they would be uncomfortable without it. But, if you're the kind of person who always enjoyed self-started and self-executed projects in the past, the world of the entrepreneur might be for you." If you are unsure about yourself, a pleasant compromise between security and independence can be found by acting as a consultant to several large firms.

Attend to your interests before attending to your bank account. Although they are sometimes hard to separate, job satisfaction and large paychecks are not the same thing. Think hard about what you enjoy in life and firmly make yourself narrow your job search to positions that honestly fit your interests. Only after finding that segment of the job market that answers your needs should you incorporate the dollar factor.

Don't forget your biggest assets. Those assets are age and the sublime experience that goes with it. The ability to solve practical problems tends to increase with age, says Dr. Steven Cornelius, associate professor of human development at Cornell University. In addition to hard job skills, you've probably acquired a kind of second sense for correct social maneuverings in the workplace. "These qualities make you perfect for supervisory positions, handling younger employees, and mediating relationships between workers," says Dr. Cornelius.

Relationships

Marriage in the middle years is a unique proposition offering you an unparalleled chance to discover your mate all over again. At the same time, it is also a period of upheaval, change, and doubt. For years the relationship has been running on a kind of cruise control set for raising and launching the children. The kids are gone now and both you and your spouse are facing a slightly frightening freedom, and wondering what to do with it.

Renewal

We need to go through a personal and marital renewal every five years, according to Dr. Paul Welter, professor of counseling at Kearney State College, Nebraska. "What I mean by renewal is taking an inventory of our lives and asking ourselves not 'What do I expect from life?' which is a question of happiness, but rather 'What does life expect from me?' This is a question of meaning and of mission."

During the midyears, marriages and people are often looking for new purpose and meaning. "Inner renewal means that we understand the meaning of our existence and are ready to pay the rent on it by reaching out, by helping and encouraging the world around us," says Dr. Welter. "In

a marriage, it can be as simple as giving your spouse your full support."

Burnout

"Boredom is the number one cause of marriage burnout in these years," says Dr. Welter. "It occurs when a person feels that he or she knows everything there is to know about his or her spouse and explores no further. Additionally, outer renewal takes the place of inner renewal."

Signs of outer renewal, which can sometimes serve as markers of marital burnout, consist of multiple job changes, a sudden need to relocate, and the desire for new gadgets and toys. Another sign of burnout is increasing amounts of time spent in front of the television. "It's often called the electronic fireplace, but unlike a real fireplace, no talking or sharing goes on in front of it," says Dr. Welter.

Here are three questions you might want to ask yourself to determine if you are experiencing marital burnout. These same questions can also serve as a starting direction to rectify the situation.

Do I know my mate's purpose in life? If the answer is no, this might be a good starting point for some very interesting discussions with your spouse.

Am I trying to control this marriage? If the answer is yes, not only are you denying your mate an equal share, but you are cheating yourself as well. The relationship formed by equal partners has more possibilities than the imagination of one dominant partner could conceive alone.

Can I think of one really interesting thing my mate said to me last week? If the answer is no, you either don't listen as

132

well as you could or you haven't learned to appreciate your spouse's interests.

Discovery

"Shared tasks are a good way to initiate discovery of each other," suggests Dr. Welter. "Chores often get segmented into solitary duties in which he takes out the garbage and she washes dishes (or vice versa). Find things to do together such as painting the den or cleaning out the garage." Here are other ways to discover your mate.

Share your friends.   Cultivate friends you both can enjoy rather than relying on separate circles of friends for each of you. People behave differently in social settings than they do at home. You may get to see a facet of your spouse you never saw before.

Share a mission or a service. Whether it's volunteering for soup kitchen duty on Saturday afternoon, saving the whales, or co-chairing the neighborhood crime patrol, do something you both can work on for the betterment of the world.

Share a sense of wonder.   Explore the world together. Share the moment when you both see the Grand Canyon for the first time or watch the sunrise over the Acropolis in Athens.

Ask seed questions.   Ask what caption was under your spouse's high school yearbook picture. What is the best thing your spouse remembers about being 9 years old? Seed questions such as these begin a conversation in one subject that grows and crystallizes into another. You may discover, completely by accident, new facets of your mate's personality that were

formerly hidden. Go one step further. Think of and then ask your mate a question you've never asked before.

Mental Acuity and Creativity

Midlife is that time when you finally put away those thoughts of writing the great American novel, winning the Nobel prize, or composing a number one chart buster. You suspect that what used to be a creative bonfire is now nothing more than smoldering coals. Well, nothing could be more removed from the truth.

IQ does not decline with age in the midyears.   "People used to think that one's mental peak was around the age of 20," says Dr. Mary Howell, director of the Kennedy Aging Center in Chatham, Massachusetts. "But there is now a large body of IQ testing data that suggest that for people who stay mentally active, IQ will at least stay the same in some areas, and may even increase in others."

Mental stimulation is a must for acuity in the midyears.   If you don't continue to utilize and stimulate your mind, you will find yourself losing your abilities. "Mental fitness is maintained by learning new things, applying old information in a new way and by combining things we know to form new ideas," says Dr. Howell. Other fine ways of toning your mental muscles are through crossword puzzles, reading, and board games, such as chess, Scrabble, and Pictionary. On the other hand, the easiest way to lose your mind is by watching too much TV. "TV is one of the great thieves of mental acuity because it is a totally passive form of entertainment that makes no demands upon the viewer."

Creative inspiration is no stranger to midlife. "While there is some evidence that creative productivity is highest in the early twenties, it may be due more to an abundance of energy and a conquer-the-world attitude rather than a higher abstract or cognitive quotient," says Dr. Howell. "I'm not at all sure that whatever it is peaking at that time is the most important aspect of creativity. Many authors, painters, inventors, and composers actually find advantages in their later years as they gain further technical skill and the ability to make grand thematic connections in their art."

Midlife is no time to slack off. Here, from *The Book of Ages,* by Desmond Morris, is just a small list of what other people have done in the neighborhood of the midyears.

● At age 35, Italian scientist Evangelista Torricelli invented the barometer.

● At age 36, Edgar Rice Burroughs wrote *Tarzan of the Apes.*

● At age 37, Ingmar Bergman's film, *Smiles of a Summer Night,* brought him international fame.

● At age 38, Edwin Herbert Land invented the Polaroid camera, which developed pictures in 60 seconds.

● At age 39, Coco Chanel produced Chanel No. 5, the cornerstone of her fragrance empire.

● At age 40, Paul Revere made his famous ride.

● At age 41, Johann Strauss composed "The Blue Danube."

● At age 42, Al Jolson starred in the first feature-length talking film, *The Jazz Singer.*

● At age 43, Donald Campbell broke the land speed record, traveling 403.1 mph in a car named Bluebell.

● At age 44, Ian Fleming wrote his first James Bond novel, *Casino Royale,* and Roger Moore was 44 when he began playing the part of James Bond.

● At age 45, Christopher Cockerell obtained a patent for his new invention, the hovercraft.

● At age 46, Shirley Temple Black was appointed ambassador to Ghana.

● At age 47, Alexander Fleming discovered penicillin.

● At age 48, Henry Wadsworth Longfellow published his most successful work, "The Song of Hiawatha."

● At age 49, William Booth founded the Salvation Army.

● At age 50, Charles Darwin published his famous book, *The Origin of Species.*

● At age 51, William Faulkner, America's voice of the Deep South, won the Nobel prize for literature.

● At age 52, American civil engineer and architect William Jenney designed the Home Insurance Company Building in Chicago, thus inventing the first skyscraper.

● At age 53, Margaret Thatcher became British prime minister.

- At age 54, Alfred Kinsey published his first "Kinsey Report," *Sexual Behavior in the Human Male*.

- At age 55, Johann Gutenberg typeset the famous Gutenberg Bible.

- At age 56, Nikolai Rimsky-Korsakov composed "The Flight of the Bumblebee."

- At age 57, American explorer Charles William Beebe descended to a record depth of 923 meters in a bathysphere off the coast of Bermuda.

- At age 58, Fyodor Dostoyevski wrote his masterpiece, *The Brothers Karamazov*.

- At age 59, Jonathan Swift's *Gulliver's Travels* was published.

PODIUM PANIC: HOW TO BEAT PUBLIC FEAR NUMBER ONE

There was a famous opera star whose stage fright was so intense that she became convulsed with stomach pains before each performance. She didn't complain.

Fear, she claimed, added emotional wallop to her voice.

If you've ever been the focus of group attention—whether to sing an aria, make a speech in a packed auditorium, or present your ideas to a few business associates—you probably know what stage fright feels like. And, unlike the diva, you probably don't think it helped your performance at all.

Experts say that most people are afraid to speak in front of a group. According to one survey, public speaking is the premier fear of Americans—followed by fear of heights, bugs, money problems, deep water, sickness, death, flying, loneliness, dogs, cars, darkness, elevators, and escalators.

So, if you coast through one-to-one situations but fumble when several pairs of eyes swerve toward you, you're hardly alone. And there is hope. You might not conquer stage fright completely—many fine performers never do—but you *can* learn to keep it under control.

It's the physical symptoms that are the most distressing: the pounding heart, the flushing face, the wavering hands, the quavering voice, the knocking knees. At that point, you may think you're panicked. You're not—yet. The way you react to your body's reaction makes all the difference.

Believe it or not, many people who love public speaking have the same physical symptoms as nervous people—but while nervous people allow themselves to be scared by those symptoms, extroverts find them exciting, like riding a roller coaster.

Dr. Michael Beatty, a professor of communication at Texas Christian University, has discovered in his research that shy people interpret their pounding hearts as a communication to themselves that something is wrong, while extroverts experiencing identical symptoms say they're thrilled. For both, "it's a natural response, a signal that you feel an important event

136

is occurring. Tell yourself that you're physically excited, not terrified. It's true, and it will calm you," says Dr. Beatty.

You can relax by consciously changing the way you think about speaking. "There's no such thing as a formal speech," says Ralpha Senderowitz, a Philadelphia area consultant who helps corporate executives improve communication skills. Senderowitz tells clients to direct their energies toward this thought: "I am going to have a conversation *with* people."

Relax the Audience First

Concentrate on relaxing the audience, Senderowitz advises. You'll benefit, too. She recommends that speakers begin with an "introduction to the introduction"—a few informal remarks that address the audience's concerns directly. For example: "Over luncheon just now, Ms. Jones told me an inspiring story about her personal success with foundation and fund raising. Her experience illustrates the winning techniques I want to discuss today." You might also begin your talk by relating to a point the last speaker made. You'll feel less like you're giving a speech and more like you're involved in a dialogue.

Don't think about speaking as a win-or-lose proposition. That's what Sandy Linver, author of *Speak Easy* and head of an Atlanta consulting firm, Speakeasy, tells clients to help them control their nervousness. "If you're thinking in terms of a battle," Linver says, "you provoke your body's extreme response to battle conditions. Instead of viewing speaking as oppos-

ing forces clashing, see it as a coming together. The aim is not to win as much as it is to connect, to make contact."

You can do that through the content of your speech. For example, if you're talking to members of a firm that's had a bad experience with your company, level with them from the beginning, suggests Linver. "Say, 'I know that you'd like a perfect solution, but that's not going to be possible today. What we can do is look at our alternatives together.' "

One client calmed himself down in front of a hostile audience by beginning his speech with an impromptu review of their complaints. Both he and the audience felt better.

The key, says Linver, is to "let out what you are most afraid of. Much physical tension is caused by being afraid of revealing yourself." Another example: You're angry at your supervisor. When you confront her, you hear, to your horror, that your voice is shaking. Don't let that rattle you more! "Instead, say, 'I'm so upset about this situation that my voice is shaking.' Putting too much effort into control will only increase the tension."

Many shyness experts recommend admitting your anxiety in certain situations. It can relax both you and the audience, and put the audience on your side. When in uncomfortable situations, one speaker begins by saying, "I feel like I'm diving into the deep end of the swimming pool! And I never dive. I always start swimming by putting my toe in on the kiddie side."

Admitting your anxiety "may sound like Pollyanna-ish advice," Linver says, "but I've seen very tough executives use it successfully."

Think Positive

Your thoughts have a direct impact on your nerves. If you're anticipating a public speaking situation and are telling yourself, "I'm a lousy speaker; I always panic," you will hurt your performance. That's why psychologists use a technique called cognitive restructuring to help people cut off the negative self-talk that panics them.

Dr. Barry Lubetkin, a psychologist at the Insitute for Behavior Therapy in New York City, uses the technique with patients at the institute's shyness clinic. They are taught "coping self-statements" to strengthen their confidence.

For example, many people are afraid of public speaking because they are perfectionists. They tell themselves, "I must be the best or I won't try at all." Dr. Lubetkin suggests that when they catch themselves thinking negatively, they say, "*Stop.* I don't have to be perfect." Other coping self-statements to practice are, "My nervousness is normal and natural; I know more about this topic than my audience, that's why I'm here." Senderowitz tells her clients to remember Eleanor Roosevelt's famous words, "No one can make you feel inferior without your consent." With enough practice, the positive thoughts *will* relax you.

Calming Images

People who have never had a good experience in talking with a group have no positive memories to draw on when they must speak. To deal with that problem, behavioral psychologists use powerful tools called systematic desensitization and imagery rehearsal. The techniques are used to treat all types of phobias. And Dr. James McCroskey, chairman of the speech communication department at West Virginia University, says they help a large majority of the students in his shyness clinic get over their fears.

His students are taken through a relaxation procedure similar to hypnosis or meditation. They are instructed to progressively tighten and relax all their muscle groups. Once they feel completely tranquil, they visualize themselves successfully going through the troublesome situations. They start with the least threatening scenario (like asking a question at a small meeting) and work up to the most fearsome (like giving a speech to a large group).

Ideally, Dr. McCroskey says, imagery rehearsal should be guided by a professional. Some therapies do teach clients to do it themselves, however. Dr. Barbara Powell, a Connecticut psychologist, and author of *Overcoming Shyness,* suggests this procedure: "Sit down, take a few deep breaths and relax all the muscles progressively, beginning with the toes and moving up. Let your imagination carry you to a relaxing situation, like lying on a beach. Then, when you feel relaxed, imagine yourself in the situation you are afraid of. Imagine going through it in as relaxed a way as possible."

With enough practice—it may take several weeks—you can learn to mentally rehearse the scariest scenes while remaining completely relaxed.

This imagery procedure is more than just dreaming, says Dr. Richard M. Suinn, chairman of the psychology department at Colorado State University, who has helped the U.S. Olympic team practice for competition with this technique. "Imagery is an experience rather than a thought process." It's closer to real life than role-playing, and "the emotions you experience in the imagery do carry over" when the real situation comes up.

Dr. Suinn used imagery to help one businessman whose voice weakened whenever he had to speak to a group. Dr. Suinn led him, in imagery, through speaking situations, with the man imagining his voice strong and clear. The problem cleared up.

Be Prepared

Experts agree that a good speaker, like a good scout, is always prepared. Knowing your audience, and what you want to say, is basic. But you should also rehearse physical aspects of your speech.

Gestures and movement liven up your performance and channel your nervous energy, says Dr. Gerald Phillips, head of the Pennsylvania State University shyness program and author of *Help for Shy People*. "The best performers are terribly nervous. The thing that distinguishes them is that they find ways to involve the whole person. They don't depend on just their voices. They find ways to use their hands and bodies."

Dr. Phillips tells his students to structure their notes for a speech in the form of a visual diagram that they can use physically: "The boss wants you to explain why your idea is good. Draw one box and write in it 'saves money.' In another, write 'shortens working time.' In another, 'makes peo-

ple happy.' Write three reasons for each under each box. As you talk, put your finger on the box, talk about box one, and read the three reasons." Not only will you be organized but you can "use the diagram to keep your hands active," Dr. Phillips says.

Visual aids can be a big plus, too. They add excitement to a presentation and will help you feel less like everyone in the room is staring at you. You can even do this in a small group or an individual situation. One client presented an idea to a supervisor with a miniature "flip chart" he had made from a pad of paper.

Bruce McKinney, a formerly shy person who was trained through Dr. Phillips's program, now teaches speaking skills at James Madison University in Virginia. He tells his students to set behavioral goals. "We have the students turn their feelings away from thinking about nervousness by focusing on the behavior needed to present a speech."

McKinney tells them not to think, "I will be a success if I remain calm," but to practice thinking along these lines: "If I look at the audience 75 percent of the time and at my notes 25 percent of the time, I know I will have accomplished something. I will speak loudly so nobody asks me to repeat myself. I will look at each member of the audience at least once." You can try this, too. Ask yourself what a dynamic speaker does, and then set behavioral goals.

One technique that all the experts recommend is deep breathing whenever you feel jittery, especially when you're about to speak. "Some people are so nervous that they almost forget to breathe," says Dr. McCroskey. "Then they feel light-headed, and they think it's because of nervousness."

There's no doubt that you can learn the skills you need to be a better speaker, and the more you practice, the better you'll become. Dr. Phillips adds that if you must do a great deal of public speaking for your job, you should take a public speaking course. But check out the class carefully before you sign up. Teachers who tear down students in class can do more harm than good.

Nerves Don't Show (Honest!)

You may find some comfort in the fact that the audience probably can't see how nervous you are. "We did a little study of people who said their hands shake and they blush when they give a speech," says Dr. Phillips. After they gave a speech, Dr. Phillips reports, the audience reported that they couldn't detect any signs of nervousness at all!

With enough practice, you may even reach the point where you find you enjoy public speaking. Bruce McKinney was so shy that he dropped out of college temporarily because his professor asked him to make a class presentation. But now he enjoys standing up in front of 200 students to teach speaking skills. "The more I do it, the more I like it," McKinney declares. "I'm not an extroverted person, but I've found I really like standing in front of a group."

USE YOUR BRAIN
TO LOSE YOUR BELLY

Of all the faculties and talents of the human brain, the most undependable, the weakest, and the wimpiest is *willpower*.

We hear the word a lot, and we seem to admire the idea of willpower, but in reality, what is it? A purely *negative* faculty. The ability to resist doing things we have an itch to do. To hold our tongues when we feel compelled to speak out. To hold our tears when we feel like crying. To stay in the house vacuuming when the first beautiful day of spring wants to shower us with sun.

That doesn't exactly sound like a great resource for positive living, does it?

Yet it's the resource that nearly all of us rely upon exclusively when we need to lose weight. We lean on it like a crutch. And it snaps under our weight like a toothpick.

Think for a minute of some really meaningful dialogues you've had with yourself—maybe about a new project, or the direction of your life. Now listen to *this* dialogue: I shouldn't eat this . . . I really shouldn't . . . Oh, well, I guess I ate it.

That little bit is about the full extent of our mental vocabulary for willpower. You have probably had more profound conversations with the clerk at 7-11.

Because all willpower can say is *no*. And that gives *you* no room to negotiate, no chance to use any of the wonderful mental abilities this book is all about.

I asked a very successful but very pudgy marketing executive at one of my weight loss workshops: What talents, what mental techniques do you use in your work?

There were so many it took 5 minutes to draw them all out. Daydreaming . . . brainstorming . . . long-term planning . . . exquisitely detailed record keeping . . . staff retreats and pep rallies . . . all sorts of motivational techniques and reward schemes . . . communication skills galore, from body language and birthday cards to screaming at the top of his lungs and setting fire to memos at staff meetings.

And what do you do to lose weight? I asked.

Willpower, he said.

Only, it didn't work. Maybe, he added

on reflection, "because I don't have any."

So here we have a person who is absolutely loaded with positive skills and attributes, using the one he has least of to try to control his weight.

All overweight people, almost by definition, have very puny willpower when it comes to eating. That goes too for those of us who aren't overweight but need to watch ourselves lest we quickly get that way.

But isn't willpower what weight loss is all about? I hear someone asking.

No! (I scream at the top of my lungs). All those mental techniques our executive used in his work, and many more that you and I use everyday, can all be harnessed to get the job done and *keep* it done.

Weight control, after all, is basically a management challenge. You have to *manage* your weight. You can't wrestle it to the ground with one big effort of willpower and then walk away the victor.

Well, actually you can. Probably you've already done it. For a week or two. And then what happened?

That's the second problem with the force of willpower. Weak to begin with, it also has a short life. It lives in bursts, but then dies without warning. And your weight comes back long before your willpower does.

The positive living approach is just the opposite. For one, you'll be using the *strongest* parts of your brain and personality to successfully manage your weight — not your weakest.

And your progress, instead of coming in bursts, will be slow, steady, sure, and secure. It will build on its own success. And it will gradually fall into a system that will become part of your everyday habits and reflexes. You will always need

to be conscious of the challenge. But you will soon get to the point where weight control is no longer a major, nagging problem in your life.

Which of These Strengths Do You Have?

Each of us has different strengths, inclinations, and talents. The ones you will use to accomplish your weight loss goal are those you have the most confidence in.

Below we have listed six strengths of mind and personality. No one has all of them (I know I don't!), but each of us has *some. Read the descriptions and decide which of them most nearly sound like the real you.* Your results here will determine which weight loss techniques — described later — are most likely to work *for you.*

Sherlock Holmes

You love to get to the bottom of things, especially things that are causing trouble. When your car engine kicks out, you want to know which exact part of it, and what *part* of that part, is the real problem. When your grass fails to thrive, you want a chemical analysis of your soil, not a quick delivery from the sod farm. When Johnny's school grades slip, you don't just lecture him, you read his assignments, check his homework, talk to his teacher. When there's a problem at work, you spend hours studying data sheets, more hours observing things first-hand, and then interview everyone concerned. Basically you believe there is a reason for everything, and that you can discover it.

141

142

Quick Change Artist

You thrive on novelty. You're always moving around your furniture, redecorating, planting new and exotic flowers. At work, changes that dismay others are like a fresh breeze to you. Ideas like trying a vegetarian diet, vacationing in Japan, or learning to sail a boat strike you as perfectly reasonable. Every couple of years, you try a new hobby. When traveling, unfamiliar foods and schedules that put others out of sorts only give you pleasure. Basically, you like changing things because it's exciting—and you never know what good result may come from it.

Regular Guy

You thrive on schedules. If given half a chance, you'll make them for others, too. You pay all your bills on time and file your taxes in February. You keep an extensive list of telephone numbers handy and keep a calendar that has writing under every date. It would take a major earthquake to make you late for an appointment. You never run out of postage stamps and always keep a six-month supply of toothpaste. You eat at the same time every day and make restaurant reservations a week in advance. When you find a hotel you like, you stay there every time you visit the town. Basically, you like being highly organized because it makes your life simpler and happier. And it comes easy to you.

Leg Shaker

You love to use your body. Repetitive motions that bore others—like swimming, walking, turning over a garden—give you a deep sense of contentment. Perhaps you don't do it much, and perhaps you don't call it exercise, but when you feel your pulse beating faster, when you feel the sweat on your skin, when you feel the warmth of blood coursing through your muscles, you feel good. You belong to a health club—or would if your time and money allowed. Dancing? You're crazy about it. Basically, you consider yourself a physical person. You express yourself by what you *do* at least as much as you do by what you say.

Great Cook

Recipes? You've got a million. You try new ones all the time. You make notes on them, and keep them for future reference. You've modified many, too. Or maybe invented some from scratch. You understand well the terms and tools of the trade. Your kitchen is neat and well organized. You know what fennel and cardamom taste like, and when to add the chopped tomatoes. Given a piece of fish or chicken, you could go to your pantry and refrigerator this very minute and come up with the wherewithal to serve them six different ways. A great new cookbook is your idea of a great gift. Basically, you enjoy expressing yourself through your skill and creativity as a cook, and you're proud of it, too.

Positive Thinker

Once you set your mind on something, you seem to be drawing on sources of strength deep within you. You know from experience that you are capable of doing things that—on first impression—seemed very difficult. You frequently fantasize about future accomplishments or exciting projects. When you begin a project, you have great persistence because you feel certain there will be a good outcome. Ideas like taking up bodybuilding at the age of 50, or planting trees in your backyard to help protect the ozone layer, strike you as perfectly reasonable. You are deeply inspired by people who succeeded in their goals against enormous odds. Basically, you believe that you can accomplish anything you set your mind to.

Techniques by Type

Now that you have some idea which "types" are most like you, read the following weight loss tips. Pay special attention to the ones listed under the heading that are "you," however many or few that may be. *They are the techniques and ideas you'll most easily be able to use on a long-term basis.*

Sherlock Holmes Tips

● Write down on a piece of paper all the reasons you want to lose weight. Underline the most important. Now look at what you wrote. Your primary reasons should be *serious, personal,* and *positive.* If they aren't, there is no point in trying to lose weight. You should be losing only for yourself—not your spouse or friends. Not for special occasions. Not even because you hate being fat. Hate is too negative a reason; your motivation will soon fall apart.

● On that same sheet, write down whether or not you truly believe you can succeed. If the answer is "yes!" then

you've got the prime ingredient: belief in yourself.

● While eating in your usual way, begin to keep a food diary. In it, write down everything you eat or drink, from meat to mint, even a glass of water. Also write down *when* you ate or drank these items, and exactly *where* (standing at the kitchen counter, for instance). After three days, study your diary. Look for patterns. See any?

● Continue your diary for another three days, but now also write down how you *felt* when you ate, and *why* you ate (e.g., starving, bored, to be polite).

● Determine from your diary how often, and where you're eating *when you're not really hungry.* And notice where you are when you're really going overboard—in front of the TV, for instance.

● Devise ways of simply doing something else at those times and places. Or simply avoiding them. You may decide, for instance, not to go near a table stacked with doughnuts, to listen to records instead of watching TV, to quit looking in the fridge, to never eat in the kitchen. Now you're using strategy, instead of sheer willpower.

● Scout around your home (and office) for food stored in the wrong places. Like on the coffee table, the kitchen counter, your office desk. Food should be kept out of sight.

● Your detective instincts will be glad to discover that your plate can affect how much you eat. Place settings with intense colors such as violet, lime green, bright yellow, or blue are thought to stimulate appetite. The least appetite-arousing plates are dark and elegant looking.

143

Quick Change Artist Tips

● Here's a little trick called carbohydrate preloading. The point is to cut down on dietary fats and make up the difference with carbohydrates. *This strategy can produce a 5-pound weight loss in just four to six weeks.* The first thing you eat when sitting down to a meal should be a starch or carbohydrate. Soups made with rice, barley, potatoes, noodles, or beans are perfect. A small serving of pasta with tomato sauce will fill the bill, too. Eat the rest of your meal as slowly as you can. According to Harvard University weight loss expert Dr. George L. Blackburn, that should give the "carbos" enough time to activate hormones that will diminish your craving for fat.

● Because you may well have a streak of impulsiveness, you might be able to keep on the right track better by joining a weight loss group. Choose one, though, that works by encouraging behavioral change, not special foods or radical regimens. You, especially, need to change your behavior so that good habits become second nature.

● Don't let your enthusiasm for new projects get out of hand. Cutting back drastically on your food intake is almost always followed by a major relapse — and then feelings of guilt and disgust. Instead, change your eating habits and food intake gradually.

● Once a week, try going vegetarian. If your culinary imagination is running low by 5:00 P.M., eat dinner at a Chinese, Indian, or Thai restaurant. The point is not so much to lose weight that one day as it is to introduce you to how satisfying a low-fat, high-fiber meal based on grains and vegetables can be.

● If you drink a lot of beer, cut way down. One a day is enough. Some people — men, particularly — find this one change produces dramatic results in just a few weeks.

● If you're really experimentally oriented, try eating dinner with your fork in your left hand (or your right if you're a lefty). That will automatically slow down your intake and cause you to experience the "full" sensation sooner.

● Try chewing your food at least ten times before swallowing it. Same reason.

Regular Guy Tips

● Because you're well organized, you should be able to shop from a list. Allow yourself one or two treats. But don't improvise on the spot. And don't shop on an empty stomach.

● The treats you allow yourself to buy shouldn't be your "weakness foods." If you positively feel you need them, make a special trip to the store. Often, you'll decide it's not worth the effort.

● Eat only at scheduled times in scheduled places. Most overeating occurs in the kitchen or in front of the TV.

● Don't eat foods out of their original containers. You usually wind up eating more than you do when you serve a measured portion and eat from a plate.

● Eat a relatively large breakfast and a good lunch every day. Research has clearly shown that eating most of your calories earlier in the day — as opposed to large, late dinners—can result in weight loss even when the calories remain the same. Evidently, our activity during the day causes more of the incoming calories to burn away.

● Try a little mood music to help you lose weight. Before sitting down to eat, put on some slow, relaxing tunes. You may find yourself eating less. That's what researchers at the Health, Weight, and Stress Clinic at Johns Hopkins Medical Institutions observed when they watched people eat to both fast and slow music.

When slow, classical music was playing, people took fewer bites per minute, chewed more, and swallowed before taking another bite. Even though their meals were about 15 minutes longer, they ate less. They also apparently had a happier time, for they talked more with their dinner mates and were more likely to say they'd enjoyed the meal.

● Drink four to six glasses of water a day.

● Is one of your regular guy habits eating dessert every day? Replace it with a 45-minute after-dinner stroll, and you can lose 10 pounds or more in three months.

● Since you've a penchant for structuring your life, build in a lot of pleasurable activities that can substitute for the pleasure of eating. Work on your photo album, look through a seed catalog, listen to music, walk the dog, browse through a bookstore, or plan your next vacation. Make a list of the things you really enjoy. How many are you enjoying now? Maybe that's why you have a weight problem!

● Are you a regular snacker? Keep a plastic container of raw veggies in the fridge and dive into them when you need a good munch.

Leg Shaker Tips

● You might be able to forget all about dieting if you're not more than about 20 pounds overweight. In one classic, year-long study, chronic dieters who couldn't keep their weight off lost an average of 22 pounds just by walking every day. Begin with a distance that's comfortable and work up to 45 minutes to 1 hour a day.

● Divide your exercise into two shorter sessions instead of one long one. That approach burns more calories, a result of revving up metabolism more often.

● Don't feel compelled to jog. Walking burns up the same number of calories per mile: about 100.

● Find more excuses to dance. Each hour burns up 300 to 500 calories. Best bet: square dancing.

● If walking or other exercise causes chafing, use Vaseline. Even slender runners use it as a preventive.

● Rejoice in the fact that the weight you lose with physical activity is nearly all fat. The dieter, who may be losing weight more quickly, is losing lots of valuable body protein along with fat. Incredibly, even the heart muscle shrinks on a diet.

● If you have trouble staying on your exercise regimen, vary it. An absolutely

146

ideal program would probably combine several weekly sessions of walking, dancing, and weight training.

● Don't go overboard on sit-ups. A reasonable number will give you the muscle tone you want. Hundreds, however, won't melt the fat off your tum. The best way to burn fat *anywhere* is whole body exercise—especially those that use the large muscle groups in the legs and back.

● If you're more than 40 pounds overweight, exercise before you eat. That seems to change the way the body handles insulin, and results in a higher metabolism rate for your food.

● If you're only moderately overweight, you burn more calories by exercising *after* you eat. But on a full stomach, don't do anything more strenuous than walking.

Great Cook Tips

● For a sweet but low-fat dessert, make an angel food cake and top it with strawberries.

● Don't feel you must make meat, which contains a hefty portion of fat calories, the centerpiece of every meal. Cut the usual portion by one-third to one-half; then up your servings of vegetables, pasta, grains, and potatoes accordingly.

● At the stove, lighten up your use of butter and oil. Rely on no-stick sprays and low-sodium broths for sautéing. Heighten flavor with aromatic vegetables like onions, leeks, garlic, and chili peppers. Try different herbs and vinegars, too.

● Spices can do more than simply replace butter and oil. At least the *hot* ones. In England, researchers found that adding chili peppers and mustard to food produced an internal "after-burn" effect. Not heartburn, but calorie-burn. After each meal, people eating the spicy food lost an average of 45 more calories to metabolism than people eating a bland meal. Some people burned up as much as 76 extra calories.

● Here's a cute little tip sent in to the Rodale newsletter, *Lose Weight Naturally,* by Lori Sugar of Buffalo. "I love fresh corn on the cob oozing with fresh butter. But when I tried to use less butter to cut down on fat, I'd run out of butter before the corn was gone. Then I found a better way—I fill a water glass with *hot* water and put a teaspoon of butter or margarine on top. I dunk in the ear of corn, and when I pull it out, there's a thin layer of butter evenly coating my ear of corn."

● Try substituting plain yogurt for sour cream; lite or skim milk for regular. On sandwiches, begin cutting the mayo with mustard until you like the taste of just mustard. Develop a taste for the new low-fat cheeses. If you must use butter or margarine on bread, soften it first; you'll get by with 75 percent less.

● When cooking chicken, use only skinned breast meat. Grill it slathered with mustard for Chicken Diablo. Stir fry in chicken broth with vegetables and herbs. If you don't overcook it, chicken won't need any added fat—not even from its skin.

Positive Thinker Tips

● Got a sudden craving for some food you know you don't need? Use your positive thinking to get yourself past the challenge. People who believe their urge to eat will only get worse until they douse it with chocolate are wrong.

"Gratifying an urge by eating only makes urges stronger and more frequent," says Dr. G. Alan Marlatt, director of the Addictive Behavior Research Center at the University of Washington. "In contrast, letting the urge pass will weaken it. If you can outlast enough of the urges, they will fade to obscurity."

● Congratulate yourself every day that you eat in structured, sensible ways. You are doing your health a big favor. Take pride in that.

● Set a goal, yes (you *love* to do that!), but make it realistic and long term. It doesn't matter how much you lose this week. In two months, yes.

● Remember that it's perfectly natural to hit a weight loss plateau or two on the road to slenderness. Tell yourself it's part of the territory. You'll soon be past it.

● Be assertive. Don't let friends or your host or waiter tell you what to eat. No need to talk about a diet, just say, "I'm sorry, I'm full."

● Frequently, imagine yourself as slender. Not too slender—let's be realistic! But looking good. And feeling good. Impress that image into your mind. Tell yourself, "This is the real me."

● Frequently and vividly imagine yourself doing the things you want to do—eating sensibly, exercising, shopping carefully. Tell yourself, "This is how I act."

● If you aren't a leg shaker, use your mental powers to move in that direction. Exercise is the perfect approach for a person with little willpower but lots of *positive* energy.

● When you exercise, have a goal. One good one: "walking" from your hometown to an exciting place you've never been. Just figure out how many miles are involved, and walk them over a period of time in your own neighborhood. Stationary bike enthusiasts get a big kick from such journeys. Many mark their progress on a map.

● Put signs of encouragement around the house. And especially on the refrigerator door. Signs like "How about a nice glass of water?" or, "Am I really hungry?" One woman swears by the phrase, "Nothing tastes as good as being skinny feels."

M. B.

THE EMOTIONAL PHARMACY

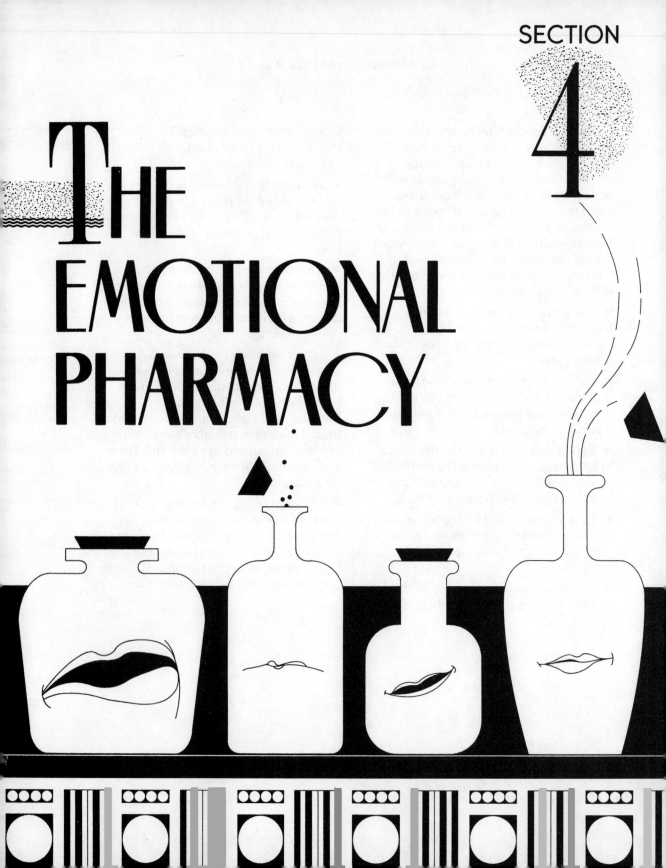

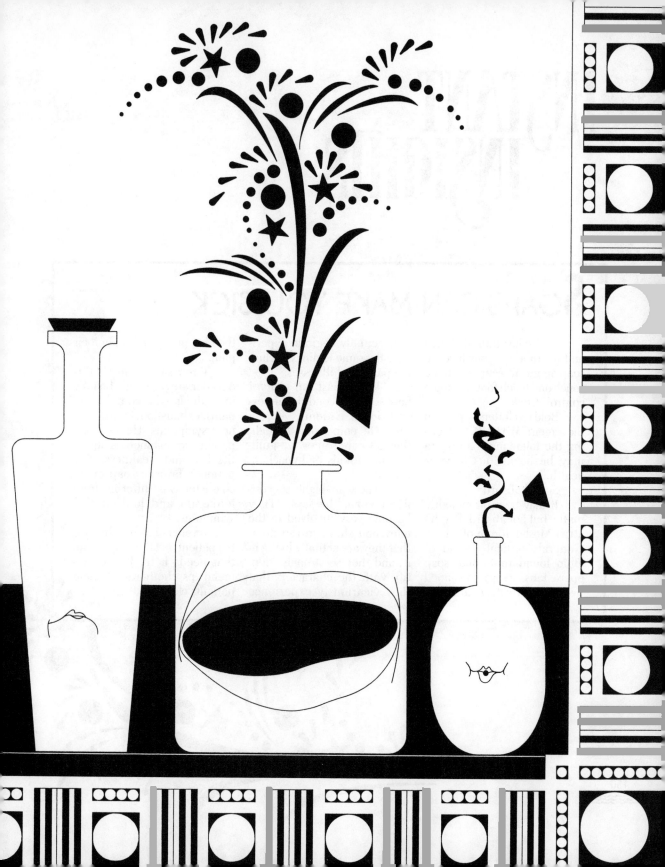

INSTANT INSIGHTS

Soaps can make you sick

You've just finished lunch and it's time for your favorite soap opera. You curl up on the couch and reach for the remote control. *Click.*

Bold red letters appear on the screen: *"WARNING:* Viewing the following soap opera may be hazardous to your health."

Sound absurd?

It may be a bit melodramatic, but not absurd. Psychiatrist Moshe Torem of Akron General Medical Center of Ohio found that some soap opera fans are so consumed by their favorite characters, they actually begin to experience the same feelings, including pains and illnesses.

"In the past ten years, I have seen this condition in several dozen patients," Torem says. He points out, though, they also are somewhat gullible individuals or hypochondriacs.

"These are highly suggestible people," he says. "They become very involved in the television show, to the point that they are actually living in it, and they so strongly identify with the characters that they vicariously experience their happiness and suffer their pain."

Torem says victims of this disorder are physically healthy individuals who complain of pains, exhaustion, or other illness symptoms. He said one patient complained of appetite loss and weakness. The patient's favorite soap opera character was suffering from leukemia and had similar symptoms.

Torem points out that it is the patient, not the soap opera, that needs help. He recommends psychotherapy to help patients clean up their acts.

THE CHEMISTRY OF COPING

Your confidence in any given situation—or lack of it—can determine just how much epinephrine and norepinephrine is circulating in your blood. That's right. Your perception of how capable you are can actually alter your body chemistry.

Epinephrine and norepinephrine are potent brain chemicals that stimulate the heart muscles, accelerate heart rate, and increase blood pressure. Consistently high levels can lead to anxiety, hypertension, and cardiac rhythm disturbances.

What can you do to maintain optimal levels? Learn to cope with your fears.

That's what Stanford University Medical Center researchers found when they investigated the effect of perceived coping skills on the body's stress response system. The study followed 12 women with spider phobias through their treatment programs.

Whenever the women found themselves in situations they felt unable to handle, their levels of epinephrine and norepinephrine shot up. But when they felt capable, levels of both brain chemicals declined. When treatment ended, and the women could calmly handle the spiders, their epinephrine and norepinephrine levels decreased accordingly.

They also reported fewer frightening thoughts and dreams, researchers said.

HEAVY SWEATERS LIGHTEN MOODS

A heavy sweater feels better after a rigorous workout than a light sweater.

People, that is, not articles of clothing.

How good you feel after a tough aerobic workout depends partly on how much you sweat, suggests Dr. Robert Brown of the University of Virginia. Heavy sweaters tend to have greater feelings of well-being than light sweaters. Dr. Brown explains that a chemical exchange in the bloodstream takes place during a workout. When you sweat, your body loses some sodium and other chemicals as well. When this new mix of blood reaches your brain, your mood lifts. "Poor sweaters," says Dr. Brown, "don't report an increase in well-being."

Body, you old traitor

You've heard of psychosomatic illness, physical ailments born of emotional distress. But did you know that the reverse is also true? Disturbances in your body can create disturbances in your head.

So reported Dr. Norman Geschwind, former director of the behavioral neurology unit at Beth Israel Hospital in Boston. His unit uncovered a number of physical ailments that produce psychological symptoms.

Nutritional deficiencies or your body's reaction to drugs can bring on depression. Too much caffeine, very high blood-fat levels, or cerebral allergies caused by such foods as milk, wheat, peanuts, or food additives can add up to anxiety. And undiagnosed epilepsy sometimes produces bizarre behavior rather than seizures.

Studies at Pittsburgh Western Psychiatric Institute, by Dr. David J. Kupfer and colleagues, have shown that a substantial percentage of depressed patients, including those considered suicidal, have underlying physical disorders. Once the disorder is treated, depression usually subsides.

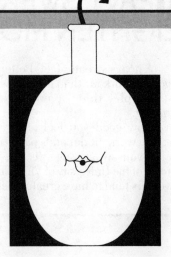

WEEP THAT WOUND AWAY

Cuts and scratches are really something to cry about.

Shedding tears actually speeds up the healing process of skin wounds, claim Soviet researchers from the Academy of Medical Sciences.

When laboratory rats with skin wounds were given eye irritants to induce crying, their wounds healed quicker and scar tissue formed up to 12 days faster than usual. When the tear glands were removed, the healing process not only slowed, but actually reversed: The rats' wounds began to open again.

The Soviet scientists concluded that some sort of healing chemicals are secreted through tear glands and are carried through the bloodstream to all parts of the body.

Scientists have not yet identified the chemicals, but are convinced of their healing powers and positive effects on skin repair.

WORRY LESS, HEAL FASTER

Being too realistic may be the worst thing for a person about to undergo surgery. Researchers have found that patients who avoid thinking about pains and problems they may encounter after an operation don't experience many.

Two different coping mechanisms, avoidance and vigilance, may be used by patients, say researchers H. Asuman Kiyak, Peter P. Vitaliano, and Jeffrey Crinean of the University of Washington. *Avoidant* copers anticipate few problems with their surgeries; *vigilant* copers generally expect many problems to crop up.

The research team hypothesized that vigilant copers would heal quicker and be more satisfied with their operations because they faced the fact that problems might arise. But, after studying 114 surgical patients, it turned out that those who expect nasty complications will get them. Those who expect only a few complications or avoid thinking negatively have very few postsurgical problems.

Scientists point out that patients' presurgical expectations about complications are usually more pessimistic than actual typical results would warrant. What's more, patients who expect many problems end up healing slower than those not expecting many problems.

For all these reasons, patients are advised to find a happy medium in their expectations. The researchers also suggest surgeons become aware of patients' expectations and help the patients develop an informed, at-ease attitude to speed up the recovery process.

DON'T LET LONELINESS BREAK YOUR HEART

Can you really die from a broken heart? Perhaps, recent research shows.

Loneliness and social isolation helped trigger 20 deaths in research patients with ischemic heart disease, claim researchers at Sweden's Karolinska Institute in Stockholm. One hundred fifty middle-aged men were monitored and evaluated for ten years. By then, 20 had died from their heart conditions. But the study shows that the amount they smoked or drank had little to do with their deaths since none of them overindulged in either activity. Instead, social isolation seemed to be a leading factor in their deaths.

The researchers speculate that loneliness creates neuroendocrine effects possibly leading to atherosclerotic problems. They suggest engaging in some light social activity—like bowling or playing bridge—at least once a week to lighten up your lifestyle.

SLEEP A LITTLE LONGER, LIVE A LITTLE LONGER

If you feel you just can't drag yourself out of bed some mornings, don't! That's what Harvard Medical School physicians advise. Rolling over and catching a few more winks may send you on a guilt trip, but it could save your life.

It's more likely you will suffer a heart attack in the early morning, rather than at some other time of the day. Prime-time heart attack hours are between 6:00 and 9:00 A.M., notes Geoffrey Toffler of the Harvard team. He says that blood clotting, a common cause of heart attacks, seems to occur more in the morning. When this is combined with the body's responses to waking up and becoming active, the result may be a heart attack. Toffler explains that bracing yourself to face the day is physically similar to the symptoms leading to a heart attack: your blood pressure rises and you pump extra adrenaline needed to get up and go. Blood clots, if present, get a head start on their trip to the heart.

Toffler says taking life less seriously and sleeping longer may help ward off heart attacks, especially if you are heart attack prone. He cautions that smoking also increases the blood's clotting tendency.

TRUSTING SOULS GET TO HEAVEN LATER

Suspicious minds cut short the songs of their own lives, a Duke University study shows. In a 15-year study of 500 older men and women with similar health and lifestyle patterns, those scoring high on hostility tests had 6.4 times the death rate as those with low scores.

This significant difference shows, says Duke psychologist John Barefoot, that hostile or cynical attitudes may lead to premature death.

The Duke study began in 1969 by giving the 500 participants a hostility test. They were asked to agree or disagree with statements like "People are basically honest" or "In a time of crisis, people will generally look out for themselves." In 1984, Barefoot and his colleagues checked up on the subjects; 143 of the 500 had died. Barefoot says that further analysis of the findings indicated that the survivors were generally the ones who were less suspicious. He says this shows a definite link between attitude and physical health.

Barefoot says it's not suspicions that cause deaths, but rather the way suspicious people live their lives as a whole. He believes cynics tend to rely less on others and shoulder more burdens alone, leading to increases in stress and stress-related deaths.

AGELESS Rx: WALK TO CHURCH

Religion is a kind of fitness activity for elderly churchgoers, claim researchers at Rutgers University.

Responses to a Yale University Health and Aging Project survey show elderly people who actively and publicly participate in religious services are less likely "to be functionally disabled or to show signs of depression."

One reason for the religion-health connection, speculates Ellen Idler of Rutgers University, is that religiously oriented people are more likely to lead healthier lifestyles: They eat less meat, drink less, and smoke less.

But the most likely reason, she suggests, is that religion may foster a more positive approach to illness, pain, or disability.

DEPRESSION CAN BE EXHAUSTING

Tired all the time? You say you can't pinpoint a physical cause? Daily exercise and healthy eating haven't helped?

Better examine your feelings then.

A large-scale population study, conducted by the National Center for Health Services Research, found that the most powerful predictors of exhaustion were not physical factors but psychological ones. Individuals who reported feelings of depression or anxiety were seven times more likely to suffer from chronic fatigue than people with no such emotional problems.

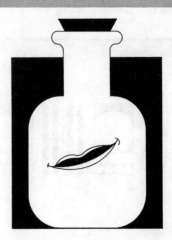

Care for a pet
If you care about yourself

Senior citizens are happier, healthier, and better tenants when they have a pet to care for, claim researchers at the University of California at Davis.

Once they were given the opportunity to own pets, elderly residents in federally assisted housing not only improved their own well-being, but improved the overall living conditions of their homes, reports Dr. Lynette Hart, acting director of the Human/Animal Relations Center at the university.

She and assistant Bonnie Mader studied 50 housing authorities in California after a 1982 state law permitted pets in government-aided residences. Some 84 percent of managers said conditions actually improved or at least stayed the same. They also said pet owners were more secure, had a better and more positive outlook on life, and exercised more.

Bad moods are bad medicine

You've heard the phrase, "You'll worry yourself to death." Whoever coined it wasn't kidding.

A University of California at Riverside study suggests that people who suffer from chronic anxiety, long periods of pessimism, and unremitting tension and hostility are twice as likely to contract some kind of illness.

In fact, psychologists Howard Friedman and Stephanie Booth-Kewley say their data suggest that constant hostility is as dangerous to health as smoking or following a high-cholesterol diet.

In their analysis of 101 previous studies investigating the connection between personality traits and specific diseases, the pair found links between some or all of the "neurotic" traits and susceptibility to four disorders under study: asthma, peptic ulcers, arthritis, and heart disease.

What's the antidote? Psychotherapy may foster physical as well as emotional well-being.

MIND OVER IMMUNITY

Hungry white sharks swim toward their prey, their gleaming dorsal fins slicing through a blood red sea. The prey, a sick-looking green globular fish, flails about helplessly. More sharks appear on the horizon; there are hundreds of them. Their jaws open wide as they approach their victim. Their sharp teeth glisten. The red ocean churns. The green glob is mercilessly killed.

Believe it or not, this image may improve your health.

At least, it might if you were to imagine that the sharks are really your white blood cells (the general term for the cells that run the immune system), that the blood red sea is your bloodstream, and the green glob an invading virus or possible cancer cell. Like participants in a recent test of immune function, after a visualization as powerful as this one, you'd probably find that the number and strength of your white blood cells would go up.

Why might it work? According to the new science of psychoneuroimmunology (PNI), your health may be intimately connected to your state of mind. Scientists developing this revolutionary new field study the connections between states of mind (*psycho-*), the brain (*neuro-*), and the system that protects the body from illness, called the immune system (*immuno-*). Their findings may soon turn health care as we know it completely upside down.

"The old notions of how we understand mind/body relationships are much more complicated than we ever thought," says the scientist who conducted the shark-imagery test, Dr. Howard Hall, assistant professor of pediatrics at Case Western Reserve University School of Medicine. "We know that people can regulate their physiology through biofeedback and meditation. But we are soon going to learn more about that. We will have a whole new model of how the mind affects health.

"Right now, we are trying to find out how people can voluntarily enhance their immune systems," says Dr. Hall. "In the shark-imagery test," he explains, "researchers asked about 20 healthy people to imagine their immune systems filled with white blood cells that function like sharks swimming around scavenging for germs. Then we told them to imagine that there were even more sharks swimming around.

"We had them practice that for a week, and found practice helps a lot. Those with good images who can relax often have an effect," continues Dr. Hall. The result of the test: There was a statistically significant increase in the numbers of lymphocytes, one type of white blood cell, in the people who were able to do the visualization.

While most scientists contend they don't know enough yet to say that doctors should be prescribing visualization to their patients, the results of Dr. Hall's study do suggest that this may be one way your state of mind can affect your immune system. And making the immune system stronger is one way to avoid and cure disease.

The Lowdown on Feeling Down

PNI research has progressed during the past five years to the point where most scientists firmly believe that pessimistic, helpless, hopeless feelings can weaken your immune system and harm your health.

One of the studies that led scientists to this belief was conducted on 1,337 medical students. The researchers separated those who weren't that close to their parents and weren't very satisfied with their personal relationships from those who were healthier psychologically. The first group was eventually found to have a risk of cancer later in life that was three to four times higher than that of the healthier students, reports Dr. Ken Pelletier, associ-

Your Love Is Showing

A good marriage may be the best heart protector a man can have. Two Israeli researchers, Dr. Jack Medalie and Dr. Uri Goldbourt, learned this when they studied 10,000 men who showed signs that they might develop angina pectoris. The researchers gave the men a battery of psychological tests and questionnaires to fill out. When they later compared the results of the psychological tests with a list of which men actually developed the chest pains, they found a telling trend.

The men who were most likely to develop angina were also the most likely to answer "no" to the question, "Does your wife show you her love?"

Another study of married men conducted by Dr. Harold Morowitz of Yale University, found that a male heavy smoker who is married stands about the same chance of dying prematurely as a male nonsmoker who is divorced. The married man's relationship with his spouse compensated for the health threat posed by his cigarette habit.

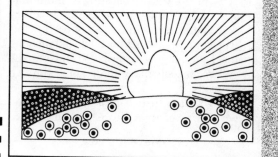

SOME POSITIVE PRESCRIPTIONS

Why do people get sick? Generally, it's because they are exposed to a bacterium or virus. But not everyone who's exposed to a virus catches it. The difference between those who do and those who don't? Today, more and more scientists believe that an inability to handle stress, not enough social support, and a negative outlook on life may make you more susceptible to disease.

And lately, scientific evidence suggests that a positive state of mind may be able to strengthen your immune system. In fact, studies show that people who stay healthy longer tend to have an optimistic outlook, a sense of control and commitment in their lives, and plenty of loving social contacts.

All the answers aren't in yet, but you can take advantage of this seminal research by following the advice of the scientists themselves.

Dr. Howard Hall, assistant professor of pediatrics at Case Western Reserve University School of Medicine. "Get very, very relaxed using some relaxation technique. Then imagine anything that would make you feel as if you are boosting your immune system. Do this for about 10 minutes every day. There's no definitive proof yet that this will work, but it can't hurt. I do it. I imagine that I am charging up my blood and immune system. It feels like energy going through my body."

Dr. Blair Justice, professor of psychology at University of Texas Health Science Center and author of *Who Gets Sick.* "If you are feeling as if you're coming down with something, listen to music that really moves you. It won't guarantee that you won't get sick, since illness isn't caused just by the mind. But the mind can help resist illness, and exposing yourself to beauty is one of the best ways to develop resisters."

George Solomon, M.D., professor of psychiatry at UCLA. "There's good stress and there's bad stress. Distress is what is likely to have more of an effect on immunity than others. Learn to handle stress."

Sabina White, director of the Laughter Project of student health services at the University of California at Santa Barbara. "If you are under stress, try to look at the situation and find some humor in it. When I'm stressed, I try to laugh about it. It gets me moving. Laughing doesn't always eliminate the problem, but it does make me feel

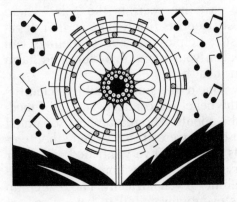

a lot lighter than I would be if I didn't try it."

Dr. Kelley Madden, research fellow in neuroimmunology at the University of Rochester in New York. "Take very good care of yourself. Eat right and exercise. If you're sick, don't let it get you down emotionally. All this helps strengthen health."

Dr. Justice. "Get regular physical exercise. Not just for what it does directly to the body, but rather, for what it does for the head as well. Those who exercise regularly are less likely to get depressed. And those who are less likely to get depressed are less likely to get sick."

Dr. Solomon. "Change medical education and change the reimbursement (insurance) system so doctors get paid for spending time with their patients and understanding them. You can't separate physical well-being from mental well-being. If you promote mental well-being, there will be more physical well-being."

Dr. Justice. "Don't see every problem as a ten on a scale from one to ten. Seeing problems as the end of the world elevates stress chemicals in your body and keeps them there. The body responds more beneficially when you say to yourself, 'This is bad so I'm going to change it,' rather than, 'This is awful and I can't stand it.'"

White. "Laugh at what's available. Seek out things to laugh at. I deliberately seek out funny movies, just so I can laugh."

ate clinical professor in the departments of medicine and psychiatry at University of California, San Francisco, School of Medicine and author of *Mind as Healer, Mind as Slayer.*

"There is a link between disease and depression, loneliness, and hopelessness that's been shown in research," says Dr. Pelletier. "Sleep deprivation and unemployment have also been shown to make people more susceptible to disease."

Many types of illness have been weakly correlated to mood, continues Dr. Pelletier, including allergic diseases, autoimmune disorders, and infectious diseases. People who feel they don't have enough social support are more likely than the average person to get arthritis, tuberculosis, high blood pressure, and heart disease, for instance. These people also have a shorter than average expected life span, he says.

These kinds of links are circumstantial; they say that people with certain personality characteristics are more likely to have certain diseases than people without those character traits. Of course, that doesn't mean that everyone with those traits will get ill, or that everyone with the illness has those traits. As a result, the conclusions scientists can draw from these kinds of studies are limited.

Other studies involve taking blood from people before, during, and after they are in a stressful situation. The blood is analyzed and certain types of white blood cells are counted and measured. That is another way to test the effect of mood on the immune system.

Several studies of this kind have shown a decrease in lymphocytes among students during exam periods, reports Dr. Pelletier.

And husbands whose wives recently died of breast cancer also had fewer lymphocytes than normal.

In her studies, Dr. Janice Kiecolt-Glaser, psychologist, of Ohio State University, tested the effect of loneliness on the immune system. She studied two groups of people: medical students and psychiatric patients. She gave them psychological tests to ascertain how lonely they were. Then she tested their blood to measure the activity of natural killer cells, a type of white blood cell believed to be important in the control of viruses and cancerous tumor formation.

Dr. Keicolt-Glaser found that those who were lonelier than average had much lower levels of natural killer cell activity, which could make them less able to fight cancer should they need to.

A Booster May Be Just What You Need

All these studies are probably making you think it's pretty dangerous to be in a bad mood. Well, don't worry too much—no one ever died of a blue day. But they do show the importance of positive living.

So what should you do if you feel really down, and no amount of positive thinking is going to change that, at least for the moment? Is there any way you can counteract the possible negative effect your mood is having on your immune system's strength?

Joining a support group or just being around friends while you're down may give your immune system the extra boost it needs, says Dr. George Solomon, professor of psychiatry at UCLA and one of the

PROJECT LAUGHTER

A good laugh—the kind that makes your eyes tear and your stomach hurt—can de-stress you just as well as relaxation can, says Sabina White, of the Laughter Project at the University of California at Santa Barbara.

In a study by the project, White learned that people who spent an hour participating in a laughter workshop dealt with psychological stress just as well as another group that just relaxed.

As a result of her study, White conducts laughter workshops for students under stress at college. The workshops focus on sharing embarrassing moments and laughing about them, learning ways to find humor in distressing situations, and talking about the kinds of humor that are healing—like jokes about life—and the kinds that aren't healing—such as jokes that put down groups of people.

"I realized that if you don't value laughter, you may just stop doing it," says White. "That happened to me and I missed it. Life is a lot lighter now that I laugh again."

founders of PNI. And exercise may increase your production of natural killer cells, he says.

When he makes these recommendations, Dr. Solomon is operating on the belief that if a negative state of mind can weaken the immune system, then a happier one—like feeling cared for by your friends—might strengthen it.

The Healing Power of Your Mind

This positive outlook is the cutting edge of PNI research, and is already turning up encouraging results. It just may be that laughter, love, and optimism can help prevent or cure disease. Dr. Hall's shark visualization study, with which we started off, is just the beginning of this upbeat research. Other studies have produced some even more surprising and promising results.

● Students at Western New England College in Springfield, Massachusetts, were found to have dramatically higher salivary levels of a virus-fighting component known as immunoglobulin A after watching a videotape of funnyman Richard Pryor. No such rise was seen after the students watched a chuckle-free documentary.

● Psychologist Kathleen Dillon found that college students who reported using humor as a coping device had higher levels of virus-fighting immunoglobulin A in their systems than students of a stodgier ilk.

● Tests done at the Menninger Clinic in Topeka, Kansas, showed that lovebirds

MADE IN JAPAN: HEALTHY SOCIAL TIES

People in Japan have the longest life expectancy in the world, and certain scientists are tripping over each other to figure out why. Is it the food? The climate? Or maybe it has to do with the emphasis the Japanese place on community, suggests Dr. Ken Pelletier, of the University of California, San Francisco, School of Medicine.

"Community support groups and close personal relationships have been linked to better health and lower absenteeism, lower incidence of cancer and heart disease, and reduced hospital stays," says Dr. Pelletier. Human companionship may be one of the most important factors in health.

Studies of Japanese people, says Dr. Pelletier, have pointed out the importance of community and intimate social bonds in their cultures. These bonds may be a protective factor that allows them to live so long, he says.

fly higher. People in love suffer fewer colds and have white blood cells that more actively fight infections than the cells of nonlovers.

● Patients at a convalescent home in the San Francisco Bay area were able to reduce substantially their doses of painkillers after four weeks of participating in a game in which they took turns making each other laugh.

● Happily married women have stronger immune systems than those who are less well-matched, found Dr. Kiecolt-Glaser

THE HARDINESS FACTOR

A hardy plant can grow in just about any weather and any soil. A hardy person can stay healthy under lots of stress and unhealthy conditions, say Dr. Suzanne C. Ouellette Kobasa of City University of New York, and Dr. Salvatore Maddi of the University of Chicago, both psychologists.

What makes a person hardy? According to Dr. Kobasa, it's a set of beliefs about oneself and the world and how the two interact. After more than a decade of research, Dr. Kobasa and Dr. Maddi have found that people who hold this set of beliefs tend to be unusually resistant to many kinds of illnesses.

What are the beliefs? A sense of control over your life, a personal commitment to what you are doing, and a feeling of challenge. Dr. Maddi describes a hardy personality: "You feel self-confident, and that the world is rather benign. You have commitment, or the knack of finding something important about whatever it is you are doing. You also have control, or the belief that you can influence what is going on around you. . . . Further, you think your life is best led in pursuit of development. Pressures and disruptions, however painful, appear to be something you can learn from and grow [from]."

and Dr. Ronald Glaser of Ohio State University.

● When taught relaxation and guided imagery techniques three times a week for a month, 45 geriatric residents of an independent-living facility showed a significant increase in disease-fighting natural killer cell activity. That was compared to another group who merely had "social contact" visits—and didn't show the same increase, found Dr. Kiecolt-Glaser.

● Dr. G. Richard Smith, Jr., associate professor of psychiatry and medicine at the University of Arkansas Medical Sciences, studied 28 experienced meditators. After explaining how the immune system works, he gave them skin patches of the chicken pox virus and asked them to control their responses to it. One group was told to have a stronger than normal response, one group a weaker than usual reaction, and one group a typical reaction. The results showed that more people were able to control their responses than weren't.

"This suggests that certain experienced meditators may have some ability to modulate their immune systems," says Dr. Smith. "If this turns out to be true across the board, then other people may have that same potential." And that could mean deciding to fight a disease with more power than you normally have at your disposal.

Why do scientists think these positive immune boosters work? It might have

FEMININE PROTECTION

Need a health boost? Spend some time with a woman.

Scientists have known for a while that social contact helps sick people get better and healthy people stay healthy. New research now tells us that social contact with a woman is the most helpful for both men and other women.

Married men are healthier than unmarried men, for instance. Widowers are not as healthy as men whose wives are still alive. And men with female friends are healthier than men with just male friends.

Married women, on the other hand, are not healthier than unmarried women. In fact, some studies show they are less healthy. Women get their health benefits from social contacts with other women. They tend to be in better health if they have close female friends or relatives, for example.

"There's some evidence that women are just more effective at providing support," explains Dr. Debra Umberson, assistant professor of sociology at the University of Texas in Austin, who reported this research in *Science*. "Women know how to do it better than men, perhaps because they are put in a position of providing care more often than men. Men could probably learn to be better at it than they are."

---

less to do with what you do, and more to do with *doing* almost anything at all, some say. "Watching a funny movie may have an effect on your immune system simply because you are doing something for yourself," says Dr. Solomon. "The fact that you are taking an active role in your health and taking control clearly has a positive health effect."

Others, like Dr. Pelletier, think it may have more to do with social interaction than control: "Evidence is accumulating that positive social support is necessary to good health," he says. "Supportive interactions among people, cultures, and possibly our interdependence with the planet may affect our ability to resist illness. Social support presumably works to prevent illness by keeping the immune system in homeostasis [balance] or by enhancing it."

Dr. Bernard Siegel, assistant clinical professor of surgery at Yale University School of Medicine and author of *Love, Medicine and Miracles,* thinks that the positive living effect on the immune system is due to nothing less than love. "I am convinced that unconditional love is the most powerful known stimulant of the immune system," he says. "If I told patients to raise their blood levels of immune globulins or killer T-cells, no one would know how. But if I can teach them to love themselves and others fully, the same changes happen automatically. The truth is, love heals."

So . . . control, social support, and love. If those are the things that make our immune system healthier, we are still left with another question. How does the immune system "know" you're doing something for yourself? How does social support "get into" the body?

To answer that question, first we have to discuss how the immune system works.

Your Built-In Self-Defense System

"Your first line of defense against viruses and bacteria that invade the body is the phagocyte, or cell-eater," explain Dr. Nicholas R. Hall, associate professor of neuroimmunology, and Dr. Alan L. Goldstein, professor of biochemistry, both at the George Washington University School of Medicine in Washington, D.C.

"When the skin is breached, swarms of these scavenging white blood cells descend upon the scene and devour the transgressors one by one until the phagocytes literally eat themselves to death. They are completely indiscriminate in what they eat.

"The second type of defense is able to recognize particular invaders and to tailor highly specific counterattacks," they explain in *Science* magazine. These more skilled white blood cells are called lymphocytes.

Lymphocytes are grown in the bone marrow and are stored in the lymph, a clear fluid that flows throughout the body. There are two different types of lymphocytes: B-cells and T-cells. These cells have different jobs to do to keep you healthy.

The B-cells stay in the bone marrow until they reach maturity. Later, they circulate in the bloodstream and eventually land in the lymph systems of certain organs:

the spleen, the tonsils, and the adenoids. They rest there, inactive, until a call to duty. Then, they rush to the site of attack and use their special sensing abilities to identify the foreign body. Using this knowledge, the B-cells synthesize and release certain proteins, called antibodies, that are designed to identify and destroy the specific attacker they are fighting.

The other type of lymphocytes, called the T-cells, leave the bone marrow early on and migrate to the thymus gland. Later, the T-cells, like the B-cells, enter the bloodstream and eventually land in the tonsils and the spleen.

Unlike the B-cells, the T-lymphocytes don't produce antibodies. Instead they act as a support system. There are different types of T-cells: helper T-cells, which help the B-cells; killer T-cells, which produce lethal substances of their own to kill off attackers; and suppressor T-cells. The suppressor T-cells are important because they keep the immune system in check. Without them, your self-defense cells could literally destroy your body from the inside.

The T-cells and B-cells protect you from different diseases, explains Dr. Joan E. Cunnick, associate research professor of pathology at the University of Pittsburgh School of Medicine, in the journal *Advances.* "People who cannot produce antibodies [because their B-cells aren't functioning properly] are susceptible to infection with bacteria. They may develop pneumonia and meningitis," she says. On the other hand, "people whose T-lymphocytes are not functioning optimally are susceptible to infection with fungi and viruses."

Everyone comes into contact with the bacteria, fungi, and viruses that cause disease, continues Dr. Cunnick. As long as your immune system is functioning properly, the dangerous attackers aren't likely to have any effect. It's only when the immune system lets down its guard that the foreign bodies go into action and cause diseases.

The important question to answer, then, is when and why would the immune system let down its guard.

The Head Bone Is Connected to the Immune Bone

Until recently, scientists believed that the immune system functioned entirely separate from the brain. They did have some good reasons. If you put white blood cells in a test tube, far away from any brain, they are still capable of killing off attackers.

But with the advent of PNI research, scientists realized that there are lines of communication between the brain and the immune system. There are receptor cells on the white blood cells that are primed to detect certain neurotransmitters from the brain, for instance. And there are nerves that travel from the brain and end in immune-related organs like the thymus and the spleen. Especially significant are the connections between the limbic area of the brain, which controls emotions, and the immune system.

POLLYANNA'S LEGACY

Pollyanna was right—it's better to be optimistic. New studies show that pessimism can make you get sick more often and even die young. Of a group of 99 Harvard University graduates followed for 35 years, those who explained their misfortunes and disappointments in an optimistic way tended to have better health than pessimistic classmates later in life, according to a report in *Journal of Personality and Social Psychology*.

What counts as pessimistic? The researchers say that seeing a stable, long-lasting cause for misfortunes, assuming that the cause of a bad event will have a ruinous effect on many areas of your life, and blaming yourself for the cause rather than other people or circumstances are all earmarks of a pessimistic style.

If you were to explain why you didn't get promoted this year by saying, for example, "I seem to be unwilling to face reality," and then went on to note that you never face reality and that's why you'll never be able to maintain a happy marriage, you'd be pessimistic. A more healthy reaction, suggests the research, would be to say, "I guess I didn't get promoted this year because the company isn't doing well and doesn't have much money to spend."

GROWING HEALTHIER

Which of these activities can improve your health?

- Taking control of your life.
- Giving care to a living being.
- Growing parsley.

Actually, all three will help. When nursing home residents were given plants of their own to take care of and were urged to assume more responsibility for themselves as well, they said they felt more in control of their lives. Researchers soon noticed that the residents were healthier and more active. It was later found that they also lived longer than residents who didn't have plants or responsibility for themselves, according to a study reported by Dr. Blair Justice in his book *Who Gets Sick.*

Since communication between the brain, which controls our states of mind, and the immune system is possible, many scientists think it stands to reason that such communication actually occurs. And if that is true, then it is reasonable to suspect that the messages from the brain actually affect the function of the immune system.

Let's return to our earlier question. When and why would the immune system let down its guard and allow foreign bodies to attack our health? The answer suggested by PNI research is that, even though the immune system can function perfectly well without any input from the brain, it does respond to the brain's messages. Its function is modulated by these messages. So when the brain says, "I feel down, weak, and out of control," the immune system may respond by becoming down, weak, and out of control itself.

Of course, even people who are never down emotionally still get sick sometimes. That is because illness isn't *all* from the mind, says Dr. Blair Justice, professor of psychology at University of Texas Health

I WANNA HOLD YOUR HAND

Remember when you were really little and had to go to the doctor's office to get shots? Remember how holding your mother's hand seemed like the only way to survive the ordeal? By now, you can probably stand a needle without Mom, but your body never outgrew the need for a hand to hold.

A recent British study learned that having your hand held can help you recover from surgery faster. The researchers tested two groups of women who were having the same surgery. "In one group, a nurse held the hands of the women while their blood pressures and temperatures were being taken. In the other group, their hands were not held," explains Dr. Blair Justice in his book *Who Gets Sick.*

The women whose hands were held were able to leave the hospital sooner and recovered faster at home than the other group of patients. "This should work for men just as well," says Dr. Justice.

Science Center and author of *Who Gets Sick*. "There are three arenas that control our health," he explains. "The mind is one. The environment and genetic predispositions are the other two."

You might get sick, therefore, because your genetic makeup says that you will always be susceptible to a certain virus. Or you might get sick because you are in a sick environment, and are coming into contact with many bacteria or viruses. "No matter how positive a person is, if there is an overpowering environmental or genetic reason for him to get sick, he will," says Dr. Justice.

The key to staying healthy is to keep the areas you can control strong, and not to worry about the areas you can't control. You can't change your genetic makeup, but you can spend time in clean, healthy environments and you can certainly strengthen the messages your mind sends to your immune system. "It's important to have as many resisters as possible in the cognitive brain area," says Dr. Justice. "It's no guarantee that it will keep you from getting sick, but it surely can't hurt, and it may help a lot."

SMILE YOUR WAY
TO A LONGER LIFE

Confess: You're not the mild-mannered person people think you are. Secretly, you have a Type-A personality and it's as plain as day when you get behind the wheel of a car. When you drive down the street, others better get the heck out of your way.

According to Dr. Meyer Friedman, you're a typical case. He's the San Francisco cardiologist who, along with Dr. Ray Rosenman, first studied behavior marked by impatience, aggressiveness, and hostility, labeled it Type A, and offered evidence hinting that it may hurt your heart enough to kill you. (Some experts agree that Type-A behavior is as big a risk factor for your heart as smoking or high blood pressure.) Dr. Friedman points out that this crazed-driver syndrome is just 1 of 30 or more dead giveaways for the Type-A personality (some surprisingly subtle)—and 1 is all it takes to label you Type A.

Do you interrupt or hurry the speech of others? Vigorously tap your fingers or jiggle your knee? Turn every game into an intense competition? Frequently try to do more than one thing at a time, like think about three different problems at once or talk on the phone while writing letters? If so, you're a suspected Type A, says Dr. Friedman.

But you are not alone. Three fourths of urban males and an increasing number of women, Dr. Friedman says, are Type A's.

But the big news is that there may yet be hope for us Type A's. It has been widely assumed that it's easier to make pigs do pirouettes than to alter Type-A behavior. Yet in their recent landmark study of Type A's, Dr. Friedman and his colleagues present evidence that Type A's can change their ways and that the change can cut their risk of heart disease.

A Change of Heart

For the new study, known as the Recurrent Coronary Prevention Project, Dr. Friedman and his fellow scientists recruited over 1,000 Type-A men and women who had had at least one heart attack. The researchers gave over half these people special counseling on how to alter their Type-A behavior. Then they monitored all participants for 4½ years to see who suffered recurrent heart problems and who altered their Type-A behavior. And when the researchers finally analyzed the results, they were elated.

"There was a significant decrease in Type-A behavior in the people who got Type-A counseling." Dr. Friedman says. "But more important, this group had *half* as many heart attacks as those in the other group. No other therapy—not diet, drugs, surgery, or exercise—has ever achieved such remarkable results. We had demonstrated that Type-A behavior isn't just associated with heart disease, but helps cause it."

But deterring doom, Dr. Friedman says, isn't the only by-product of reversing Type-A behavior. "In our study," he says, "when people modified their Type-A habits, they gave themselves a fuller, more productive life. They granted themselves the freedom to listen, to play, to take pleasure in friends and family, to mature, to regain self-esteem, to give and receive love. These advantages alone make altering Type-A behavior worthwhile, even in people who don't yet have heart disease."

Now Dr. Friedman and colleagues at the Meyer Friedman Institute in Mount Zion Hospital and Medical Center in San Francisco are busy using the same Type-A counseling to banish Type-A habits in business executives, army officers, and others. And in *Treating Type A Behavior: And Your Heart,* Dr. Friedman and coauthor Diane Ulmer insist that Type A's can even apply this Type-A couseling on their own to change their ways.

So for all of us Type A's, here's how to use this self-counseling to get out of the world's deepest behavioral rut.

Not Me, Not Me!

The first step, says Dr. Friedman, is discovering for yourself that you're really Type A. But if you are Type A, wouldn't that fact be perfectly obvious to you?

"Not necessarily," Dr. Friedman says. "The main exterior signs of Type-A behavior are aggravation, irritation, anger, and impatience—what we abbreviate as AIAI. They're overt but still often hidden from the Type A. Generally, Type A's are great at spotting Type-A behavior in others, but awful at detecting it in themselves."

So if you're Type A, how can you accurately assess your own behavior? Be honest with yourself, says Dr. Friedman, and get a second opinion from your spouse or friends. Then take their comments seriously, even if you don't like what you hear.

Some of the questions you should ask yourself (and the people who know you) are:

● Do you have a compulsion to win at all costs, even in trivial contests with children?

● Do you clench your fist during an ordinary conversation?

● Do you have easily aroused irritability or anger, even in minor matters?

● Do you have a ticlike grimace in which the corners of your mouth are twitched back, partially exposing your teeth?

● Do you sigh frequently?

● Do you have trouble sitting and doing nothing?

● Do you detest waiting in lines?

● Do you eat, walk, or talk fast?

172

- Do you often angrily defend your unshakable opinions?

- Do you grind your teeth?

- Do you nod your head while speaking (rather than while listening as many other people do)?

"Few Type A's exhibit *all* the Type-A signs," Dr. Friedman says. "But most Type A's have several. We have found that exhibiting even one of them (mild Type A) increases your risk of having a heart attack before age 65."

Axing Type A

So are you Type A or not?

If you are and you admit you are, you're halfway to kicking Type-A habits, says Dr. Friedman.

The next step is to deal with the cause of your Type-A behavior. And guess what? The cause is not rush-hour traffic, your blockhead boss, your neighbor's yappy dog, or the guy in the White House. It's low self-esteem and insecurity, Dr. Friedman says.

"We observed, " he says, "that every 1 of the 592 people who received Type-A counseling in our study harbored insecurities and in most cases low self-esteem. Every single one of them doubted that they possessed the necessary abilities to perform present and future duties well enough to merit promotion.

"Typically, Type A's struggle to achieve more and acquire more in less time, thus bringing on all the AIAI symptoms. And this struggle is a way of compensating for these feelings of insecurity and inadequacy. Eradicating the feelings is sometimes a

matter of discovering what past events triggered them, or ensuring that your expectations do not vastly exceed your capabilities, or even getting professional counseling."

Along with wrestling with the sources of your Type-A behavior, you also have to change the false benefits that feed it. Here's a hard-core Type A talking: I don't want to be anything but Type A. Type A's make the world go round. Their aggressiveness gets things done. Their impatience kicks butts and makes things happen. Besides, I have to expect a lot from myself to get ahead. And even if you put a gun to my head, I couldn't change one iota.

Here's the voice of realism talking back: Since when does your tendency to become easily irritated, aggravated, and angered about innumerable things and persons help you succeed? And does your impatience really help you make timely decisions—or force you to jump the gun with half-baked bunk? If Type A's get things done, they do so in spite of their Type-A behavior, not because of it. Fact is, Type A's don't run the world; plenty of Type B's (calmer, less-harried people) dominate, too. And high expectations don't help you get ahead. They doom you to fail. Most important, you *can* change. So say science and hundreds of reformed Type A's.

This kind of point and counterpoint has to happen in your head, says Dr. Friedman, until you've replaced every bit of Type-A nonsense with hard facts.

■ Drilling for Life

Now comes the hard part: the repetitive drills. These are behavioral exercises designed to root out Type-A habits and replace them with healthier ones.

"Old habits die hard, as our study participants discovered," Dr. Friedman says. "It took months of doggedly executing the drills to kick the ingrained harmful habits. At first, the participants just went through the motions. Then slowly the repetitive actions began to change how the participants felt, until new habits seemed as natural as breathing."

There are two types of drills, says Dr. Friedman, general and specific. You do the general ones as often as possible, on no particular timetable. You do the specific drills according to schedule—a different drill once a day for seven days, then repeat the sequence week by week throughout the month. You try a different set of drills for each month. For best results, select specific drills from the list below and schedule them throughout a full year.

If you're a die-hard Type A, these drills will drive you nuts—at least at first. On the other hand, they can't be any worse than a heart attack.

General Drills

Be sure to do these drills often.

● Announce to your spouse and friends that you intend to turn over a new leaf, to whip your AIAI.

● Start smiling at other people and laughing at yourself.

● Stop trying to think or do more than one thing at a time.

● Play to lose, at least some of the time.

● When something angers you, immediately make a note of it. Review the list at the end of each week and decide objectively which items truly merited your level of anger.

● Listen, really listen, to the conversation of others.

Specific Drills

Combine these drills into seven-day schedules, a different drill per day, repeating each schedule throughout a month.

● For 15 minutes, recall pleasant memories.

● Don't wear a watch.

● At the supermarket, get in the longest checkout line.

● Do absolutely nothing but listen to music for 15 minutes.

● Buy a small gift for a member of your family.

● *Cheerfully* say "Good morning" to each member of your family and to people you see at work.

● Carefully, slowly scrutinize a tree, a flower, sunset, or dawn.

● Walk, talk, and eat more slowly.

● On two different occasions, say to someone, "Maybe I'm wrong."

● Tape-record your dinnertime conversation, then play back the tape to see whether you interrupt or talk too fast.

So, Type A's, how long must we strive to be Type B's? Always, says Dr. Friedman. "I beg you to continue to save your life—year after year."

173

BAND-AIDS FOR THE SOUL

At some time in life, everyone suffers the type of emotional wound that can take months or years to heal. The loss of a friend, the death of a loved one, or a divorce all modify life in far-reaching and unalterable ways.

The vast majority of life's emotional hurts, though, are little ones — the garden-variety upsets that can leave you rattled for a day or two. Still, who wants to waste even one day on negative emotions? And the more hassles we have to deal with, it seems, the more disturbed we are likely to be by the *next* little incident that comes along.

How can you stop those emotional cuts and scrapes from turning into a major malady? By stocking your mental medicine chest with a handy supply of Band-Aids for the soul.

Here is a list of some typical, every-day upsets, and some tips from psychologists on how to make a quick recovery. Their suggestions are specific, but the underlying principles can be applied to most of the common hassles you might encounter.

Going Nowhere Fast

When you get caught at a traffic light, does your face turn red?

"There are three general strategies for dealing with that type of situation," says Dr. Robert D. Kerns, Jr., assistant clinical professor of psychology at the Yale University School of Medicine who is also chief of the counseling and health psychology section at the Veterans Administration Medical Center in West Haven, Connecticut. "The first is behavioral — *doing* something to minimize the frustration. If you're caught at a traffic light, for instance, you can turn on the radio to distract yourself, or roll down the window to get a breath of fresh air.

"The second type of strategy is called cognitive, and refers to what you *think*. For example, tell yourself positive statements. If you're late for an appointment and get caught at a traffic light, you can tell yourself, 'I'll make it, it's only one light, it only lasts 60 seconds.' You can even count the seconds.

"Another cognitive strategy is to distract yourself by thinking about a different, more pleasant scene. You can imagine what you'll do to relax at the end of the day, or imagine walking in your yard, looking at the garden."

If you really are going to be late, you might want to take a slightly different approach. "In that case, it's probably not the traffic jam that's causing you distress, but anticipation that something awful or catastrophic will happen later because of being late," says Dr. Kerns. "Rehearsing how you're going to cope with that future situation is a positive way to distract yourself. You might decide to make a joke about catching every light, make a simple apology, or just be ready to get down to business when you do arrive. That's a useful way to spend that time.

"The third strategy is to use relaxation techniques to minimize your emotional distress or the physiological arousal associated with it. Sit comfortably in your seat and relax all of your muscles very quickly until you become like a rag doll, or close your eyes for 15 seconds."

The Left-Out Feeling

Have your friends ever forgotten to invite you to an outing? Have you ever had a birthday that nobody remembered? Or has your son or daughter ever forgotten to send you a card on Mother's Day?

"It's important to recognize that one time or another everyone has forgotten a date, forgotten to send a card or to call," says Dr. C. Eugene Walker, professor of psychology at the University of Oklahoma College of Medicine and author of *Learn to Relax*. "We all fall down. There probably isn't a person who hasn't done it or had it happen to him. You have to realize that it's just a part of life."

"It's not the fact that you didn't get the card that's so upsetting," says Dr. Kerns, "but the negative thinking that goes along with it. A person prone to becoming distressed by those situations will go into a whole internal tirade about the event — all of the awful things that are meant by it. They'll say, 'This means they don't think of me, don't care about me, don't love me.' They'll think back to similar situations in the past that brought about similar feelings and they'll dwell on them. Psychologists refer to that type of thinking as negative cognitive distortion. It's common in people with depression.

"The strategy for dealing with that is to catch yourself early on in the phase of negative thinking and try to stop it," Dr. Kerns says. "Not by saying, 'Don't think that', because as soon as you say, 'Don't think about X', you're going to think about X more and more. What you really want to do is think of positive statements — a different way of evaluating the same situation. You can say, 'Maybe the card is late. I've sent late cards before. I can probably expect it later in the week. And if I don't get one, it's not the end of the world'. The idea is to minimize negative thinking by thinking more rational thoughts."

Coping with Overload

When your schedule has you swamped and you're ready to set fire to your office, you can use these pointers to get you back on an even keel.

"First, you need to be realistic about

what you can get done," says Dr. Robert Felner, director of training in clinical psychology at Auburn University in Alabama. "Don't say 'I'll work 40 hours straight and finish everything.'

"One of the best ways to approach a work overload is to map out exactly what you've got to get done and prioritize the list. There's no way to deal with a general work overload, but you can deal with each of ten tasks individually. That way, at the end of the day you can look at what you've accomplished instead of feeling like you've failed. There are too many people who spend a day being very productive and go home feeling like they didn't get anything done because everything isn't finished."

"Schedule in breaks—periods of reward to gather each step along the way," suggests Dr. Kerns. "Tell yourself that you will make it through. Appreciate that you've made it through similar situations before and that you'll do it again."

Marital Spats

If a fight with your spouse ruffles your feathers for a whole day, you may want to learn some strategies for smoothing things out more quickly.

"I can really be affected by marital spats," says Dr. Stephen D. Fabick, a clinical psychologist from Birmingham, Michigan. "One thing that helps me is just realizing that it's going to happen every so often. You can't have your happiness totally dependent on whether you and your spouse are getting along that day. And you can't judge your relationship by it either."

"It's important to make plans for solving the problem," says Dr. Walker. "It's very disturbing to leave a problem open or unsettled. Propose a strategy and make a date to discuss it later." That way, it's easier to get on with your day.

"You might want to plan to do something special when you get home to make up," says Dr. Kerns. "That's a more positive way to think about it."

Butterflies

Most people are familiar with that fluttery feeling they get in their stomachs when they have to give a speech, take a test, or go to a party at the boss's house. That feeling is often more distressing than the actual event.

"That's referred to as anticipatory anxiety," explains Dr. Kerns. "It's not so much the doing of the task that's so anxiety producing, but the anticipation of it—the ruminating about it. We tend to think about the event in ways that provoke intense anxiety. The result is butterflies in the stomach, a headache, or other symptoms.

"A good strategy is to realize that you are responsible for what you're doing to yourself, and that you have the ability to control those feelings," he says. "You can say, 'It's not the situation—it's my thinking about it that's generating the anxiety. I'm responsible, I'm in control, and I'm able to do something about it.'

"If it's a speech you're giving, you can organize your talk and practice it. If it's a social engagement you're dreading, you can think about who'll be there, and mentally rehearse what you might say to them.

"You can also use relaxation techniques," recommends Dr. Kerns. "They'll reinforce your feeling of control because you'll see that you have the ability to do something. But there's also a physiological rationale for doing them. They literally loosen your muscles, slow your heart rate, and control your blood pressure."

The most widely prescribed relaxation technique is progressive muscle relaxation. You do it by systematically tensing and relaxing the various muscle groups in your body to generate a sense of total body relaxation. Deep, regular diaphragmatic breathing can also help you relax. The shallow chest breathing we do most of the time seems to go along with anxiety.

Another good relaxation technique is called positive imagery. That's where you imagine a relaxing scene, using as many senses as possible. "A beach scene works well for me," Dr. Kerns says. "I imagine being alone on the beach, watching the waves rippling, hearing the sound of the waves breaking on the shore, tasting a hint of salt in the air, and feeling the warm sun and sand. Some people like to imagine walking through the woods on a crisp fall day. For others, sitting in a rowboat on a lake with a fishing line is very relaxing. Whatever your scene is, the more elaborate and detailed you make it, the more relaxing it will be."

"You should also recognize that anxiety is part of life," says Dr. Walker. "That's much less upsetting than having the attitude that it's terrible and you shouldn't have to feel it."

In fact, you may even be able to put that anxiety to good use. "Up to a point, anxiety can really help people," says Dr. Fabick. "If we realize that, we can use it

to our advantage. Many actors and actresses say that they get nervous, but it helps them get up for the performance. If you accept the normalcy of the anxiety and harness the energy in a positive way, it can help you."

Big Plans Fall Through

Have you ever looked forward to something, like a vacation or a visit with your family, and had it fall through at the last minute? Maybe you were planning for it, dreaming about it, and when it fell through it left you feeling a little blue.

"It's important to realize how understandable it is that you would feel disappointed," says Dr. Kerns. "You don't want to cover it up with Pollyanna-ish statements. But it's also important to put it in perspective."

"You can do things to be good to yourself to reduce the disappointment," suggests Dr. Felner. "Try doing a couple of little things that are fun. Sometimes peole punish themselves after a disappointment and don't do anything. That just makes things worse. You can say 'Gee, I won't get to go to the Bahamas this year, but I can take a couple of side trips. And there are a lot of fun and productive things that I can do around here.'"

"It's great to get excited," says Dr. Fabick. "But with any expectations you've got to keep in mind that you can't count on things always working out. You don't want to go to the other extreme, though, where you never get excited about anything. The healthiest people seem to be able to find some balance of realistic expectations, keeping in mind that Murphy's Law [if anything can go wrong, it will] is always operating.

"Another preventive measure is having several options. Many times we become so focused on just one possibility that if it falls through we become despondent."

You've Lost Your Temper

Have you ever gotten so angry that you've felt dangerous? Or has one of your outbursts left you feeling shaken, scared, or even guilty?

First off, step back. "Instead of trying to justify your anger, take steps to reduce it," suggests Dr. Felner. "Don't act on that anger. Instead, sit down, take deep breaths, and try to relax. Most people find that when involved in an argument, if they can get out of the same room for 15 minutes they're okay. They just need that time to pull back and calm themselves."

"It's a good idea to discharge the energy physically by taking a brisk walk or by participating in some other form of exercise," says Dr. Fabick. "And realize that it's normal sometimes to want to choke somebody. Don't feel guilty about it, just don't do it."

Teenage Tussle

Anyone who's lived with a teenager probably knows what life on a roller coaster is like. One minute everything's fine and the next minute your child is screaming, "I hate you!" Maybe you even scream back.

"At times like those, your strongest link is with the other parent," says Dr. Kerns. "It's important to reach out to that person for support and to align with them.

"The pain you can feel in that situation is not simple to deal with. You might be able to minimize it, though. If you know full well it's a temporary thing, tell yourself that. Don't overdramatize it—keep it in perspective. You can say, 'He's not lost forever. We'll get over it in the next few days.' You can see it as just one upset in a long line of events and seeming catastrophies in raising a child. It starts in infancy and continues all the way through."

"If *you've* gone overboard, acknowledge your own regret. And address it if the teen has, too," says Dr. Fabick. "Kids do well with parents who have the strength to admit mistakes."

Dr. Felner agrees. "It's unfortunate that parents have been fed all that stuff about consistency being more important than everything else. If you've lost your temper, you can apologize. Sometimes, in a rage, a parent might tell a kid that he's grounded for a month. If it's unreasonable, you can go back and say, 'Look, I was angry and upset. I said the wrong thing. You're only grounded for two days. I'm sorry.' You'll both feel better."

LOVE YOUR NEIGHBOR: THE LIFESAVING COMMANDMENT

Vince Ward will be the first to tell you that high blood pressure can be one of the unwelcome perks of his high-tension job. Ward, 52, is advertising and public-relations director—"flak-catcher"—for one of the nation's largest telecommunications firms.

But Ward says his blood pressure is fine. In fact, everything is fine. He's fit, doesn't lose sleep worrying, "and my kids like me." In his spare time, Ward works with parolees from the Kansas State Penitentiary, raises money for a children's home, and has donated more than 14 gallons of blood to the Community Blood Bank of Greater Kansas City. All in all, he says, "I'm a pretty happy guy."

When she was a child, they called her Dummy. And Kay Arnold grew up believing they were right. But the 48-year-old homemaker knew she had musical talent and she knew she wanted to help people. So, she joined a troupe of entertainers called SENSE, in Newington, Connecticut, that performs for the disabled and elderly. Today, Kay Arnold has a different opinion of herself.

"This gives me a sense of worth I never had before," she says. "It's like therapy that works both ways." And she noticed something even more remarkable. "I have arthritis," she explains, "and when I perform, it seems to make that pain go away."

Vince Ward and Kay Arnold are more than just a couple of do-gooders. Their lives—full and healthy—illustrate a little-known corollary to The Golden Rule: Doing unto others can do wonderful things unto you.

Though there weren't stress tests and electrocardiograms in the days of St. Luke, he was medically accurate when he wrote, "It is more blessed to give than to receive." We've always known that people with generous spirits tend to be happier, but now doctors are saying they're healthier and live longer too. Generosity comes naturally to us, they say. In fact, it may be nature's way of keeping us well.

Most people know that stress has been implicated in diseases as diverse as trench mouth and cancer. Stress is a definite factor in hypertension and coronary heart

180

disease. Recent evidence indicates it suppresses the immune system, the body's first line of defense against disease.

So what does stress have to do with the charity that begins away from home? Some prominent scientists believe that giving yourself to others is an effective antidote to stress.

One of them, the late Dr. Hans Selye, who was responsible for the early studies tying stress to illness, called the concept altruistic egoism. Biblical scholars might call it the as-ye-sow-so-shall-ye-reap syndrome. It seems generosity has some valuable paybacks: the love and gratitude we inspire in those we help. Like stress, love has a cumulative effect, Dr. Seyle said. We can weather the storms of life if we have hoarded good feelings for bad times, in much the same way squirrels hoard food for the winter. Those feelings are perpetual reminders that although everything else might be bad, we aren't. Knowing that can make life easier.

Dr. George Vaillant, psychiatrist and director of a 40-year study of Harvard University graduates, identified altruism as one of the qualities that helped even the most poorly adjusted men of the study group deal successfully with the stresses of life.

Does all this mean selfishness could make you ill? Dr. Larry Scherwitz thinks it might. A social psychologist at the Medical Research Institute of San Francisco, Dr. Scherwitz turned up a startling fact in a major study for risk factors in coronary heart disease: The people who referred to themselves using the pronouns I, me, and my most often in an interview were more likely to develop coronary heart disease, even when other health-threatening behaviors were controlled. "The more self-centered people were much more likely to die of heart attack than the less self-centered," says Dr. Scherwitz.

The reason for that may be quite simple, suggests Dr. Dean Ornish, author of *Stress, Diet, and Your Heart*. "This exaggerated focus on the self may further reinforce the sense of isolation and separateness," he says. In other words, looking out for number one isn't enlightened self-interest at all. It's just lonely. And loneliness kills.

So says Dr. James Lynch, a leading specialist in psychosomatic medicine from the University of Maryland School of Medicine. Dr. Lynch documented the connection between loneliness and heart disease in his book *The Broken Heart*. What he discovered is that most loneliness-prone people in American society—the divorced, widowed, and elderly—are more likely to die from heart disease than other segments of the population. Loneliness, he says, is the number one cause of premature death today.

"The mandate to 'Love your neighbor as you love yourself' is not just a moral mandate. It's a physiological mandate. Caring is biological," Dr. Lynch says. "One thing you get from caring for others is you're not lonely. And the more connected you are to life, the healthier you are."

Dr. Lynch goes the phone company slogan one better. He warns: Unless you reach out and touch someone, you'll die. He has plenty of support for his claim.

Love and Death

In a well-known study of residents in Alameda, California, Dr. Lisa Berkman, of Yale University, and Dr. S. Leonard

Syme, of the University of California at Berkeley, both researchers, discovered that the most socially isolated people were more susceptible to disease and had death rates 2.3 to 2.8 times higher than those with a large number of social relationships.

An elderly volunteer worker in suburban Baltimore puts it another way. "Involvement makes you keep well so you can keep giving. It makes you take care of your health. It's a blessing to ward off old age."

Alfred N. Larsen sees evidence of that firsthand. Larsen is national director of the federal Retired Senior Volunteer Program (RSVP), which has placed hundreds of thousands of elderly people in community volunteer jobs. He says he's convinced of the value of volunteer work for the elderly, who lose family, friends, and often a purpose for life as they grow older. "Doctors always tell us that elderly people who engage in volunteer work are a lot better off, visit the doctor less often and have fewer complaints," he says.

It keeps you young. It keeps you healthy. The experts are saying that caring for others keeps you alive. And Dr. Linda Nilson, researcher and sociologist at UCLA, goes so far as to say altruism may be a part of our survival instinct.

While poring over data on 100 natural disasters, Dr. Nilson began to discern a strong pattern of altruism among disaster victims. Even when their own lives were disrupted, victims almost invariably lent helping hands to their neighbors. It seems to be part of the recovery process. In a disaster, she says, "we go back to a sense of tribal cohesiveness, having to reconstruct the society around us under tremendous survival pressure. We realize our survival depends not only on our own

happiness but on the survival and happiness of others."

The community that evolves out of disaster is called a therapeutic community, says Dr. Nilson, and it is so nurturing, it wards off psychological problems later on. In fact, disaster survivors report an exhilarating sense of well-being and feel better not only about themselves but about their neighbors.

Help Me, Help You

These therapeutic communities are, in essence, makeshift self-help groups. But self-help, with its implications of individual effort, is a misnomer. What self-help groups like Alcoholics Anonymous offer is the solace of mutual aid. "Their members get help from helping," says Frank Riessman, director of the national Self-Help Clearinghouse, City University of New York.

It's no simple idea. Self-help group members give one another a special kind of human companionship. "There's a strong sense of connectedness with people who really understand you because they share your problem," says Riessman. For those with health problems, there's a bonus. Self-help groups literally can be a form of health care. Riessman says this is nowhere more apparent than among victims of high blood pressure, who reinforce their own good health habits—sticking to a low-salt diet and exercising—by giving the same advice to others.

Like Dr. Nilson's disaster victims, people helping others in the proverbial "same boat" are practicing a survival skill. Lending a helping hand makes the vulnerable feel less vulnerable, says Riessman. "They

182

feel they have some control over their lives."

That measure of control may be the difference between sickness and health, according to a study by Colorado researchers. They subjected rats to identical electrical shocks, but allowed one set of animals to control the jolts. When they examined them, they discovered the animals that couldn't escape the shocks showed a reduced disease-fighting ability in their white blood cells. Having control over stress, postulates one of the researchers, Dr. Steven F. Maier, can prevent the suppression of the body's immune system, which might otherwise leave you vulnerable to everything from bacteria to cancer cells.

And being a helper can really puff up your ego, says Dr. Lowell Levin, professor of public health at Yale University and an expert on the health benefits of mutual aid. "When you're a helper, your self-concept improves. You are somebody. You are worthwhile. And there's nothing more exhilarating than that," he says. "That can influence your health."

That's exactly what the California Department of Mental Health learned five years ago when it surveyed 1,000 Californians. Those who cared most for themselves and others regarded themselves as being much healthier, both mentally and physically, than those with little concern for themselves and the next guy.

One reason for that, suggests Dr. James Lynch, is that people with high self-esteem take better care of themselves. "Really caring for yourself includes caring for your body," he says. "And that becomes the foundation of caring for others."

Other people also help us establish our own identities, he says. "When you say 'I,' 'I' has no meaning until you look into my eyes and see 'you.'" The people who give to others generally find themselves in eyes brimming with gratitude and love, and there's no greater ego boost than that.

So, you want to be happy, healthy, and to live a long life. Does that mean you should march right out like Vince Ward and give a pint of blood, or belt out a song in a nursing home, as Kay Arnold does? No, not if you're only giving to get something in return. The only way a giver can really reap the benefits of giving is if the urge comes from the goodness, not the need, in his heart. Says Dr. Larry Scherwitz. "If you're altruistic because of the goodies you get out of it, you're not altruistic. If the person you've helped doesn't thank you and you get angry, you're not altruistic. You've become too attached to the fruits of your labor."

THE PEN IS MIGHTIER THAN THE ANALYST

Okay, it's confession time. When frustration or depression has shoved you to the breaking point, do you rant and rave like a 4-year-old when no one is looking? Do you make kamikaze nosedives on Boston cream pies at midnight? Or do you just sit in the dark wondering whether the simple life of a Himalayan shepherd is not the true road to peace? I won't tell you which one I'm guilty of but, after talking to Dr. James Pennebaker, author of *Confessions in Health*, I've traded in my subscription to the Pie-of-the-Month Club for a much more effective antidepressant — a pen.

"All of us have upsetting experiences or troublesome thoughts that we tend to worry about a great deal but don't want to mention to others," says Dr. Pennebaker. "Writing is a great way of unburdening ourselves in private. It's a way of putting our problems into a more manageable form, making understanding, and perhaps even solving, them a little easier."

Writing off your worries has physical benefits as well as emotional ones. We all know that mental stress has a way of playing havoc with the body. According to Dr. Pennebaker, as his writing class participants relieved themselves of their anxieties, they experienced bonus dividends in the form of lowered blood pressures and improved immune functions. "The end result for many of my students was a considerable reduction in doctor's office visits for illness."

Before we learn how to turn a dollar's worth of pen and paper into a healthier and happier life, let's keep in mind two things. First, you don't need to be one step away from an analyst's couch to benefit from this technique. I think we can all admit to a spare problem or two, which, though small, still could use a good putting to bed. Second, don't hesitate to try this just because you haven't written a great novel lately. You don't have to be F. Scott Fitzgerald. You just have to be honest.

Getting Started

"The first thing you'll want to do is find a place where you won't be inter-

184

rupted," suggests Dr. Pennebaker. "If possible, make it an interesting spot where you don't normally go." This place could be a quiet corner in the stacks at your local library, or somewhere scenic such as under an old oak tree by a creek. Don't just head on into the kitchen and plop yourself down under that humming fluorescent tube light. You are embarking on a unique psychological session with yourself. You're worth a nice setting.

"Set a time limit with which you are comfortable," continues Dr. Pennebaker. "Twenty to 30 minutes should do it to start. But the important thing to remember is that you *must* write for the entire time. No stopping and losing yourself in thought is allowed. If you need to repeat yourself to fill up the time, do it." Interestingly enough, in all the time Dr. Pennebaker has run his sessions, not one participant has repeated themselves.

What to Write About

A blank piece of paper can be an uninviting host. How do you make the initial leap? "Your first impulse might be to write about what you've done today or what's new at the office," says Dr. Pennebaker. "Don't give in to that impulse. That type of writing is not the cathartic experience you're looking for. Focus on thoughts and feelings. How do you feel right now? Start right there and you may be suprised at what comes out next."

If you have a specific problem in mind, you can also start there and get to the heart of the matter. If there's no problem and you're feeling fairly placid, try a trick Freud used with his patients. Write about the last thing in the world that you'd want to discuss.

Anonymity and Dotted i's

"Your writings should be for your eyes only," says Dr. Pennebaker. "This is a very important point. If you think that someone else is going to read it, it's very likely that you won't be as honest or as daring as you could be. And if you rein in your thoughts, this technique won't work." If you want to save your writings, make sure from the start that you have a locked drawer to keep them in. These are your innermost thoughts and no one else should see them or happen upon them by chance.

"Also, since these writings are not for publication, don't worry about spelling, grammar, or punctuation," says Dr. Pennebaker. "Nothing should stop your flow. It's the content of what you're writing that's important, not the gift-wrapping."

Why Does It Work?

"Some people hypothesize that just the mere expression of our emotions provides a healthy release, but I think it goes a little deeper than that," Dr. Pennebaker says. "Troubling thoughts have a way of recurring without our actually understanding or pinpointing the underlying problem. The nature of writing motivates us to put our thoughts into words, clarify them, and explore them in some type of linear order. In that way, the problem eventually emerges on paper. Having discovered it, we can start solving it."

Also, a problem that seems large, untidy, and multifaceted in our minds can suddenly appear much smaller, neater, and more manageable when it's broken down into smaller components and turned into four or five paragraphs on a page. It's rather like those days when it seems that there are 75 million things that need to be done and you just can't begin to tackle them. But as soon as you make a list, suddenly you find yourself saying, "Well, I can do this one and this one right now, then . . ." And suddenly you've gotten everything done.

A word of advice: Don't try doing this every day. According to Dr. Pennebaker, too much writing can become a substitute for action. But apply it occasionally when needed. At first you might feel a little self-conscious about it; with practice you'll find it gets easier to explore yourself through writing. As you get better at it, your body and mind will find greater relief with each session. And quite frankly, at under a dollar a session, psychoanalysis has never been more of a bargain!

M. G.

ADVENTURES IN RUBENFIELD SYNERGY

Laughter rings through the rec hall on this chilly May night and the effusive, wise-cracking New Yorker at the center of it all is beaming like a den mother. Ilana Rubenfield, teacher, innovator, healer, has just finished telling the one about the Jewish woman from Brooklyn who schleps all the way to Nepal to tell her son, the big-shot guru, to come home.

It's evident from her delivery that the lady loves to clown. But watch her eyes work the room as the laughter crests. Forty-five adults, some lounging on floor cushions, others upright on wooden benches, in a semicircle around her. She takes us all in. Within minutes, she knows volumes about us.

Rubenfield, you see, has spent the last 25 years learning to "read" the body for clues to the emotional state and life attitudes operating within. And for the last several of those years, she has taken her knowledge on the road to places very much like this cozy Unitarian camp and conference center in the Berkshires of Massachusetts, where we've gathered for the weekend. She has a new therapy to promote and potential teachers to recruit.

In the audience tonight are massage therapists and psychologists, a university English teacher, a neurologist, a business consultant, a nurse, and a potter. We've each paid up to $230 in program fees and board to Rowe Conference Center to spend the next 2½ days acquainting ourselves with the Rubenfield Synergy Method, Ilana Rubenfield's trademarked blend of psychotherapy and bodywork.

To people who follow trends in the human potential movement, this is cutting edge stuff. Rare are the therapies that let you work through your emotional hurts, and your physical aches and pains at the same time, while showing you how they're related. This is perhaps the simplest way to define Rubenfield Synergy. There are others.

The Rowe catalog calls the method a "powerful, elegant system for human integration, bringing body, mind, spirit, and psyche together in a present, trusting whole." It promises us we'll learn "the relationship of posture to emotion, emotion to posture," and discover "body metaphors for deep patterns in our lives."

Rubenfield herself isn't making any claims on this opening night. She'll let us judge for ourselves. Sitting there on steps of the rec hall stage, her dark hair hidden by an artfully wrapped scarf, her torso swaddled in an oversized, intricately patterned mohair sweater, she has other things in mind.

Like advice. You think she's going to drop a punchline on us without extracting its full meaning?

She waits until she has our full attention again.

"Every guru has a mother," she says, having sized up a few of us very well. "Remember that."

Good-Bye Couch, Hello Massage Table

The form the Rubenfield Synergy Method takes, typically, is a one-on-one session. Nothing unusual about that. But the traditional psychoanalyst's couch has been replaced by a massage table. Rubenfield Synergists (as graduates of the three-year training program are called) use their hands to feel what's going on in the body, and the body to bring to the fore unresolved trauma long submerged in the psyche, yet active in subtly destructive ways.

As feelings and memories rise to the surface, verbal exploration—gestalt therapy—begins. The synergist may guide the client through a dialogue with the damaged part of the self, engage him in role-playing or in any number of cathartic activities.

What makes Rubenfield Synergy different from many forms of bodywork is that practitioners don't concern themselves with loosening tight muscles or massaging out "stuck" places. Instead, they focus on the parts of the body that relate to the emotional issue that has come to the fore. The idea, says Rubenfield, is to enable the client to "consciously let go of whatever they're holding in their bodies."

To see the work unfold is riveting. During my weekend at Rowe, Rubenfield did four demonstrations for us, using separate volunteers. Part stand-up comic, part consummate Jewish mother, she always seemed to know just how to play it, to deliver exactly what the person on the table—or we in the healing circle—needed.

From what we saw, Rubenfield Synergy is Rubenfield stroking the contours of Nancy's feet and telling us that these are feet that wear high heels often and do a fair amount of dancing. (Nancy confirms this.)

It is Rubenfield stiffening momentarily as she passes her hand over Joel's left knee, and asking him to tell her more about the major knee injury he suffered a few years back.

It is Joel's body slowly twisting to the right, the way a plant reaches toward the sun, when Rubenfield conducts a little experiment in which Joel hears praise in his right ear and criticism in his left ear.

■ How She Got Here

Rubenfield's starting point for her current work was, curiously enough, the

RUBENFIELD'S MIRACULOUS BACK RELAXER

Ilana Rubenfield, creator of the Rubenfield Synergy Method, shares this quick, simple, and effective back relaxer whenever she gives workshops.

What makes it unusual is that it uses an element of surprise. The sequence causes you to break the habitual message your brain sends to your muscles. You're actually going to confuse your muscles, so they have no choice but to let go.

The steps may look complicated, but give this a try. It's fun. And the results are amazing.

1. Sit up straight on your chair. Plant both feet firmly on the ground. Move away from the back of your chair so you're not leaning against it.

2. Now roll your eyes to the right. Let your neck and body follow. Twist as far as you can go, without feeling strain.

3. Then stop wherever you are. Take a mental photograph of the wall behind you. You'll use this photograph as a reference point later, so remember it.

4. Gently return to the front. Now take your left hand and pass it over the top of your head. Cover your right ear with that hand.

5. Lean gently to the left a few times. Do it in a quiet, soft way. Imagine that your spine and the muscles attached to it are soft and flexible. Maybe you'll see yourself as a flower stalk, a soft piece of elastic, a bamboo tree. Use whatever image comes to mind. And, as Rubenfield is fond of saying, "Think soft."

6. Now come back to the middle. Take a moment to tune in to your body. How do the ribs feel? The neck? The spine?

7. Let go of that awareness. Now take your right hand and pass it over the top of your head, so that the hand covers your left ear.

8. Now bend a few times to the right. Bring your "softening" image to mind again and use it.

9. Take several breaths. Slowly straighten up.

10. Take your left hand and again pass it over the top of your head. Cover your right ear.

11. This time, roll your eyes to the left and twist around as if you're looking at someone behind you. Then allow yourself to gradually face front again.

12. Twist again to the left. Only this time, look out of the right corners of your eyes. Look to the right, while you twist to the left.

13. Come back to the front and let everything go. Let your arms hang loosely at your sides.

14. Now roll your eyes to the right. Let your head, neck, and body follow. Continue to twist to the right until you feel strain.

15. Take another mental photograph. How does that compare with your first one? Quite a difference, right?

Julliard School of Music where she trained to be a conductor, and, inadvertently, a near cripple.

The problem, as she looks back on it, was that no one ever taught her how to stand properly so she wouldn't injure her back when she worked. And so, she did. So badly in fact, that she thought about giving up conducting. The best doctors could do for her was inject her with a Novocainlike substance that made the pain bearable just long enough to allow her to get through a performance.

Nothing changed until a friend suggested she try the Alexander Technique. As Rubenfield remembers it, the conversation went something like this:

RUBENFIELD: What's that?

FRIEND: I don't know.

RUBENFIELD: You don't know?

FRIEND: I don't know, but it works.

RUBENFIELD: You expect me to try something you can't explain to me?

FRIEND: Right. I can't put it into words, but it's terrific. Go try it.

What Rubenfield would learn later is that the Alexander Technique was created by a nineteenth-century Australian actor who needed to cure himself of *his* chronic affliction so he could continue working. F. M. Alexander's problem was that he kept losing his voice. When doctors couldn't help, he set out to observe himself with mirrors to see if he could figure something out.

In time, he realized that the way he moved when he performed compressed his neck, jamming down his vocal chords. When he taught himself new movements

respectful of his body's structure, his voice returned to normal. Eventually, he incorporated his discoveries in a movement reeducation system, which now has teachers around the world.

One of those teachers was Judith Liebowitz, whose gentle, healing touch set Rubenfield on a brand new course.

"I go to her apartment and this woman, who is not a doctor, asks me to lie down on the massage table," she tells us. "And this is the experience that changes my life: She put her hands on my face and head and I never felt anything like that in my life. It was unbelievable! And then she says to me, 'Ilana, relax. Let me move your head.' And I said"—here she grits her teeth, hamming it up—"I am relaxed and you can move my head.' And she said, 'I can't move your head. You're not letting go.' We had a little difference of opinion."

Later, Liebowitz asked Rubenfield what kind of work she did. When she said she was a conductor, Liebowitz handed her a pencil and wanted a demonstration. No one, during all the years she sought treatment, had asked her to do that before.

In minutes, Liebowitz knew the answer. "Of course you have back pain and spasms."

"Of course?" asked the mystified conductor.

"Of course," said Liebowitz, and she pointed out to Rubenfield how her stance threw her ankles and knees off balance, and what happened to the rest of her body when she craned her neck and head so far forward.

Rubenfield, fascinated, decided to continue the lessons a couple of times a week. One day, an odd thing happened. Liebowitz touched her in her usual gentle way, and Rubenfield wept, as deep reservoirs of memory from her past flooded her consciousness. Several tear-filled sessions passed, and Liebowitz suggested that Rubenfield see an analyst.

Bodywork theorists explain the phenomenon by saying that the nerves and muscles of the body bear the imprint of every emotional trauma since birth. They maintain that if you release tension in the part of the body that "holds" the trauma, the details of the incident, and any unresolved feelings attached to it, are likely to surface.

Rubenfield found an analyst she liked, but considered the setup awkward at best. "She touches me, but she won't talk to me. He talks to me, but he won't touch me." Why, she wondered, isn't anyone integrating the two?

And so necessity, that mother of invention, threw a new project in her path. Like F. M. Alexander before her, she was about to leave behind the performing arts to become a health guru.

The 1960s and 1970s found her extremely busy. She became a certified teacher and board member of the American Center for the Alexander Technique. She met Fritz Perls, studied Gestalt Therapy under him, and experimented with using bodywork techniques as he verbally counseled a client. In 1971, she joined the first United States training class of Moshe Feldenkrais, a physicist who grew up in her native Israel and devised his own system for freeing the body and brain from its fixed habits.

And in 1977, she offered her first training class in the Rubenfield Synergy Method, which integrated all of those therapies. Twenty-two students graduated from it. These days, Rubenfield divides her time between training synergists, assisting private clients (Judy Collins has been one), and promoting her method, as she's doing right now.

An Emotional Roller Coaster

Weekend workshops with Rubenfield are an emotional roller coaster. How carefully she orchestrates the rise and fall. One minute you're dabbing at your eyes with Kleenex, moved by a stranger's pain as she works through some hurt from her childhood. The next minute, you're dancing tush to tush with someone you hardly know, reggae music blaring from an almost-always-on cassette player, and you're laughing yourself silly.

But don't let the roller coaster effect fool you. There is a tight logic to the way the workshop unfolds. Friday night, we break the ice with a simple hand-to-hand contact exercise, designed to make us more aware of how much information touch can yield. Saturday we experiment with Feldenkrais body awareness exercises, learn to give and accept feedback from a partner, and experience the drama of Rubenfield in a one-on-one session. Sunday she reserves for the more spiritual exercises in her repertoire.

Throughout, she shares with us her accumulated wisdom. Caring for the caretaker is a priority with her, and a point she makes often. She also tells us we can't force change on another; we can really only offer encouragement and support to our partners and let them decide how much change is comfortable. And she advises us against honing in on the sore spots at first. Any point in the bodymind is an entry to where we want to go.

Avoiding Burnout

All of the lessons of the day culminate Saturday night in the one-on-one work Rubenfield does with Mara, a softspoken Maine lawyer who's active in the new underground railroad. As a volunteer advocate, it's Mara's job to help Guatemalan refugees apply for political asylum in Canada—and to listen to their heart-rending stories.

Friday, when Mara took her turn at the microphone to introduce herself, she told us she was on the verge of burnout and scared. One of her co-volunteers was already in bed with back pain; another had been hospitalized for the same thing. Mara didn't know who would take over for her if something happened to her.

So Rubenfield wants to troubleshoot, to see just how Mara works. She places two folding chairs in the middle of the room; the group arranges itself in a circle around this "stage."

Mara takes a chair in the center and at Rubenfield's invitation, sets the scene. The man she is about to counsel fled from his home after a neighbor boy warned him the authorities were after him. The boy was shot to death as a consequence of his actions.

Mara picks Michael, a genial blond activist who, conveniently, speaks Spanish fluently. They converse in that language, Michael pressing on about his worries,

Mara trying to explain the procedure for asylum.

Rubenfield stands behind Mara, observing. "Freeze, Mara," she says suddenly. "There's nowhere for your movement to go." And she shows Mara, and the group, how stiffly Mara is holding herself. She adjusts Mara's posture, then steps back to watch.

"All right, stop," she says, minutes later. "You hardly breathed. When you keep explaining the procedures to him, you hardly take care of yourself." She works on Mara's neck.

"Don't worry about him right now," Rubenfield adds. "He's so worried about himself, he doesn't know the difference. Between you having to speak a foreign language, and the subject matter, your neck gets very tight."

"Yes," Mara says, sounding relieved that Rubenfield understands.

"Try to be a little more sing-song," Rubenfield suggests. "And move your shoulders a bit more." She helps Mara to feel what she means by moving Mara's shoulders back and forth in an exaggerated fashion.

"Something tells me this is going to send mixed messages," Mara says, in just the right tone to crack us all up.

But before the demonstration ends, Mara is crying, and a few women in the group are teary-eyed with her. They understand the weariness she feels in the face of this constant stream of tragedy. It's gotten so all that Mara really *wants* to do is spend time puttering in her garden. But isn't that selfish?

Rubenfield helps Mara to understand that her desire to garden isn't selfish, it's healthy—her body's way of taking time off to revitalize. To help Mara firm up her resolve, Rubenfield has her compose—out loud—a resignation letter to the Superwomen of America Club.

Rustic Rowe

The work Rubenfield does with Mara is of particular interest to Doug Wilson, our caretaker at Rowe this weekend. Ordained as a Unitarian minister, Wilson is not unfamiliar with the problems that beset peace and social justice activists. In fact, a private room in the recreation hall, the book-lined room in which I slept, is dedicated to the Ploughshare Activists.

Wilson took on the executive directorship of Rowe Camp and Conference Center in 1973, a job he now shares with his wife, Pru Berry. The camp itself has been in existence since 1924.

These days, the facilities, which are set in a pine woods and at the edge of a 14,000-acre forest preserve, include a renovated 200-year-old farmhouse, assorted cabins, a rec hall, and meditation chapel. Things here are still a bit rustic. Guests are expected to bring their own linens. Some private rooms with bath are available, but most of the accommodations are dorm style. Program fees are reasonable, and vary according to family income.

Probably the most sophisticated part of Rowe's operation is its restaurant-quality vegetarian meal service. The standing ovation that cook Alice Cozzilino got at the close of the Rubenfield weekend was plenty enthusiastic.

A family feeling pervades mealtime. The weekend I was there, we held hands before meals and joined Pru in a Shaker hymn, and Doug in a not-so-reverent rendition of grace. And we guests helped clear the table, wash the dishes, and put them away.

Creating Healing Energy

Sunday, the activities take a metaphysical bent. Rubenfield teaches us to work with the healing energies in our hands.

John, Joel, and I team up, as the rest of the crew forms groups of threes. Trusting soul that I am, I even volunteer to be first in my group.

John's hands gently land on one shoulder, Joel's on the other. And then I feel two pairs of hands tapping, patting, a wave of soothing motion traveling down to my feet and back up again to my shoulder.

At Rubenfield's direction, John moves in front of me, Joel behind me. They massage my head and neck and sweep accumulated tension—what Rubenfield calls negative energy—away from my face.

And then my buddies raise their hands above my head and imagine a chalice filled with golden light, which they'll spill over me. They keep their hands out a few inches from my body and I can feel their downward motion. The air between their hands and my body feels charged, electric.

Two pairs of hands touch ground and travel back up again, their owners chanting my name, softly first, then louder and louder as the hands move toward my head. Names echo in the room, bouncing off each other. It's pretty intense.

After everyone has had their chance, we spend a few minutes chanting "om," the universal sound. The group sound is resonant, clear.

And that brings us to our final one-on-one demonstration, this one with Linda, a sweet-natured woman in her forties who lost her teenage son to suicide within the last year.

This one is particularly wrenching. The boxes of tissues make their rounds.

At the conclusion of the piece, Rubenfield leads Linda back out to the circle and asks her to affirm to a few of us that she is a strong woman, capable of standing on her own.

Linda's eyes meet mine briefly, and I notice that her face—like that of the others who have had their turn on the table—

seems a good ten years younger. Cleansed of tension and pain, it now has an appealing, soft, open expression.

It isn't until I get home and join some friends at a dance that I realize I'm presenting a different face to the world, too. "You look great," a friend says. "Really relaxed. What'd you do this weekend?"

But the best thing: I wake up the next morning and my jaw feels odd. It takes me a while to figure out that this strange sensation is how my jaw feels fully relaxed. During tense weeks, I sometimes grind my teeth in my sleep. But that night, even though I never had my turn "on the table," my body had no need of that bad habit.

D. G.

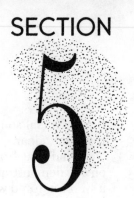
SECRETS
OF SERENITY

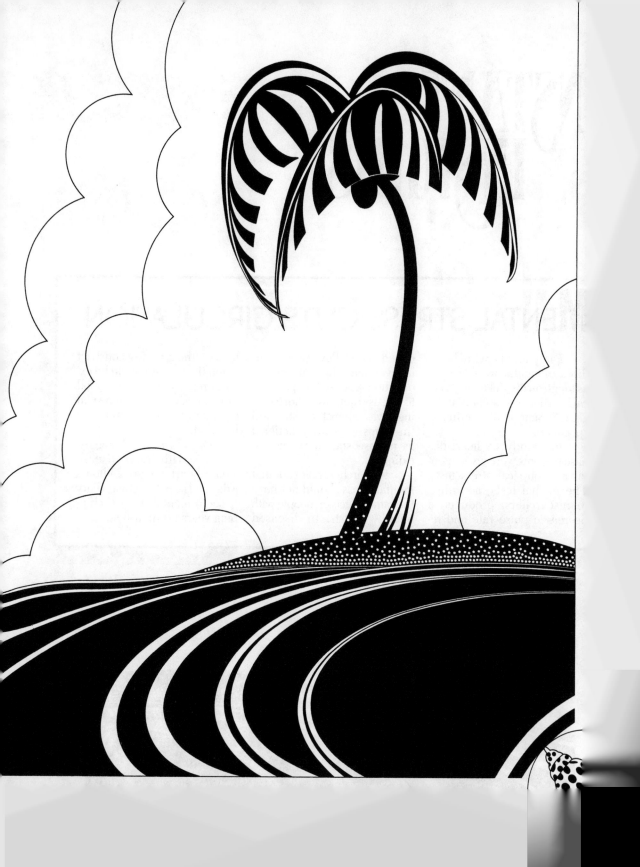

INSTANT INSIGHTS

MENTAL STRESS CUTS CIRCULATION

For patients with heart disease, mental stress can be as tough on the ticker as physical exertion, researchers at the UCLA School of Medicine speculate.

In a study, 39 heart disease patients were given mental and physical stress tests. The mental tests, according to researchers, produced a decreased pulse rate and reduced blood flow (ischemia) in over half the patients. A question asking the patients to discuss their own shortcomings was almost as stressful (in terms of heart reactions) as intense stationary bicycle riding.

Researchers point out that mental stress should not have the same effects on people with healthy hearts. In diseased hearts, the arteries constrict when they really should be expanding; the increased blood flow necessary for physical or mental stress cannot be handled.

Doctors at UCLA suggest patients with heart disease wear a heart monitor 24 hours a day and keep an activity diary to see if mental stress is chipping years off their hearts.

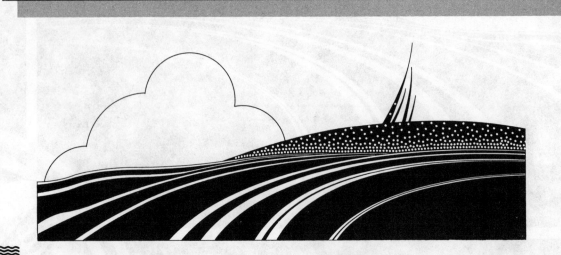

INOCULATE YOURSELF AGAINST STRESS

A simple restructuring of your exercise program may be what you need to inoculate yourself against stress.

Dr. Irving Dardik, a founding chairman of the U.S. Olympic Sports Medicine Council, has developed an approach to exercise that exploits the natural relaxation process you feel after a workout. He calls it cardiocybernetics. You might just want to call it relaxercise.

How does it work? Well, forget your continuous ½-hour workout. Instead, divide your routine into 8 to 16 segments. The segments should be 3 to 5 minutes each. During each segment, you exercise and then allow yourself to recover, using imagery and relaxation techniques.

Dr. Dardik claims that the recovery/relaxation period helps your cardiovascular and immune system learn to adapt to the physiological changes associated with the stress of exercise. When you encounter stress in real life, you can cope with it better.

GREAT DAY, GREAT SLEEP

Want to sleep unusually well? Make sure to have a stimulating day. And if you can't manage that, take a warm bath before bed.

Researchers at Loughborough University in England found that restful, slow-wave sleep does increase after a "behaviorally active day."

They tested volunteers who spent four-day periods in a pretty uneventful sleep lab. On one of the four days, they took the volunteers on an outing in a distant city, where they visited a shopping center and museum, an amusement park/zoo, a scenic spot, and then went to a movie.

The night of the outing, the volunteers conked out earlier than usual, and experienced longer-than-usual periods of restful slow-wave sleep. They awoke feeling refreshed. REM (rapid eye movement) sleep was not affected.

In another trial, the researchers confirmed that a warm bath makes people sleepier at bedtime and produces slow-wave sleep.

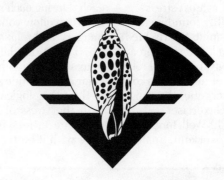

RELAX YOURSELF WELL

Master the art of relaxation and give your immune power a boost.

An Ohio State University study of 45 healthy senior citizens found that seniors who were taught relaxation techniques and guided imagery by a visiting medical student showed a significant boost in natural killer cells—a special type of white blood cell that helps fight tumors. Seniors who were visited by the medical student without receiving lessons in relaxation showed no such change. Nor did members of a control group, who were not visited.

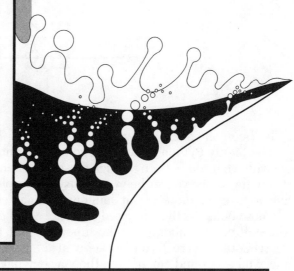

HAIR DRYERS: YOUR PASSPORT TO THE LAND OF NOD

A bonnet-style hair dryer can induce sleep similar to that brought on by a hot bath or exercise. The dryers, report scientists in England, increase the brain's temperature, which increases energy consumption and makes the brain sleepier. Research shows, however, that it may not work when aspirin is taken, because the drug blocks the warming effects on the brain.

MAKE YOUR OWN RELAXATION TAPE

It's been one heck of a week.

The Monty Python crew could go to town with what you've been through these last few days, but you've been too busy living it to even *think* about laughing. With those boulders they dropped on you at the staff meeting today, and the super-hero schedule you're trying to keep at home, you're wound up tighter than a yo-yo string. From where you sit, the next person who asks you to do something had better be prepared to write his own obituary.

Is there any relief for the weary, you wonder?

Would you believe there's a one-word cure? (Drum roll, please) *Relax*.

"That's easy for you to say," you lob back.

To which we reply: It's also easy for you to do. What'll make it nearly effort-less is your own, custom-made relaxation tape. For under two dollars, you can write your own ticket to the greater realms of serenity and lower blood pressure. We'll show you how, step-by-step.

The great thing about relaxation tapes is that you can use them wherever and whenever you have some free time. Add earphones to your tape player and you can even relax on the bus or train during that commute home. The other benefit is that the tape tells you what to do. You never have to stop and strain to remember what comes next.

Just about any relaxation tape on the market can do that for you. So why bother making one?

For one reason, it's cheaper—the price of a blank cassette versus $5 to $25 or more. For another, a homemade tape can be just as effective. You're doing the relaxing, not the tape. If you can believe your own voice, no sweat. (Let's face it, though. Some people don't trust them-selves with anything. They'd do better to learn relaxation skills from an expert, who can assure them that they're doing it right.) If you're a do-it-yourselfer, read on. The best thing about making your own tape is that you can tailor it to your specific wants and needs.

What Will You Gain?

Experts say that deep relaxation will help you lower your oxygen consumption, rate of respiration, pulse, and blood pressure. At the same time, you increase your immune power and shift your brain wave production to the mellower frequencies. In short, you cut your body a break. Grateful being that it is, it's likely to reward you with a much-needed sense of well-being.

Dr. Rene Mastrovito teaches relaxation skills to patients at Memorial Sloan-Kettering Cancer Center in New York. He finds patients can learn to relax enough to sit serenely through a bone-marrow aspiration, which requires a frighteningly large-size needle. Others can relax enough to curtail anxiety-related nausea.

"If you teach people to relax their musculature, you can reduce anxiety, pain, and discomfort," he says. "There seems to be an inverse relationship between muscle relaxation and anxiety. It's almost impossible to feel anxious and nervous without the body being tensed in some way."

Just imagine how your week would have felt had you managed to keep all your muscles loose. Better yet, don't imagine it. Experience it.

Select Your Script

Below are two basic scripts for you to choose from. One is more active and involves tensing your muscles and then releasing them. The second is more passive and is best suited for those of us who are very imaginative and highly susceptible to suggestion.

We've also included a variation to show you how you might create your own add-on to the basic script. This addition will help you deal with a specific anxiety-producing situation.

Remember that the tape is yours to create as you wish. Jazz it up if you want. You can read it into a tape recorder yourself, or ask the help of a loved one who has a really soothing voice. You can even experiment with recording this script while very soft, relaxing music plays in the background.

Don't be afraid to make changes in the basic script. If, for instance, you opt for "Basic Script I" and want to adjust the amount of time you keep your muscles tense, go through the script and make those changes. Or if you opt for "Basic Script II" and want to increase the pauses, go through the script and make those changes. As your body awareness increases, you may find you want to decrease the pause periods because you can relax in much less time.

For now, if you feel you need to go through the whole sequence twice to really relax, you can do that, too. Be sure to take enough time for yourself.

Ready, Set, Record

All you need spare is 20 to 30 minutes. You'll also need a tape recorder and a blank cassette tape. (A 60-minute one will do for the basic script. You'll want a 90-minute one, just to be sure, if you want to experiment with variations. Be sure to get a good-quality tape that the manufacturer says is suited for voice recording.) If your watch has a reliable second hand, or if you can switch to the mode on your

201

digital watch that counts seconds, you'll find that helpful, too.

Basic Script I

"(Insert name), this is your time to relax. Whatever you've been thinking about, whatever worries you have, let go of them now. Deposit them in an imaginary lockbox across the room from you. They'll be there when you return, if you want them. This time belongs to your body. Let your mind be at peace.

"This is your time to relax. Each time you give yourself time to relax fully, it will be easier and easier for you to feel deeply relaxed.

"Take a moment now to settle yourself comfortably on a bed, or sit up straight in a straight-backed chair. Slip off your shoes if you haven't already done so. Loosen anything that is tight. (Pause for 15 seconds.) Good.

"Say to yourself, 'I can relax now and breathe comfortably. This is my time to relax.' (Pause.)

"Now take a deep, deep breath. Good. Hold it. Count silently to five. (Pause for 5 seconds.) Now exhale, counting to ten as you do. (Pause for 10 seconds.)

"Let's try that again. Deep breath, hold it, count to five. (Pause for 5 seconds.) Now release it, counting to ten as you exhale. (Pause for 10 seconds.)

"This third time, hunch your shoulders up, as close to the ears as you can get them, and hold yourself still. Count silently to five. (Pause for 5 seconds.) Now exhale, pushing all the air out of your lungs. Let yourself inhale slowly.

"Good. This is your time to relax. Breathe deeply and slowly. Feel your breath expand your belly and then feel your belly sink back down as you exhale. Stay with this for a few minutes. (Pause for a few moments.)

"Now, close your eyes.

**"With your mind's eye, bring your awareness down into your feet. Inhale, and at the same time, tense your feet, curling your toes up. Hold the position while you silently count to six. (Pause for 6 seconds.)

"Now exhale and relax your feet. Feel the exhalation leaving your feet. See how good it feels to let go. Inhale again and then exhale slowly, while you say to yourself gently, 'Relax, feet, relax.'

"Now inhale and contract your calves. Make them as tight as you can. Good. Hold for a count of six. (Pause for 6 seconds.) Exhale slowly and relax the muscles. Experience how good that relaxation feels. Inhale and exhale slowly again. Say, 'Relax, calves, relax.'

"Now inhale and contract the muscles in your thighs. Hold for a count of six. (Pause for 6 seconds.) Excellent. Now exhale slowly. Focus on how wonderful that feels. Inhale again and exhale slowly. Say, 'Relax, thighs, relax.'

"Now inhale and contract the muscles in your buttocks and your stomach. Hold for a count of six. (Pause for 6 seconds.) Very good. Now exhale slowly. Enjoy the sensation. Feel the exhalation leave your buttocks and stomach. Take another breath and release it slowly. Say, 'Relax, stomach; relax, backside.'

"Now do the same with your chest and breathing muscles. Contract your muscles and hold. Count to six. (Pause for 6 seconds.) Now exhale slowly. See how pleasurable this is. Feel the exhalation bathe your chest. Take another breath, and gently release it. Say, 'Relax, chest, relax.'

"Now focus on your shoulders and chest muscles. Tighten your shoulders by pulling them up and back. Contract the muscles and hold. Count silently to six. (Pause for 6 seconds.) Good. Now exhale slowly, let all the tension drain away. Yes, this is wonderful. Take another slow breath and then release it. Say, 'Relax, shoulders, relax.'

"Now inhale and tighten your neck and neck muscles. Hold, while you silently count to six. (Pause for 6 seconds.) Exhale and release. Focus on the sensation. Inhale again and then exhale slowly. Say, 'Relax, neck, relax.'

"Now do the same thing with the muscles in your arms, from your shoulders to fingertips. Inhale and contract your muscles. Tight. Tighter. Hold for six. (Pause for 6 seconds.) Great. Exhale and relax your arms from the shoulders right down to the fingertips. Tune in to how that feels. Take another slow breath. Exhale. Say, 'Relax arms; relax hands.'

"Now inhale and tighten up your whole face. Tighter. Tighter yet. Hold it for a count of six. (Pause for 6 seconds.) That's good. Now exhale slowly and relax your face. Good. You feel great. Inhale again and then exhale. Say, 'Relax, face, relax.'

"Now focus on your breath down in your belly. Feel your belly rise and fall with your breath. Stay with this until you feel even more deeply relaxed. (Pause for 3 minutes.)

"Now count backward from ten. When you reach one, you will feel deeply relaxed and invigorated. 10 . . . 9 . . . 8 . . . 7 . . .

6 . . . 5 . . . 4 . . . 3 . . . 2 . . . 1. Open your eyes. Thank yourself for taking the time to relax."

Note: If you feel you need to do the relaxation exercise a second time, substitute the following paragraph for the last paragraph.

"Now you will sink even deeper into relaxation. Begin with your feet." (At this point, return to ** and read the script all the way through a second time.)

Basic Script II

"(Insert name), this is your time to relax. Whatever you've been thinking about, whatever worries you've had, let go of them now. Deposit them in an imaginary lockbox across the room from you. They'll be there when you return, if you want them. This time belongs to your body. Let your mind be at peace.

"Take a moment now to settle yourself comfortably in a straight-backed chair. Kick off your shoes if you haven't already done so. Loosen anything that is tight. Get comfortable. (Pause for 30 seconds.)

"Close your eyes now. Just breathe slowly. Concentrate on inhaling deeply. (Pause.) Then concentrate on exhaling. Do this for a few minutes. Feel your mind clear. (Pause for 2 minutes.)

Now let's work with the right hand and arm. Bring your attention to the right hand. Make a mental note of how much tension you find there. (Pause for 10 seconds.) Will it to leave. Push it out through the fingertips, out through the pores of the skin. (Pause for 15 seconds.) Keep going until your right hand and wrist feel loose and limp and floppy. (Pause for 15 seconds.)

204

"Now concentrate on your right forearm and elbow. Make a mental note of how much tension you find there. (Pause for 10 seconds.) Let your forearm feel heavy and your elbow feel loose. Your arm is like a rag doll's arm. Loose and limp and floppy.

"Now let's focus on the upper arm and shoulder. Search your shoulder and upper arm for tension. (Pause for 10 seconds.) Will it to leave. Let it run right down your arm and out your fingertips. Your whole arm feels very loose and very light. (Pause for 15 seconds.)

"Let's work now with your left hand and arm. Make a mental note of how much tension you find there. (Pause for 10 seconds.) Now, will it to leave. Push it out through the fingertips, out through the pores of the skin. (Pause for 15 seconds.) Keep going until your left hand and wrist feel loose and limp and floppy. (Pause for 15 seconds.)

"Now concentrate on your left forearm and elbow. Make a mental note of how much tension you find there. (Pause for 10 seconds.) Let your forearm feel heavy and your elbow feel loose. Your left arm is like a rag doll's arm. Loose and limp and floppy.

"Now let's focus on your left shoulder and upper arm. Search the shoulder and upper arm for tension. (Pause for 10 seconds.) Will it to leave. Let any remaining tension flow right down your arm and out your fingertips. Your whole arm feels very loose and light. (Pause for 15 seconds.)

"Let's move down from the shoulders to the back. Let that wonderful relaxed feeling in your loose, limp arms flow into your back. If there is any tension to be found in your back, let it flow out through your waist. Let the tension bubble out from your pores. Keep feeling those bubbles moving out until your back sinks into relaxation. (Pause for 25 to 60 seconds.) Your back is the back of a rag doll. Soft and comfortable. See how good that feels.

"Let's move all the way down to the feet and ankles. Can you feel the tension in your feet and ankles? Make a mental note of it. (Pause for 10 seconds.) Now, will it to leave. Push it out through your toes, the pores of your skin. Let your ankles be soft and limp. (Pause for 15 seconds.) See how good that feels.

"Let's try to move that feeling up into your calves and knees. Let your calves become really heavy and your knees loose and limp. (Pause for 15 seconds.) Your calves are like a rag doll's leg. Loose and limp. See how that feels.

"Now, we move up into the thighs and pelvis. Search the area for any tension. Make a mental note of it. (Pause for 10 seconds.) Now, will the tension to leave. Push it out through your knees, the pores of your skin. Let your thighs become really heavy and sink into the chair. Your legs are like a rag doll's legs. Soft and limp.

"Let that loose, relaxed feeling move from your pelvis into your hips. Let your hips become heavy and sink down into the chair. Really, really heavy. (Pause for 5 seconds.) Be aware of any tension in your hips. (Pause for 10 seconds.) Will it to leave. Push it out through the pores of your skin. (Pause for 20 seconds.)

"Let the relaxed feeling move up from your hips into your back. (Pause). Up through your shoulders. (Pause) Into your neck. Make a mental note of any tension in your neck. (Pause for 10 seconds.) Let your neck become very heavy, very limp.

Will the tension to drain out of it. (Pause for 15 seconds.) Your neck feels loose and floppy.

"Now focus on your jaw and cheeks. Make a mental note of any tension. (Pause for 10 seconds.) Will that tension to leave. Send it out through your breath. (Pause for 15 seconds.) Let your breath draw out any remaining tension in your nose area, your eyes, your forehead. (Pause for 25 seconds.)

"Now concentrate on your skull. Make a note of any tension. (Pause for 10 seconds.) Will that tension to leave. Push it out through your scalp. When you get one layer of tension out, inhale (pause), exhale (pause), and start pushing out the new top layer. (Pause for 25 to 60 seconds.) Now let your head sink easily down into your neck.

"Now let your awareness slowly travel through your body, searching for any places that are still tight. (Pause for 10 seconds.) One by one, will the tension to leave each area. (Pause for 25 seconds to 2 minutes.) Your body feels heavy, heavy, heavier and soft like a rag doll. Feel yourself sink even more deeply into the chair.

"Take a few minutes now to experience the deep sense of relaxation. Make a mental note of this feeling so you can return to it whenever you need it."

The Special Challenge Variation

"Now that you feel totally relaxed, let's go on a little journey together to a place inside where you are all-knowing, confident, and capable. This journey will energize you and increase your sense of well-being.

"You see before you a beautiful glass staircase. This staircase leads to the higher reaches of your mind, that place inside of you where all your potential is stored.

"Ascend to the first step. It's clear red, and you can see through it, as if it's a piece of hard candy. If you find anything on the step that doesn't belong, clear it off before you move on.

"Climb higher. This step is orange, a beautiful, stained-glass orange. Pause on this step. If you find anything here that doesn't belong, clear it off.

"Climb up again. You find yourself on a yellow step. Make sure the step is clean. When it is, let the clear yellow light from the step flow up through your feet into your spine and out through your head. See the yellow energize your brain.

"Climb up again onto a sparkling clear step of green. Pause here and clear off anything that doesn't belong. Feel the green under your feet and around you and see how good you feel about yourself.

"Climb higher, onto a step of blue, the radiant blue of a pure, clear lake. Remove anything from the stair that doesn't belong there. Pause here for a moment.

"Next, step onto a step made of shining violet. Clear off anything that doesn't belong. Pause here and see how open and expanded you feel standing on this step.

"The top step is made of indigo. It's a dark indigo, but you can still see through the glass. Clear off anything that doesn't belong. Then pause here. See how powerful you feel on this step.

"Before you now is a white corridor. This corridor connects you to the executive suite in your mind, the place where you are powerful, confident, and capable, where all of your potential is stored. Step inside this room. What does it feel like to be here? (Pause for 15 seconds.) Can you see anything? (Pause for 15 seconds.) Spend a minute or two in your command center, really getting to know it. Get a good feel for the room. (Pause for 2 minutes.)

"Now that you have a good feel for the room, be confident in your ability to carry this feeling with you. It's there inside you, and it never leaves you. All you need to do is remember it.

"Now, in your mind's eye, replace the furnishings of the executive suite with an image of where your special challenge will occur. The final job interview, for instance. See yourself sitting in a chair, answering questions. Feel how easily you do this, how relaxed and at ease you are. From this place in you where your brightest potential is, where you are confident and capable, you easily retrieve the information you need.

"Spend a few minutes here, seeing yourself answering questions with confidence and assurance in your abilities. Your body is relaxed, your breathing is slow and natural and you feel good about your performance. (Pause for a few minutes.)

"Now the interview is over. See yourself rising out of the chair, smiling, pleased with your performance. The office door leads to a white corridor. Take this white corridor to the glass staircase.

"See yourself on the indigo step at the top. Inhale and exhale slowly, then step down. Know that when you reach the red step, you will feel revitalized and calm.

"See yourself now on the violet step. Pause here. Now step down to the blue step. . . . the green step. . . . the yellow step . . . the orange step . . . the red step. Inhale and exhale slowly. Now leave the glass staircase behind you and find yourself back where you started. You can return to the staircase any time you want to."

SWING INTO EUPHORIA

Got a headache? Try some Li Shou. No, it is not Chinese aspirin. It's an ancient oriental exercise with some remarkable therapeutic benefits for our time.

Li Shou means "hand swinging" in Chinese, and that's exactly what it is.

Sounds farfetched, doesn't it? How can the simple act of swinging your hands relieve a headache? Consider: Your head throbs and aches when the cranial blood vessels are swollen. "When you swing your arms," says Dr. Edward C. Chang of Albany State College in Georgia, "you shunt the flow of blood to your limbs, thus reducing the flow of blood to your head. Result? No more headache!

"Many systems of exercise designed to prevent or treat diseases have been developed in China, but few have generated so much interest and gained so much popularity as Li Shou," says Dr. Chang, who is in the process of translating into English an ancient Chinese text describing the use of exercise as a therapeutic technique.

But you don't have to have a headache to experience a bonanza of benefits from the regular practice of Li Shou.

Done properly you can achieve a meditative state, acquire biofeedback skills, and experience the stimulation and euphoria usually associated with vigorous forms of exercise, says Dr. Chang. You also provide your heart and lungs with a freshly oxygenated supply of blood and no doubt you improve the contours of your upper arms, the area that betrays your age quicker than wrinkles.

Li Shou has the added advantage of being easy to learn and can be done by children and octogenarians alike. And, according to Dr. Chang, once you have mastered the technique you can, just by visualizing the procedure, bring warmth to your extremities without fur-lined gloves and woolen socks.

Are you ready?

1. First, the warm-up. Rub the palms of your hands against each other for a few seconds, creating a pleasant warmth. Now using both palms, massage your face from forehead to chin as if you were washing your face with dry hands.

Repeat 30 times, always massaging in the same direction.

2. Consciously relax your entire body and put on a happy face.

3. Now stand up, your feet shoulder-width apart, toes pointing forward.

4. Keeping the upper part of your body upright, let your arms and elbows sink naturally downward, spreading your fingers slightly.

5. Close your eyes partially, your lids not quite meeting, and without bending your head, mentally focus downward to your toes.

6. Now raise both hands, extending them frontward only to navel level, and swing to the back no higher than the buttocks with sufficient force so your arms bounce back and forth rhythmically, like a pendulum, 100 times. (Count on the backward swing.) Be aware of your hand movement while focusing attention passively on your toes. If your mind should wander into other pathways, like what you should have for dinner tonight, get it back on track by paying attention to your toes and fingers.

7. When you swing to the back, feel a tenseness in the muscles of both hands and feet; when you swing frontward, experience a lovely relaxation in your whole body. Gradually increase your swings to about 1,000.

After a few weeks of practicing Li Shou, you will discover a sensation like a mild but pleasant electric current drizzling downward to your fingers and toes even though your hands are not in motion. From this point on, you have the "in control" feeling you get from biofeedback.

Warning: Once you have experienced the mellow relaxation and the improved sense of well-being, Li Shou may become addictive. But, then, you don't have to brave the elements or pound the pavement to achieve its euphoric effects. You can practice it at sunrise by the side of a babbling brook or, better yet, by the light of the moon or some time during the evening hours. Because, according to Dr. Chang, it helps to neutralize the stress you have encountered during the day and induces relaxation, calming your taut nerves and, like a warm comforter, encouraging restful slumber.

ONE-DAY STRESS MAKE-OVER MADE EASY

What's a stress make-over? It's taking a long, hard look at your life and making changes. It's saying so long to merely dealing with unnecessary stress, and getting rid of the sources of stress instead. It's learning to cut corners where you can, and place priorities where you really have to. A stress make-over is getting your life in gear.

Maybelle Blum is giving herself a stress make-over. She finally realized why she has a headache by the time she gets to work each day; she doesn't leave herself enough time to feed the kids, make her lunch, get dressed, and eat breakfast. Now she sets her clock 15 minutes earlier, starts a 5-minute morning yoga routine *before* she leaves her bedroom, and revels in her new, fast-paced but doable morning routine.

Parker Fieldcraft is giving himself a stress make-over, too. He'd been listening to a relaxation tape in his car on the way to work each day. But work is less than a mile away. Now he leaves earlier, walks to work, and gets to listen to the birds singing instead.

One more. Lee Phillips used to get stomachaches whenever the mail came.

The cause: worry about bouncing checks and unfavorable bank statements. Now, with help from a financial planner and a workable budget, that cause of stress is a thing of the past.

What do Lee, Parker, and Maybelle have in common? They all said, "Why learn to deal with stress when I can get rid of it instead?"

This seems so simple, you might wonder why more people don't do it. The fact is, some people actually thrive on stressful chaos. It's stimulating, and the thrill of it can actually be addictive in some ways. But stress is destructive, too. Many doctors believe it can raise your blood pressure, increase your risk of heart disease, cause digestive distress, and possibly even help cause cancer.

This doesn't mean that all stressful situations are bad, however. Stress can have lots of good effects, too. It can invigorate you, push you on to higher levels of achievement, give you the thrills that make life exciting.

"Stress can be very useful. After all, any time you try to accomplish something, you are under stress," says Dr. Jeffrey G.

Rate Your Stress Quotient

Stress-management experts have found that some happy events, like getting married, can put more stress on your system than some unhappy ones, like losing your job. Through their research, two doctors at the University of Washington, Thomas Holmes and Richard Rahe, produced what they call a Life Change Index. It's a rating system that scores life events known to produce stress. They found that the more points accumulated, the more likely a person is to become ill due to stress.

Life changes, of course, aren't something we should avoid. They help make our lives interesting and enjoyable. But it may be useful to realize that too many at once can take their toll.

Below is the index. Mark each of the events in the list below that you've gone through in the past year, or which are about to happen. Then add up the scores for the events you marked. That's your stress quotient. According to Dr. Holmes and Dr. Rahe, those with over 300 points for the past year are at greatest risk for illness. Those with 150 to 299 are in between, and those with under 150 have the least risk. But remember, stress is only as harmful as the way you react to it. So a rating of 50 might be high for one person, while a rating of 300 is low for another.

- Death of spouse: 100
- Divorce: 73
- Marital separation: 65
- Jail term: 63
- Death of a close family member: 63
- Personal injury or illness: 53
- Marriage: 50
- Loss of job (fired): 47
- Marital reconciliation: 45
- Retirement: 45
- Change in health of family member: 44
- Pregnancy: 40
- Sexual difficulties: 39
- Gain of new family member: 39
- Business readjustment: 39
- Change in financial state: 38
- Death of a close friend: 37
- Change to different line of work: 36
- Change in number of arguments with spouse: 35
- Mortgage over $10,000: 31
- Foreclosure of mortgage or loan: 30
- Change in responsibilites at work: 29

- Son or daughter leaving home: 29
- Trouble with in-laws: 29
- Outstanding personal achievment: 28
- Spouse begins or stops work: 26
- Beginning or ending school: 26
- Change in living conditions: 25
- Revision of personal habits: 24
- Trouble with boss: 23
- Change in work hours or conditions: 20
- Change in residence: 20
- Change in schools: 20
- Change in recreation: 19
- Change in worship (church, temple) activites: 19
- Change in social activities: 18
- Mortgage or loan of less than $10,000: 17
- Change in sleeping habits: 16
- Change in number of family get-togethers: 15
- Change in eating habits: 15
- Vacation: 13
- Christmas (if approaching): 12
- Minor violations of the law: 11

Jones, medical director of the St. Francis Occupational Health Center in Indiana. "Any time you study for a test or prepare for a challenge, you use a positive aspect of stress. Stress helps us survive and motivates us. Without stress, we would be boring. We would stop growing and changing."

Good Stress and Bad Stress

So how do we know which stress to get rid of and which to keep? That's an easy one: Keep the good stress and banish the bad. They are easily distinguished.

Good Stress. It's exhilarating. It feels like riding a canoe in a swiftly flowing stream. You're under control. When it's over, you look back on the situation and you feel proud. You brought out the best in yourself. You rose to the challenge.

Bad Stress. You feel like a runaway train. You're out of control. You feel like a victim. Afterward, you are exhausted. The next day, you look back on the situation and feel you could have accomplished more had you not been under such stress. Nothing good came of it.

How Stressed Are You?

Are you under too much bad stress? Sometimes it's hard to tell. You're so used to tight muscles and that nagging worry in the back of your mind that they seem natural. But they're not. And your body knows it. If you listen to your body, it'll tell you so. "Our bodies are our best biofeedback mechanism," says Dr. Donald A.

211

212

Tubesing, psychologist and president of Whole Person Associates in Duluth, Minnesota, and author of *Kicking Your Stress Habits.*

Often, when we are under too much stress, our bodies give us signals. Maybe your stomach gets upset. Or perhaps you get a twitch in your eyelid, or a rash on your back. Is your brow perpetually furrowed? Are you tired all the time? These signs all point to excess stress.

"We as individuals have our own unique signals from our bodies," says Dr. Tubesing. "For me, it's my back. When it gets tight, I know I've been overdoing it."

Everybody has a personal list of recognizable signs that tell when the body is saying, "I don't want to go with you today," says Dr. Tubesing. He suggests you become more aware of such signals by drawing a picture of your body, and circling the areas that react to tension. If your stomach gets upset when you are tense, circle the stomach area of your drawing. If you get a headache, circle the head. You may be surprised how easy this is. According to Dr. Tubesing, he has never yet had a client who, after thinking for a moment, wasn't aware of his or her personal reactions to stress.

After you finish your picture, Dr. Tubesing suggests you make it more complete by writing, on the same paper, your personal mental and emotional stress signals. Do you have memory lapses (Ever mentally greet dinner guests with, "Are you sure I invited you?"), a dulled sense of humor, or low spirits? Does relating to friends sometimes seem more trouble than it's worth? These are typical mental signals of excess, or bad, stress.

As you become more aware of your body's stress signals, you'll be in a better position to pinpoint the causes of bad stress and get them out of your life.

Set Your Priorities

One of the main causes of bad stress is too much good stress. Odd as it sounds, that's the truth. Sure, some types of stress are good for us and other types are just plain bad. But beware: Good stress can become bad stress if it's overdone. Too much of anything is simply . . . too much. Too many tests, too many challenges, too many responsibilities will stop making you feel challenged and start making you feel burnt out.

Learn to manage your stress so you get the optimum amount, say psychologists —not too much, but not too little, either. "Managing stress is tuning it down where it's too much, and increasing it where it's too little," says Dr. Tubesing. "Nobody has enough energy and resources to do everything 100 percent. Even if you are spending all your time on things that *all* seem important to you, if your body says it's too much, you must make priorities."

And your first priority should be to simply remove as much bad stress as possible from your life. That's what a stress make-over is all about. It's not learning to relax; that would be dealing with stress once you already are suffering from it. Relaxation techniques are secondary stress management tools. What we're talking about are *first level* stress-management techniques. They must be done *before* learning to relax. Relaxation techniques are for dealing with what's left over after you've cleared away the big chunks of unnecessary stress in your life.

STRESS SIGNALS

Your body will usually tell you when it's experiencing stress—loud and clear. Here are a few of the most common signs, according to Dr. Donald A. Tubesing, author of *Kicking Your Stress Habits.*

- Headaches.
- Tightness in the neck.
- Loss of appetite.
- Excessive eating.
- Indigestion.
- Pounding heartbeat.
- Forgetfulness.
- Depression.
- Loss of interest in sex.
- Loss of self-confidence.
- Trouble sleeping.
- Feeling keyed up.
- Feeling preoccupied.
- Anger.
- Hostility.
- Quarreling.

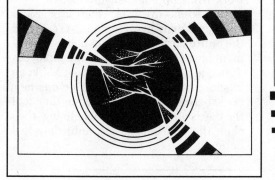

A Karate Chop to Stress

How are you going to handle those big chunks of stress, and the events and situations that cause them? The smart, quick way. Let's take a karate chop to stress, and disable it before it disables us.

How can we do that? Here are some simple suggestions you can accomplish right now, today.

1. Get a key rack and hang it near the door to your home. Make it an unbreakable rule to hang up your keys the second you come in. Then you won't have to go through the stress of frantically searching for them.

2. Get up 10 or 15 minutes earlier in the morning. Then, when things go wrong, you won't have to deal with being late on top of it.

3. Make lists. Include things you have to do, topics you want to discuss with friends, movies you heard are good, and so on. The less you have to rely on your memory, the more relaxed you'll be.

4. Don't skimp on sleep. If you're often tempted to stay up late, try setting the kitchen timer to remind you when to go to bed.

5. Leave early. If you plan to get to appointments 15 minutes early, you'll definitely be on time.

6. Make duplicates of all your keys. Keep an extra car key in the house, and an extra house key in your car, or hidden somewhere safe outside. But be sure not to hide the key with anything that could give away your address.

214

7. Be ready for an emergency. Keep a cupboard full of emergency staples, candles in case the electricity goes, and a flashlight that works.

8. Keep your gas tank at least one-quarter full. And keep your car in good repair with regular oil changes and checkups. There's nothing like getting stuck on a highway to rev up your stress levels.

9. Don't lie. And don't do things that, once they're done, will force you into telling a lie.

10. Buy an appointment book and use it. Then you won't have to worry about missing appointments or over-booking your days.

11. Learn to delegate responsibility. You don't have to be the one to do everything, whether it's at work or around the house.

12. Wear earplugs if you can't get quiet any other way.

13. Prepare for the morning the evening before. Make lunches, lay out your clothes, and make sure there's enough food for breakfast.

14. Unplug your phone when you want to take a long bath, nap, meditate, or even read without interruption. The chances of an emergency happening while you soak for an hour are almost nonexistent. But if you can't bring yourself to unplug, at least get a long extension cord and keep the phone near you, so you won't have to go running for it.

15. Organize with yourself in mind. Don't set up an elaborate filing system if you know you won't be able to maintain it. Instead, get yourself a cardboard box

JUGGLING PEACE INTO YOUR LIFE

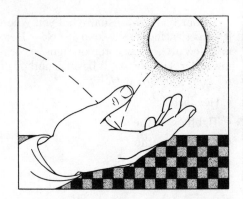

Here's the CEO's secret: When she closes her door after a harrying meeting, she's not pounding the walls or having an expensive masseuse sneak in the window. She's juggling her way back to serenity and top form.

Chances are good that Michael J. Gelb, founder and president of the High Performance Learning Center in Washington, D.C., and author of *Body Learning,* taught her how. He's pioneered this new focus-for-success technique, and his students, from top execs to salespeople to secretaries, are using it to give their minds a break from work while upping their productivity.

It's so effective, in fact, that major groups and companies like Du Pont, AT&T, and the entire northern Virginia police department have had Gelb teach their employees to juggle. "Top executives at AT&T keep juggling balls in their desks or on their bookshelves," says Gelb. "When they feel the day is about to get overwhelming, they close the door and juggle until they feel better."

Why does it work? "It teaches relaxed concentration," says Gelb. "When you juggle, you can't be trying to catch the balls. Your hand just has to interject their fall."

Juggling is so immediate, he adds, that it totally focuses even a worried mind. "It's a form of moving meditation," says Gelb, "that brings the two sides of the body into rhythmic balance. It's a moving art form."

Learn to Juggle

Follow these easy steps, remembering that attention must be freely given, not paid grudgingly, says Gelb, and you'll soon be juggling up a storm.

1. Start in a balanced, upright position, with your feet about shoulder width apart.

2. Let your arms bend so your hands rest level with your navel.

3. Begin with one ball. Throw it up so it follows an arc path, reaching a peak a few inches above your head and landing in your opposite hand. *Note:* Don't try to catch the ball. Instead, concentrate on throwing it so it lands where your hand already is. Don't reach for the ball. Remember to keep breathing.

4. After you feel comfortable with one ball (maybe a few days later), try two balls, one in each hand. Throw the first up as you did in step 3. Follow it with your eyes. When the first one reaches its high point, throw the other. Follow that one with your eyes. If you had a tracer on them, they should look like the McDon-ald's arches. *Note:* Again, don't try to catch the balls. If you don't feel like running for them, practice standing over a couch or bed. Spend your energy focusing on throwing the balls to the exact same place. If you can consistently get the balls to go to the same place, later, you can just arrange to have your hands already there when the balls fall. Don't get tense. Try to maintain a relaxed, almost casual manner.

5. Next, experiment with letting the first ball, but not the second, land in your hand.

6. Now try letting both balls land in your hands.

7. Finally, days or weeks later, move on to three balls. Hold two in one hand and one in the other.

The first ball in the hand that holds two balls is #1. The ball in the other hand (which has only one ball) is #2. And the second ball in the hand holding two balls is #3.

Throw the balls in that order, aiming for the point a few inches above your head and following them with your eyes. Let the balls drop; just focus on throwing them as smoothly as possible.

Throw each ball when the last one is at its highest point.

8. Next, experiment with letting one ball land in your hand. When that's easy and relaxed, try letting two fall in your hand. And, at last, let all three fall in your hands as they come down. Now you're juggling.

216

and put it where you can easily throw in everything important. When you need to find a paper, you'll know to look in the box, and that's a filing system that's easy to keep up.

16. Always make back-up plans, "just in case." (For example, "If we don't find each other after the concert, we'll meet at the car.")

17. Leave notes for yourself. If you have to take the car to the garage in the morning, for instance, put a reminder on the steering wheel the night before.

Use Your Head

You may have noticed that all these suggestions are things you can *do*, not new ways to think. That's because they're the absolute easiest ways to get yourself started on this new way of living. But once you get the hang of them, you may also want to try a few mental tricks that can instantly demolish a nascent stress situation.

These bits of mental magic are really no more than easy-to-accomplish attitude changes. When you're in a jam, a friend is late to meet you, or you've got a deadline breathing down your neck, talk to yourself. That's right, speak to yourself. What you say could change the outcome of the situation. That is, if you say the right things.

Learn to say, for instance, "This isn't so important," or "Maybe I'm not right after all," and you'll find yourself instantly calm and ready to deal competently with the situation at hand. If you say instead, "Darn it! This always happens to me," or "How could I be so stupid," you'll soon find yourself acting even more stupidly,

losing your head, and possibly missing a crucial opportunity.

Other good lines to feed yourself before stress gets you by the jugular are, "How important will this seem six months from now?," and "What would happen if I simply shrugged this off? Would it really make a difference?"

And here are ten more attitude changes that can help you sweep the stress right out of your life.

1. Never wait again. That is, don't get tense and irritable by focusing on when something will occur in the future. Change your attitude about waiting. Think of it as free time when you can read a paperback book or write letters. And enjoy it.

2. Take a break. Your desk at work isn't a prison and you aren't glued to your seat. So take a 2 to 10 minute stretch break every hour, especially if you sit for a long time in your job. This will boost your productivity and lower your stress levels. Also, take a lunch break—away from your desk.

3. Lower your standards. Why have a kitchen floor you could eat off of if everyone uses the table?

4. Keep a journal, or just write down your thoughts and feelings on scraps of paper. This is a great way to let out your feelings and maybe find a new perspective.

5. Value yourself. Make sure you get some time to yourself every day.

6. Mentally rehearse before stressful events. Before you ask for a raise, practice what you'll say in your mind.

Try to guess how your boss might respond, and what you could say next.

7. Value your activities. Really enjoy your meals, reading your mail, watching TV, or whatever else you do. That means doing just one thing at a time, and that's all. Don't try to eat, watch TV, and talk with your family all at once.

8. Talk out problems with a trusted friend or a counselor. You may not get the best advice from the friend, but you just might find yourself coming up with the answer during your conversation. Even if you don't, you'll feel better.

9. Rehearse with a friend before you do something difficult. Role-playing, with you acting as yourself and your friend acting like the loan officer at the bank, can make asking for a loan a lot easier.

10. Be an optimist. If you expect things to go well, they probably will.

If you believe that a stress make-over will help you make things go well in your life, it probably will.

STEP AWAY FROM STRESS

Have you ever gone for a walk when you were angry or upset? Then you know firsthand the soothing effect that walking can have on your emotions. Exercise is a great tension reducer, and walking has the added benefit of getting you out in the fresh air and distracting you with changing scenery. And *distraction* may be just what you need.

While many people report that walking provides an excellent opportunity to mull over problems, experts say you're better off leaving your concerns at home if you're trying to counteract stress. Instead, enjoy your walk and give your mind a rest.

How do you leave those problems behind when you step out the door? That's where meditation techniques come to the rescue. The beneficial effects of meditation as a stress reducer and immune-system booster have been well documented. Adding some meditation techniques to your walk may take you another step away from the negative effects of stress. While

there are no scientifically controlled studies examining the combined activity of meditation and walking, many stress-reduction specialists feel it's a winning combination.

David and Deena Balboa, New York City psychotherapists and directors of the Walking Center, suggest these simple steps for enhancing the stress-reducing value of walking.

● Release yourself from any goal or objective. This is not a fitness walk with a target heart rate goal. Walk somewhere where you can maintain a sustained rhythm without interruption — a track or long, peaceful pathway without breaks or crossways.

● Consciously relax your shoulders. Keep your head erect to avoid contracting the windpipe and shortening your breath.

● Lower your eyelids to decrease the amount of external visual stimuli.

● Allow your arms their full range of motion. You will naturally begin breathing more deeply, which automatically releases tension.

- Take a few really deep breaths. When exhaling, allow yourself to sigh gently but audibly to release tension and emotion.

- To clear your mind, focus on your breathing—not to control it, but simply to watch it. Become aware of the swing of your arms and how you move your feet.

- Periodically check your shoulders to make sure they're dropped and relaxed.

George Bowman, Zen teacher at the Cambridge Zen Center in Massachusetts, adds that focusing on your breathing and your body while you're walking brings you to a state of "mindfulness"—a mind that's open and aware in the moment, free from regrets of the past or anxieties about the future. "Pay attention to the rise and fall of the feet, of the breathing, until you reach a place where the mind quiets. Until, in the most fundamental sense, you're just walking."

MEDITATION:
THE HEALING SILENCE

Bill was the type of guy who let the morning traffic set the tone for the day. A few bonehead maneuvers, even if they didn't directly affect him and his Dodge, were enough to deepen the scowl lines on his face. These local drivers were so stupid, it depressed him. But what could he do?

That's why his co-worker was shocked the morning he took her to work, when a shrug and a bemused smile was his only response to a car that swerved suddenly into his lane.

"You're like a different person!" she said. The change was so gradual it seemed imperceptible to Bill, but she was right. A few months earlier, he had taught himself to meditate.

Six months after Anne joined a weekly meditation circle in a friend's home, a strange thing happened. The random imagery that surfaced when she focused inward began referring to a single incident: a rape seven years ago that was so traumatic she had virtually no memory of it.

One meditation produced subsequent images of a skeleton and then a small mirror in a dark frame, lying flat on its back, its glass fractured. Another image came up during several sittings—white lilies blooming from her breasts and genitals.

Meanwhile, several Pap smears confirmed the presence of a condition that precedes cervical cancer. Anne suspected this was her body's response to a trauma never allowed to heal. She underwent a procedure to remove the precancerous cells and began group counseling. Counseling showed her how the defenses she developed post-rape were getting in the way of what she wanted in her life now. Later Pap smears confirmed her cervix was back to normal.

That Christmas, a former colleague she met at a party had a compliment for her. "Wow. You've really blossomed."

His two years of Peace Corps duty behind him, Philip, the son of a career military man from the American Southwest, decided to try Vispassna (insight) meditation at a temple in Bombay.

He spent ten days in silence. First he learned to breathe in the Vispassna way and become acutely aware of his breath.

Then he learned to focus his concentration like a laser beam and explore his body —first the outer skin, then the internal organs and arteries, then the spaces in between. Then he learned to sense the energy in his body and to feel that energy extend beyond the body's physical boundaries.

When he returned to urban Bombay, with its incessant sun, its noise, its activity, he found even the dirt and the crowds touchingly beautiful. Nothing disturbed the peace he felt; all seemed perfect as it was.

Three ordinary people, three approaches to meditation, three different outcomes. Bill finds an inner calm, though his circumstances don't change. Anne finds that change is needed and arrests a potentially serious health problem. Philip has a spiritual awakening.

In each case, meditation was the tool. To see it as a tool is a good way to clear the hype that sometimes clouds it. Sure the word *sounds* exotic, but in terms of sheer utility, meditation isn't any more radica' than your common household wrench. It has lots of uses and multilevel applications. You can relearn the basic process easily.

Relearn?

Yes. Children do it naturally. Have you ever watched a toddler so absorbed in play he isn't aware of anything beyond his fascination with the toy? If you were to walk up behind him, you'd startle him. That absorption is what we're after. It refreshes and it heals.

A simple enough principle, but a powerful one. As our muscles relax, our minds quiet down and our sagging spirits revive. We find that we're once again in control of our lives.

Like Bill, we may learn that we don't need to be at the mercy of external irri-

TM PRACTICE: A FOUNTAIN OF YOUTH?

Want to shave seven to ten years off your biological age? Would you like to keep your vision and hearing intact and your systolic blood pressure down even as the years pass?

Transcendental meditation may have something to offer. Separate studies at Britian's Meru Research Institute suggest that this technique, handed down from the Indian Vedic tradition, can slow the aging process.

Michael Toomey and colleagues found that meditators scored an average seven years younger than their chronological ages, when they were tested for hearing, visual acuity, and systolic blood pressure. Researchers found that the longer a person has been meditating, the more age-resistant he is.

A later study by the same group found that the average biological age of meditators averaged ten years younger than their chronological ages.

Andrew Jedrczak, of that institute, scored 147 meditators on motor speed, reaction time, creativity, and visual memory — abilities that typically decline with age. When age, education, and sex were constant, the people who practiced meditation the longest showed the highest scores.

TM was introduced into this country in the 1960s by the Indian guru, Maharishi Mahesh Yogi. Students devote two 20-minute periods to practice each day. During this time they sit with their spines upright and their eyes closed, inwardly repeating a specific sound, which they focus on to the exclusion of all else.

222

tants (like inept fellow drivers). Like Anne, we may gain access to subconscious processes that impede us. Like Philip, we may learn to find richness and meaning wherever we are.

A Multilevel Enhancer

Meditation affects us on every level of our being. Positive physiological changes occur the very first session. Cognitive and behavioral changes often follow, if we actively use the insights meditation offers. Research suggests that benefits multiply with time, much as they do with an exercise regimen.

So, what exactly happens when we meditate?

First, we relax. Breathing slows down. We inhale and exhale about 11 times a minute, rather than the usual 16 or 20. We decrease our oxygen intake by about 5 percent. Gradually, our muscles relax. Anxiety fades, while our skin resistance rockets. If we were hooked up to an electroencephalograph, we'd see the electrical activity of the brain begin to change.

The rapid beta waves that mark our everyday waking consciousness—and which show up as a series of uneven, closely spaced peaks on the graph paper— slow down into the smoother hill-and-valley pattern of alpha waves. Communication between the right and left brain hemispheres becomes increasingly coherent.

If we repeat meditation regularly, we rack up more benefits. Studies suggest that it may slow down the aging process, lower our serum cholesterol level, alleviate pain, let us get by on less sleep, and even reduce bacteria levels in our saliva. Imagine—fewer cavities from meditating!

But that's not all. Some scientists think meditation can even make us smarter.

Among the studies pointing in this direction is one by researchers at the University of Washington, who found superior tone perception skills in people who practiced transcendental meditation twice daily for more than a year. (Transcendental meditation [TM] is an Indian Vedic-inspired practice in which you sit for 15 or 20 minutes with your eyes closed and discipline your mind by focusing on a specific sound or word, repeating it silently again and again in coordination with your breath.) Subjects new to meditation and those who don't meditate at all didn't fare as well. The results suggest that meditation gradually improves right-brain functioning, since the ability to differentiate tones is considered a province of that hemisphere.

A study done by the Iowa-based Maharishi International University, which looked for differences in brain activity during learning, also found advantages for meditators. The researchers compared TM practitioners with a group of non-meditators matched for age, sex, and entrance exam scores. As learning became evident, EEG measures showed that electrical communication between the cortical hemispheres was more coherent in the meditators than in the nonmeditators.

And a University of California at Irvine Medical Center study found that when people engaged in TM, they dramatically increased the blood flow to their brains, by an average of 65 percent. Could that account. at least in part, for the improved mental performance shown by other experiments? The researchers think so.

The effects of long-term meditation get even more subtle. Dozens of studies have found that meditation can speed psychotherapy along, lessen chemical addictions, and decrease mental anxiety. As was the case with Anne, meditation sometimes brings up the contents of the subconscious for review. Often there's gold in the seemingly random emptying of the mind.

By what power can meditation help us break bad habits? Scientists can only speculate. One view is that when our brain wave patterns shift from the rapid-fire beta rhythm to the slower alpha and theta rhythms, the waves also get larger—large enough to disturb set patterns of thinking. The disturbances may create an opening for a higher state of brain organization to occur.

Stop Your Heartbeat?

People who stick with the practice appear to develop extraordinary mind/body control. You've no doubt heard about those hard-core meditators who can perform amazing feats: The devotees who can temporarily stop their hearts from beating, or stop breathing, without any ill effects; the Tibetan monks who can raise their body temperatures so high—at will—that they can dry sheets soaked in ice water just by wrapping them around their bodies.

That is exquisite control.

Paradoxically, these hard-core meditators are just as skilled at letting go. That's what makes their reaction to stress so

DON'T MEDITATE IF ...

Let's face it. There are times when meditation isn't advisable. Just after eating is one of them. Wait at least 2 hours before you begin.

If you're being treated for high blood pressure, tell your doctor that you are considering meditation. It could change the way your body uses the medication. And if you're under the care of a psychologist or psychiatrist, consult them first.

Realize, too, that meditation is no substitute for counseling, especially when trauma or chronic difficulties are present. Meditation and psychotherapy work beautifully together, but they're not interchangeable. People inexperienced in the ways of the psyche can—innocently enough—abuse meditation by using it for escape.

If you want to transcend a problem, you've got to be willing to identify it as such and risk the personal changes the solution requires.

"Meditation, in and unto itself, isn't the instrument of change," cautions Deena Balboa, a New York psychotherapist. "It should be creative, dynamic, alive; a way to come face to face with ourselves. Sometimes that can be profoundly uncomfortable. But as we begin to feel and experience our discomfort, we can use that information again and again, take it out, question it, work with it."

Breath: The Peacemaker

Did you know that the way you breathe can directly influence your emotional state? Serenity may be just a breath or two away, but the key is *how* you do it.

Breathing from the chest is our natural response to emergencies. By moving the ribs up and out, we create the maximum amount of room in the chest for our lungs to expand. We need all that extra oxygen so we can properly defend ourselves or take flight.

But some of us breathe this way all the time. And since chest breathing is instinctively and physiologically tied to the body's emergency-response system, we can make ourselves nervous and edgy by breathing this way, even when there's nothing to panic about.

The solution is diaphragmatic breathing, says Dr. John Clark, chairman of the Himalayan Institute of Yoga in Honesdale, Pennsylvania.

"Breath is a very sensitive indicator of changes in cognitive patterns and feeling tones," says Dr. Clark. "Something as simple as having someone walk into the room can cause you to stop breathing. And disruptions in breathing can bring on a variety of physical and emotional problems. When you make someone aware of the disruptions and teach them to keep their breath even, a lot of the stress-related symptoms seem to abate."

Infants and small children naturally breathe from the diaphragm, that dome-shaped muscle that separates the chest cavity from the abdomen. Have you noticed how their bellies protrude when they breathe? That's the effect you're after. This is the most efficient way to breathe. This is also the correct way to breathe when you meditate.

To check yourself, Dr. Clark suggests you put one hand on your chest, the other on your upper abdomen. The hand on your abdomen should move, while the hand on your chest should remain stationary.

different from ours. You hook up a monk and a nonmeditator to monitors that measure blood pressure or muscle tension and then subject them to a series of short-term stressors. They perceive the potential threat and their body functions accelerate as if they were in danger.

Then something interesting happens. The monk soon realizes he's in no real danger. So he cools out. His brain, heart, and breathing rate return to baseline levels. The pattern is response/relax/normalize. Joe Average, meanwhile, remains physiologically stuck in panic city.

Fine-Tune the Immune System

For the experienced meditator, fine-tuning the immune system may even be within the realm of conscious control.

Researchers at the University of Arkansas College of Medicine found that a 39-year-old woman who's been meditating for nine years could depress her immune response at will.

Doctors injected the woman with a skin test of the viral antigen that causes chicken pox and shingles. They chose that antigen, *Varicella zoster,* because it gave them two ways to gauge her response: size of skin reaction and degree of lymphocyte stimulation. (Lymphocytes are a type of white blood cell.)

The study extended over nine weeks and was repeated nine months later, with similar results. When the woman allowed her body to react normally, her skin got red and hard at the injection site and her white blood cells marched to her defense. But when she attempted to inhibit her response, white blood cell activity was markedly reduced, as was the area of affected skin. When you think about it, that's a phenomenal ability.

Studies like these help scientists explore the mechanisms by which the mind influences immunity. Who knows? Perhaps someday, conscious control of the process—including the ability to *boost* immune defenses into overdrive—will be within everyone's grasp.

How to Begin Meditating

Learning to meditate can be fun and easy if you keep in mind three keys: posture, breath, and attitude. We've designed a starter meditation for you to try. (See the box "Ready, Set, Meditate" on page 226.)

Familiarize yourself with the three keys below before you do.

Posture. Don't worry. No one is going to close the gates of Heaven to you if you can't get your body into a full-lotus (cross-legged) position. The important thing for a beginner is to keep the spine straight. That positions your nerves just right and helps keep you alert.

Yogis and other adepts use the full lotus because they've found it to be the most stable. And that means they can sit as still as stones for hours. After a while, you'll find that even very subtle movements startle you out of the deep meditative state you were enjoying so much.

Over time, you may want to stretch your leg muscles so you can attempt a half or full lotus. Until then, you can sit up straight in a chair or use a bench or cushion to elevate your tush while your knees touch the floor. Again, be sure to keep your spine upright. Lying down is not a great idea, because you're liable to fall asleep.

Breathing. You want it to be slow, even, and diaphragmatic. Breathing is the one body function that is both voluntary and autonomic. By controlling the breath, you directly influence the autonomic processes in your body, like immunity, circulation, and digestion.

Attempt, if you can, to get an even flow between the nostrils. If you were to pay attention to your breath over the course of a day, you'd find yourself exhaling mostly through one nostril for about 2 hours. Then the breath equalizes for a few minutes, before switching sides. The period when it equalizes is when the deepest meditation is possible.

But you don't have to be a hostage to

READY, SET, MEDITATE

You say meditation intrigues you, but you don't know how to do it? Here's a basic exercise to get you started. This one is designed to help you gradually overcome the most common stumbling block—an inability to quiet your mind.

Start with a 10-minute session if you like and work your way up to 20 minutes.

Choose a comfortable chair that allows you to sit upright, or settle yourself into a cross-legged position on the floor. Loosen any tight clothing.

If you're extra tense, you can shrug your shoulders or roll your neck. Use any favorite relaxation stretches.

When you're ready, close your eyes. Let your hands rest easily in your lap, palms upturned in a gesture of receptivity. Make sure your spine is upright, and your chin is parallel to the floor.

Now take three slow deep breaths. (This is to help derail your thought train.)

Inwardly, firmly, state your intentions. ("I choose to refresh myself in the stillness," for instance.) Or insert a short prayer. Then tell yourself how long you plan to meditate.

You'll be surprised at how good you are at knowing just when to stop.

Take another deep breath. Exhale slowly. Allow this next inhalation to emerge naturally, automatically, from inside you. Focus your attention on this breath and ride it like a wave. Feel your breath flowing inside you, from deep in your abdomen to your nostrils, and back down.

Count "one" on the inhale, "two" on the exhale, "three" on the inhale and so on, up to ten. Then begin again at "one" when you inhale. Let each number completely fill your mind.

When your thoughts wander, return your attention to the count and begin again at one. Don't be angry at yourself. Simply start again.

Once you're comfortable with counting, you can simultaneously "open" yourself to a state of heightened awareness. Let your upraised palms set the tone. Imagine each cell expanding to take in the revitalizing breath you slowly and evenly draw into yourself.

the body's cycles. Teach yourself to equalize the breath by focusing on the flow of breath against the bridge of the nose. Then meditation becomes easy, rather than a continuing battle against distractions.

And if you begin feeling discomfort in an area while you're meditating, bring your attention to the area and imagine that you're sending your breath "through"

the trouble area. If you calmly keep at it a while, you may find that the discomfort goes away by itself. Or you may trigger an insight about yourself in the process. Either way, you'll probably feel even lighter after meditation as a result.

Attitude. This part can be tricky. Try to be content just to sit, without expecting much to happen. Before you start, think about something you do effortlessly well and try to bring that relaxed confident attitude to meditation. Above all, don't worry about "doing it right." There is no one right way to meditate. If you relax and keep at it, you'll discover the method that's perfect for you.

Realize, too, that it's normal for your thoughts to intrude and send your mind reeling in one direction, then another. As best you can, keep returning your attention to the object of your meditation, whether it's a movement sequence, your breath, or a pressing question. Gradually, you'll acquire mental discipline. Daydreaming, a pleasant enough diversion, won't produce the same results.

Little by little, your mind will look forward to experiencing the subtler, internal sensations of aliveness. Have you ever seen how grateful a young mother is for that first hour of quiet in the evening after the kids have gone to sleep? That's how your spirit feels about those few moments a day you succeed in putting your own restless thoughts to bed.

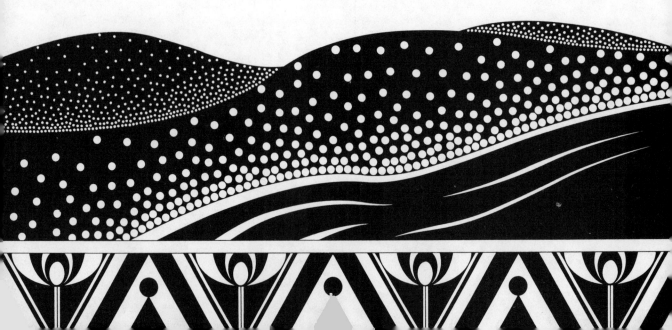

POSITIVE
HEALING THERAPY

SECTION

6

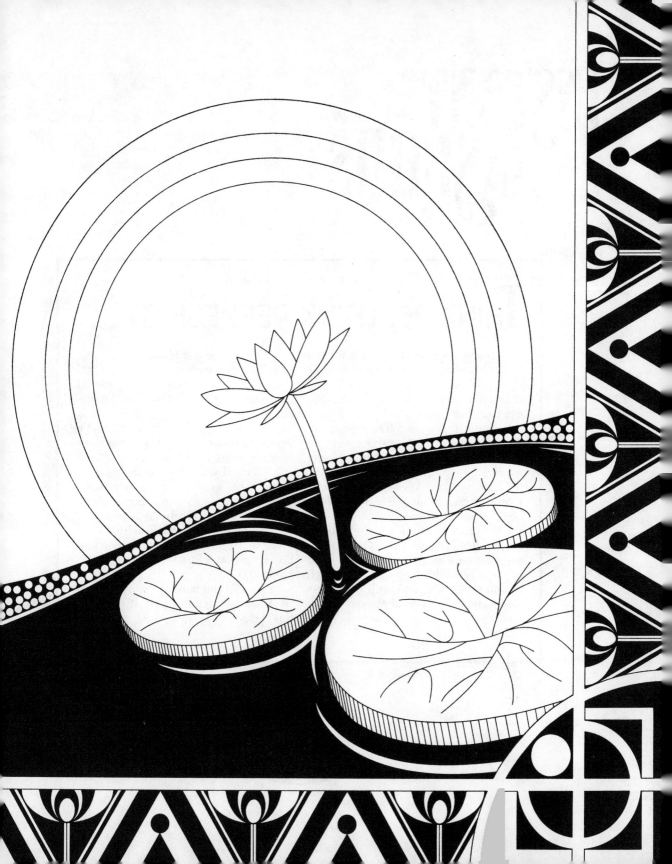

INSTANT INSIGHTS

THINK 90, THINK REFRESHED

You've been working hard for the last 90 minutes, but now your concentration is broken. A soft, sweet feeling floods your muscles, so you stretch. Your eyes get that faraway look.

It may *seem* like you're goofing off. But in actuality, your psyche may be hunkering down for some serious inner healing.

So says Los Angeles psychologist Ernest Rossi, author of *The Psychobiology of Mind-Body Healing*. He believes the body follows a basic rest and activity cycle (BRAC), which repeats itself about every 90 minutes. This rhythm is similar to the 90-minute sleep cycle, in which dream states alternate with dreamless sleep, and to the cyclical way our breath favors one nasal passage and then the other.

During the rest phase of this basic activity cycle, we slip easily into what Rossi calls the everyday trance, a special psychological state that enables the psyche to reorganize our impressions and experiences. This is when we may get a fleeting glimpse of the "big picture," or become aware of subtle discomfort.

"Basically, the body is saying 'take a rest now,' so it can do its own inner bookkeeping," says Rossi. Some of us, he adds, intuitively build a workday around this cycle: We begin at 9:00 A.M., break at 10:30, have lunch at noon and break again at 3:30 P.M., before heading home at 5:00.

Trouble can build, he warns, when we habitually ignore the rest phase of this cycle.

HELP THAT HEADACHE WITH HOPE

When it comes to headaches, more than pain is in your head. Your beliefs may be the best medication you need to chase away the throbbing, report researchers. In one study, 53 percent of the people who were told they were good at controlling their body's pain levels, even if they were not, achieved some relief from headaches. Only 26 percent of those not encouraged received relief.

STRETCH YOUR HEADACHES AWAY

Have you ever had one of those headaches that aspirin just can't seem to conquer? Try a drug-free approach to pain relief, suggests Dr. Donald Peterson, neurologist, of Loma Linda University in California.

"In my view, most headaches are due to a tightening of muscles and fibrous tissue in the back of the neck," Dr. Peterson says. "Stretching these muscles eases the tension, and helps to reduce the head pain."

Over 2,000 people have gotten results from Dr. Peter-son's neck-stretching method. And many of these people had previously not been able to find a pain-reducing drug that did the trick.

To try Dr. Peterson's exercise, "turn your head all the way to the right, place your right index finger on your left cheek and your right thumb under your chin, then gently push to the right. Simultaneously, reach over the top of your head with your left hand so that the middle finger touches the top of your right ear, then gently pull your head down toward your chest, with the head bent from the top of your neck. Hold this position for ten seconds, then reverse direction and repeat on the opposite side."

Dr. Peterson suggests repeating this exercise three times every 2 hours. When the headache pains are eliminated, do the exercise twice a day. However, if dizziness or abnormal pains occur, he advises seeing a physician.

THE HEALING POWER OF CONDITIONING: THREE GLIMPSES FROM THE FRONTIER

The unity of our thoughts and physical bodies is clearly revealed in new healing research using the power of conditioning.

What conditioning does is literally teach the body to heal itself. Used in conjunction with medical treatment, it *educates* our nervous system to mimic the effect of that medical treatment. The potential result is healing with less dependence on medical intervention—a result already being achieved in humans.

Tricked by Taste

Can your taste buds fool your immune system into delivering the response you want?

Possibly. Mice at the University of Rochester School of Medicine in New York fell for it in a big way.

These were mice with an autoimmune disease, a condition in which the immune system attacks parts of the body as if they were foriegn invaders. Dr. Robert Ader conducted the study to learn more about how placebos work.

He divided the sick mice into three groups. One group got injections of an immunosuppressive drug and were fed saccharin-flavored water at the same time. (The purpose of the drug was to lower immune response, which helps sufferers of autoimmune disease.)

Researchers conditioned the second group the same way. Except that half the time, the rats were given *only* the saccharin-flavored water. Over the duration of the experiment, the second group ultimately received only half as much of the drug. A third group also took half the dosage, but were fed the saccharin-flavored water at a different time.

The first group survived the longest, which was no surprise. What was surprising was that the second group survived significantly longer than the third group, even though they received the same drug dosage. Because they were fed the saccharin-flavored water at the same time they were given medication, their bodies were conditioned to make a connection between the taste and the effects of the drug. When the drug was withdrawn and only the taste was present, the rats' bodies automatically "assumed" they were receiving medication and made the physiological changes independently.

Can You Teach Your Body to Fight Cancer?

Imagine the fragrance of a bouquet of flowers or the melody of a favorite song signaling your immune system to fight off cancer. Far out? Researchers at the University of Alabama don't think so.

They found they could train the

immune systems of mice to rev up when the mice were exposed to an odor. They used a procedure known as classical, or Pavlovian, conditioning. Pavlov, you may recall, conditioned a dog to salivate whenever a bell rang, after learning to associate the sound with food.

The Alabama researchers exposed mice to the odor of camphor for 4 hours every 3 days for 27 days. Just before being exposed to the smell, the animals were injected with a chemical compound that stimulates interferon. This potent biochemical activates natural killer cells, our body's first line of defense against cancer.

After nine sessions, the rodents were given a three-day rest. On the fourth day, some were exposed to the camphor smell again, but without the injection.

These mice reacted with three times more interferon production and killer-cell activity than mice that were not exposed.

"We know from studies regarding stress, grief, and happiness, that the immune system is linked to the central nervous system," says the research team organizer. "Now we are beginning to see how we can influence that interaction."

"Our ultimate hope," they say, "is to be able to train the immune systems of people with cancer to mimic the effect of immune-stimulating drugs."

Migraine Sufferers, They're Playing Your Song

Beethoven may be the newest weapon in the arsenal against migraine headaches.

A recent study at California State University in Fresno found that listening to classical or "easy listening" music may do even better at keeping migraines at bay than biofeedback techniques.

Dr. Janet Lapp divided 30 chronic migraine sufferers into three treatment groups. The control group received no treatment. A second group learned progressive muscle relaxation and a visualization technique, in which they pictured the headache as something tangible they could destroy. They were also taught to intentionally raise their hand temperatures. (Hand warming helps divert blood flow from the head, which presumably helps lessen the likelihood of a migraine.) A third group also learned progressive relxation and visualization, but they listened to music instead of doing biofeedback.

After one year, the musically soothed migraine sufferers had one sixth the headaches they experienced before training, fewer than either the biofeedback or the control group. And the migraines they did have tended to be slightly shorter and less severe than those in the other two groups.

The effect may not have been related to the music itself, says Dr. Lapp. It turns out that the music group simply practiced more often. When they listened to albums at home or heard tunes throughout the day, the music reminded them to relax and practice their visualization. These constant refreshers helped them improve their skills over the course of the year.

234

THE SLEEP CURE

Feel like you're coming down with something? Are you fighting off the urge to sleep?

Don't. Sleep could be just what you need to defend yourself against the ailment.

Dr. James M. Krueger of the University of Tennessee and Dr. Charles A. Dinarello of Tufts University recently found that the same small protein that induces the most restful kind of sleep also triggers the production of interleukin-1, a key component in the body's defense system.

The proteins, called muramyl peptides, induce a deep, dream-free sleep. Dr. Krueger thinks the presence of muramyl peptides and interleukin-1 may account for the drowsiness that often accompanies disease. Whether that sleepy feeling is a sign of illness or recuperation is not yet clear.

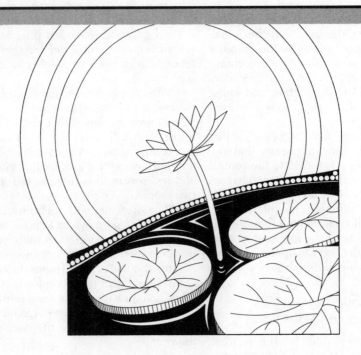

CALLING DR. LASSIE

Hospitals may soon change their two-visitors-per-bed rule to a two-visitors-*and-a-pet*-per-bed rule.

Pet visitors may speed up the recovery process for hospital patients, reports nurse Vickie Euhus. The Swedish-American Hospital in Rockford, Illinois, opened a pet visiting room at her suggestion. Euhus says if nothing else, the interaction between pet and owner/patient boosts the patient's morale. But she believes the benefits run deeper—even to the extent of improving the patient's physical recovery after surgery or illness.

For some patients, Euhus says, pets are the most important things in their lives. She believes a visit, showing that the animal is being taken care of, has a reassuring effect on the patients.

RECIPROCATE WITH NATURE

If you want to make your hospital stay as short and pleasant as possible, insist on a room with a view. And an aquarium.

Hospital patients who were able to see trees and bushes from their rooms recovered an average of 8 percent faster than those who looked out onto a brick wall, according to Roger Ulrich, author of a University of Delaware study. The nature watchers also needed fewer painkillers.

And a University of Pennsylvania study found that patients who could pass the time enjoying the antics of fish in an aquarium had lower blood pressure readings and felt less discomfort than those without fish tanks in their rooms.

How "Loud" is Your Pain?

For many people troubled by tinnitus, this affliction is more than just a simple case of ringing in the ears. "Tinnitus can be a roaring, whistling, hissing — any combination of sounds you can possibly imagine," says Dr. Laurence P. Ince of the department of rehabilitation medicine at Goldwater Memorial Hospital in New York City. "Thousands of people have these sounds," says Dr. Ince. "Imagine anywhere from 10 to 90 decibels [dB] inside your head at all times. No wonder some people get pretty desperate for relief."

Unfortunately, there has been no really successful treatment for tinnitus. Drugs, psychotherapy, and even surgery have all shown only limited value. But a new self-regulating approach developed by Dr. Ince and his colleagues shows great promise.

Patients with tinnitus were placed in a sound chamber and given headphones. They were asked to describe their tinnitus symptoms in terms of loudness, frequency, and type of sound. The sound was duplicated by an audiometer and played back to them. From then on, the matched sound was 5 dB softer than the patients' tinnitus.

"We match our sound to their tinnitus," says Dr. Ince. "Then we lowered our sound and asked patients to concentrate on lowering theirs. Each time they matched it, we lowered ours another 5 dB and just kept going. How did it work? It worked very well. Eventually we came down the scale until their tinnitus was near or below their hearing threshold."

A 36-year-old polio victim who had had tinnitus for 2½ years was able to reduce the noise 14 dB over 12 sessions. In her final session she achieved a 22 dB reduction. A 36-year-old man was able to eliminate his tinnitus completely during 6 treatment sessions, and went on to lead a normal life. A third patient, a 68-year-old woman, reduced her tinnitus from 36 dB to as low as 2 dB. Follow-up

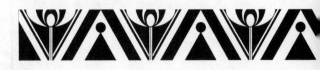

showed her tinnitus was no longer a problem.

Commenting on the self-control technique, Dr. Ince says, "I think we have a winner. Our method certainly stacks up against anything that's going."

Based on the success with tinnitus, the researchers tried a similar approach with patients suffering from chronic pain. "We decided to try 'matching' a patient's pain to a sound," Dr. Ince says. "In effect, we were saying 'You tell me how "loud" your pain is, and we'll match it in the headphones.' Then we lowered the sound gradually and asked them to bring their pain down to match the tone."

The results were encouraging. The first patient, a 70-year-old woman, had suffered with rheumatoid arthritis for many years. She had pain and deformation in both wrists as the result of a fall 11 years earlier. Gold treatments, medications, and psychotherapy had not helped. Using the self-control technique, she was relieved of pain and stopped taking all her pain medication. According to the researchers, "She was also able to wheel her wheelchair herself for the first time in years. This was accompanied by positive changes in mood, attitude, and social activity."

The second patient was a 58-year-old man crippled by multiple sclerosis. He had severe pain behind his knees that drugs had not been able to eliminate. The third patient was a 51-year-old man with multiple sclerosis and rheumatoid arthritis. Follow-up on all patients after the treatment was over indicated "no pain experiences in the areas treated in nearly all situations and during all waking hours."

Contrary to other mental techniques that ask the patient to focus attention away from the pain site, Dr. Ince and co-workers feel their method "demonstrated that, by focusing on the pain, patients can reduce or eliminate it."

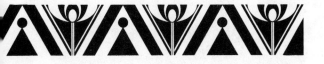

Wish Away Warts?

The patient, a disabled Boston policeman, suffered from painful, recurring common and plantar warts. Nothing seemed to help, until he entered an unusual treatment program in Massachusetts General Hospital's psychosomatic medicine unit. There he was placed under hypnosis and given suggestions that his warts would start disappearing. And sure enough, his problem was solved. When told that his health insurance would not cover this type of therapeutic intervention, the policeman requested a hearing and successfully challenged the ruling.

"Treatment of warts with hypnosis is a generally acknowledged if mystifying phenomenon," says Dr. Owen S. Surman. Although recent studies of the subject have been scarce, he points out that there is evidence the hypnotic suggestion must be "believed in" to be effective. The policeman's case, reported by Dr. Surman in *Advances,* is hardly unique.

An earlier study by Dr. Surman and several colleagues in Boston involved two groups of wart patients. Seventeen people were hypnotized weekly for five sessions and told their warts would disappear on one side only. Seven patients in a control group received no treatment. After three months, 53 percent of the hypnotized patients showed "significant improvement," in most cases on *both* sides of their bodies. Four people reported sudden and complete disappearance of their warts. None of the untreated patients showed any improvements.

According to the researchers, all the people who improved "were capable of imaging the sensation of tingling in their warts through hypnotic suggestion and three were able to experience vivid sensory imagery as well." After the initial trial ended, four of the control patients also received hypnotherapy and three showed significant improvement.

How does hypnotic suggestion accomplish such results? In the policeman's case, further studies revealed a greater activation of cerebral blood flow in the left frontal temporal areas of his brain when the wart-vanquishing suggestions were repeated. "There are great limitations in deriving meaning from a single case," says Dr. Surman, "but it is tempting to think of a cure for warts stored somewhere in the frontal lobes."

MEDITATION IMPROVES HEALTH

Transcendental meditation (TM) has been hailed as a simple means of mental refreshment, a way to regenerate your spirit after a stress-filled day at the office. Now, researchers claim, TM has shown positive long-term effects on physical health as well.

Meditators need only half the average amount of medical attention, claims Dr. David Orme-Johnson. In a study of 2,000 TM meditators, he found them to be healthier and more relaxed individuals when compared to nonmeditators. His study also showed an 87 percent reduction in heart disease and nervous system disorders, a 55 percent reduction in tumor occurrences, and a 30 percent reduction in infectious diseases in the meditators. He also found that the 2,000 visited their doctors 44 percent less often than average and were admitted to hospitals 53 percent less often.

Dr. Orme-Johnson attributes the healthful effects of TM to lower blood pressure, lower cholesterol levels, reduced stress, and reduced use of alcohol and cigarettes.

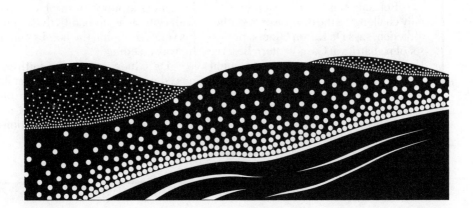

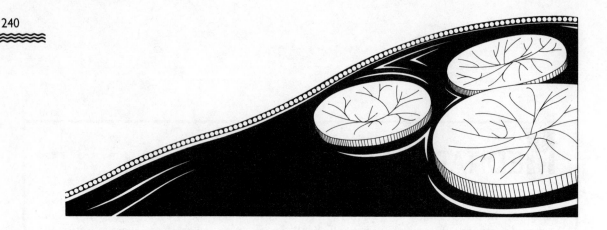

Harness the Power of Your Mental Air Force

Mind over matter works. Thirty hemophiliacs, taught to use their powers of concentration to stop their bleeding, are living proof.

Relaxation is the first step in mentally challenging the disease or any other affliction, says Dr. Karen Olness, professor of pediatrics at Case Western Reserve University. She claims to have taught the 30 hemophiliacs to relax every muscle, then imagine something pleasant. Their bleeding slows, probably due to decreased blood pressure, she says.

Migraine headaches can also be thought out, Dr. Olness says. She claims to have taught children to think away the pain of arthritis and cancer as well. And she cites an example of one 11 year old who neutralized his hemophilia by imagining a bunch of airplanes loaded with clotting-agent bombs flying through his veins, dropping the bombs wherever he was bleeding.

Dr. Olness has lots of faith in her procedures and practices mind-over-illness healing herself. She claims to have undergone a 50-minute operation on a torn hand ligament with only relaxation and positive thoughts for anesthesia.

REST BEFORE YOU ROCK AROUND THE CLOCK

When you pull an all-nighter, chances are you try to catch up on lost sleep by sleeping longer the next night. But that may not be the best solution, say researchers at the Institute of Pennsylvania Hospital in Philadelphia. A short nap *prior* to a night of lost sleep will do more to make you feel human when it's time to start your normal schedule again, they suggest.

The researchers had 40 young males stay up for a 56-hour period, only allowing one 2-hour nap. After the 56 hours, they tested subjects' alertness and feelings of sleepiness. Subjects taking a nap early on during the ordeal, they discovered, were more alert at the end of it all than subjects taking a later nap, or napping at the very end. The later the nap, researchers say, the worse the alertness scores.

Although the subjects were *less* sleepy before an early nap, they were *more* rested after. The team concluded that "preventive sleep"—timed napping prior to sleep loss—is a better alternative than napping after the loss.

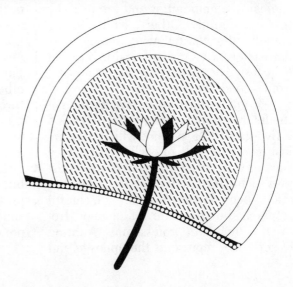

RATING SYSTEM
FOR THE POSITIVE
HEALING THERAPIES

The following therapies, while seemingly diverse, all approach the business of healing from a holistic viewpoint. In other words, what ails the body can be healed (or helped) via the mind, and vice versa. Many of these therapies have only come into existence within the last 20 years and as such, are considered newcomers to the field. Some are so powerful, their positive effects so easily documented in laboratory studies, that they have been welcomed with open arms by the medical and psychological communities and are used by them frequently. Others, while having gained a devoted following among seekers of alternative forms of health, have yet to be tested or proven effective under controlled conditions.

To guide you in your consideration of the following information, we've devised a five-star rating system, which appears just below the title of each therapy. Five stars represents a therapy of the greatest proven integrity. Not only have its healing effects been documented through careful research, but they are relied upon frequently by health professionals. A rating of zero stars represents the opposite end of the spectrum and signifies that while there are some users and practitioners of this therapy who would swear by it, its ultimate benefits have yet to be objectively proven.

The number of stars in between represent a descending scale of reliability in the eyes of the scientific community. A four-star therapy, for instance, seems to us to have a higher reliability factor than that of a two star. But again, you will find people who will swear by the superiority of the latter over the former.

The important thing to remember is that these therapies should never replace any treatment recommended by your physician. None of these therapies, on the other hand, presents an overt, physical threat to the state of your health. With proper medical approval, they can provide an interesting and helpful addition to your current treatment. As a matter of fact, the inherent self-improvement aspects built into most of these therapies may prove themselves useful to you even when you are not suffering from an illness. Why not explore and extend your horizons?

ACUPRESSURE

★ ★ ★

Think of acupressure as acupuncture without the needles. Instead, you massage specific pressure points with the tips of your fingers. The warmth you create at those points is said to convert to a minute electrical charge. By applying a charge to the right spots, you can restore the energy equilibrium in the body.

The beauty of acupressure is that once you learn the basics you can give yourself, a friend, or family member a treatment at any time. You can use acupressure to banish headaches or other minor pains, and even bring a healthy glow to your skin.

Both systems are based on the same ancient oriental concepts of health. Acupuncture, in fact, was regarded as the highest expression of Chinese medicine and was available daily to rulers. Acupuncturists were paid to keep their patients healthy; if a patient fell sick, he withheld payment.

Central to the oriental view of health is the idea that life energy flows through the body along a series of pathways known as meridians. (The Chinese call this energy *chi*; the Japanese word is "ki.") There are 14 major meridians in the body. Each one corresponds directly to certain vital organs. Energy circulating through the meridians is said to maintain harmony and balance among the organs, and energize the cells.

Cup-shaped points, just under the skin, connect to form the meridians. Chinese physicians found about 360 such points and theorized that they serve as energy conductors. You can find some of the points by just running your fingertip lightly over the skin until you feel a slight depression just below the surface. (The meridians themselves are not visible.)

The pressure points are supposed to help keep the chi circulating. But sometimes, energy stagnates at these points. The blockage could occur for any number of reasons: injury, emotional stress, poor diet, bad posture, illness. According to tradition, massaging the point helps to release trapped chi, restoring the internal energy balance needed to activate the body's own healing mechanisms.

Acupuncture gained popularity in the United States following President Nixon's visit to China. Western medicine acknowledges that it is effective in pain relief, but

243

it does not formally recognize the system because the meridians and pressure points don't correspond to any anatomical structure.

But an American osteopath was able to show that if you measure the electrical current along the skin, you can pinpoint the location of about half of the pressure points through changes in the current.

Robert Becker, author of *The Body Electric,* found the same points in every body he tested, and speculated that a more sophisticated measuring device might have enabled him to locate more of the points.

His readings indicated that the meridians were conducting current and "showed a flow into the central nervous system."

To learn more about acupressure, check with your community college or adult education program to see if they offer a seminar in basic techniques. You might also consider classes in shiatsu, a Japanese massage technique based on the pressure points.

See the entry on shiatsu, beginning on page 328.

ALEXANDER TECHNIQUE

★ ★ ★

Interested in gaining greater ease of movement, a quarter-inch to an inch plus in height, and better neuromuscular coordination? Then you might want to explore the Alexander Technique, an established approach to movement reeducation that's particularly popular with performing artists.

There's nothing fancy or mysterious about it. You learn the technique through a series of movement lessons that teach you how to make more intelligent use of your body. Over time, you replace bad movement habits with more desirable habits you've consciously chosen. Instructors say 90 percent of the correction process is mental.

As a student of the technique, you may begin by learning how to relax on a massage table, or how to sit in a chair. You'll also be taught how to adjust your walking posture and move with maximum balance. The emphasis throughout is on lengthening your body through proper positioning of your head and neck. Twenty to 30 lessons are considered optimal.

The technique was devised by F. M. Alexander, a nineteenth-century Australian actor who was seeking a way to end a series of mysterious episodes during which he lost his voice. After determining the source of his problem, he spent ten years reconditioning himself. Afterward, he came to be acclaimed for his extraordinary powers of projection.

Bernard Shaw, Aldous Huxley, and John Dewey spoke enthusiastically about the method, which was quite popular in turn-of-the-century London. Eventually, Alexander passed the technique on to several students.

Specific techniques vary among current teachers of the Alexander method. (There is now a movement underfoot by the North American Society of Teachers of the Alexander Technique—NASTAT—to standardize the training.) Currently, candidates complete about 1,600 hours of classroom instruction.

One basic characteristic of Alexander lessons, says Ron Dennis, executive director of the American Center for the

Alexander Technique, "is the gentle direction by the teacher's hand to bring about postural lengthening. In all cases the nature of the work is gentle. There is no forceful manipulation or intervention."

Instead, the lessons teach you to be self-reliant.

That's a key point, says Missy Vineyard, chairman of NASTAT. "You're given the tools and equipment by which you can fix something in yourself."

On the massage table, for example, you're likely to use guided imagery to help rid yourself of habitual tension while the instructor's hands gently coax the muscles to extend to their full resting length. As Dennis explains it, "the release of tension is done with the active participation of thought."

Alexander certainly was a believer in self-help. When his doctors couldn't do much for him, the actor decided to see if he could figure out what was happening with his larynx.

So he rigged up some mirrors in a way that would allow him to observe himself from many angles as he stood and spoke. He discovered he had a tendency to pull his head backward and down, affecting his whole body alignment in the process.

He also found he could regain his voice by letting his head move forward and up from the back, rather than by lifting his face, which compressed his neck, jamming the vocal cords.

As Alexander watched, he came to realize that what he felt he was doing was quite different from what he observed in the mirror.

Hence, teachers "try to de-emphasize this idea to feel differently or feel better," says Vineyard. "We teach people to move more intelligently by thinking differently. You grow in understanding in the use of your body."

Alexander lessons cost $24 to $45 each. Some teachers offer group instruction, but among members of NASTAT there is controversy about whether that offers enough individualized attention to make the lessons effective. Dennis says that group lessons are typically kept to six students.

He estimates that there are about 300 trained teachers of the method in the United States. They tend to be concentrated on the coasts and in the larger cities. To locate a teacher in your area, write to the North American Society of Teachers of the Alexander Technique, P.O. Box 148026, Chicago, IL 60614-8026, or call (312) 472-2404.

Dennis says the work is "helpful for the whole range of conditions you might call musculo-skeletal related tension or pain. That's not to say the condition will be helped, but the technique is definitely a resource." Beyond the absence of pain, many students report heightened body awareness, says Dennis.

Tufts University Professor Franklin Pierce Jones and his colleagues studied students of the Alexander Technique and found that the lessons expanded the skeletal frame, lengthened the neck muscles, and gave the body greater range of movement.

AROMATHERAPY

★★

The antidote to stress—or any number of ills—might be right under your nose.

Aromatherapy, an ancient art that was revived in Paris early in this century, relies on the healing properties contained in the aromatic oils of plants. Basil, for instance, is said to chase away the blues, while camomile calms. Lavender is said to heighten awareness.

The aromatic oil is the fragrant, volatile essence of the plant, extracted from either its flower, root, bark, or resin.

Usually, the oils are applied topically—through massage. But aromatherapy can also refer to the practice of inhaling certain scents. In Europe, some doctors prescribe aromatics for internal use. This is not something you experiment with at home, however; certain essences can be highly toxic in their concentrated forms.

Aromatherapy massage combines the rubbing and kneading techniques of Swedish massage with the pressure point stimulation of shiatsu and reflexology. (Shiatsu works the whole body, while reflexology zones in on the feet and hands.) The massage is said to relax the muscles, stimulate circulation of the blood and lymph, and reenergize the body.

How do aromatic oils aid the process? In several ways.

Judith Jackson, a Connecticut masseuse and author of *Scentual Touch,* an aromatherapy primer, claims that many of the aromatic oils contain antibacterial properties, which help detoxify the system. They are also capable of other effects, she says.

"The essential oils do penetrate into a few of the deeper layers of the skin. So they help do things to the tissue that are particular to that essence," says Jackson. "Juniper, for instance, is a diuretic. So if you use it where you have quite a bit of water in the tissue, it should help to flush that out. Geranium, on the other hand, is a natural astringent. It causes a certain amount of contraction."

The actual scent of the oil may also affect the body by altering brain activity. Olfactory nerves link the nose to the brain's limbic system, the seat of memory and emotion.

248

Clinical studies suggest that certain essences are valuable as antidepressants, others as natural relaxants. And recent studies at Yale University and Warwick University, London, have shown that just inhaling the aroma of spiced apple pie, or the seashore, can be as relaxing as some stress-reduction techniques.

Aromatherapy has been used to treat physical ailments, too—everything from acne to varicose veins.

The ancient Egyptians and Greeks used aromatic oils therapeutically, but the specialized knowledge of how various essences affect the body and psyche was lost over the years. Rene-Maurice Gattefosse, a French chemist who founded an essential oil house early in this century, revived the practice. He is credited with pioneering modern aromatherapy.

The practice is fairly widespread in Europe but has only recently gained much attention in the United States. Training and skill varies widely among practitioners. Your best bet, if you're interested in trying aromatherapy massage, is to find a licensed, certified massage therapist who has also undertaken study in the use of essential oils.

Most health food stores carry a line of essential oils and your library may have a guide book on aromatherapy that lists the properties of each botanical.

You'll find the aromatic oils are really closer to the consistency of water than oil. And they may be expensive. That's partly because the amount of essential oil a plant contains can range from as little as 0.01 percent to greater than 10 percent. An ounce of rose essence, for instance, can require up to a ton of rose petals.

AUTOGENIC TRAINING

★★★★★

Imagine being able to simply tell your body to relax—*really* relax—and have it respond! That's precisely what you may be able to do through autogenic training, a form of self-hypnosis you can master in minutes and use every day to help ease the symptoms of stress.

Autogenic (that is, self-regulating or self-generating) training was developed by Dr. Johannes Schultz and Dr. Wolfgang Luthe early in this century. The technique is based on their medical research (particularly in hypnosis and yoga) and has been used to try to treat a variety of maladies, including migraines. But it seems to work best as a stress tamer.

Basically it consists of getting into a passive, relaxed frame of mind while giving your body a series of self-instructions, such as, "My heartbeat is calm and regular." This hypnotic body-talking, say researchers, can somehow produce physiological changes, including deep, stress-releasing relaxation. And practicing, they say, makes it easier to get the body to "listen" and react.

Dr. Martin Shaffer, clinical psychologist, head of the Stress Management Institute in San Francisco and author of *Life after Stress,* explains the easy steps to autogenic relaxation:

As with other relaxation techniques, you need to get into a quiet room to begin. Turn the lights down low and wear loose clothing. Sit in a chair that comfortably supports your head, back, legs, and arms. Or lie down with a pillow under your head, feet slightly apart, and arms at your sides but not touching your body. Get as comfortable as you can.

Then close your eyes and slowly recite the following instructions, breathing deeply and evenly, saying the verbal cues to yourself as you exhale.

1. "My hands and arms are heavy and warm" (five times).

249

2. "My feet and legs are heavy and warm" (five times).

3. "My abdomen is warm and comfortable" (five times). (Omit this step if you have ulcers.)

4. "My breathing is deep and even" (ten times).

5. "My heartbeat is slightly calm and regular" (ten times).

6. "My forehead is cool" (five times).

7. "When I open my eyes, I will remain relaxed and refreshed" (three times).

Now perform the following sequence of body movements:

1. Move your hands and arms about.

2. Move your feet and legs about.

3. Rotate your head.

4. Open your eyes and sit up.

All this should be done with an attitude of passive concentration. Observe what's happening to your body, but don't consciously try to analyze it. By all means don't criticize yourself for having distracting thoughts. If your mind wanders, simply bring it back to your instructions as soon as possible.

Dr. Shaffer advises doing 2-minute autogenic training sessions ten times a day. "If you spend ten little times a day bringing your tension level down, it's unlikely to get up that high," he says.

And be patient: Experts say that in some cases, autogenic training can take weeks to achieve the desired physiological effect.

Unexpected Results

Be forewarned that autogenic relaxation is serious therapy and can have profound effects. There's a small chance that you may, for example, experience "autogenic discharges"—tingling or other body sensations, involuntary movements, pain, or even a desire to cry. "When that happens, simply do nothing," says Dr. Shaffer. "Tell yourself this is a normal discharge of tension in your body."

In rare cases, some people lie back, begin their autogenic rituals, but instead of feeling relaxed, lapse into a panic of anxiety. "That happens with people who need tension as a defense," says Dr. Shaffer. They're getting rid of their tension and up comes anxiety. Things they've not paid attention to are coming up to the surface." His advice is let it pass and continue the autogenic formula; if the agitation continues, stop the training and seek professional therapy to get to the root of your anxiety.

If you have high or low blood pressure, diabetes, hypoglycemic conditions, or heart conditions, consult your physician before you even start autogenics. Those with severe mental or emotional disorders are discouraged from trying the technique. And if you find yourself feeling continually restless during or after autogenic sessions—or if you suffer any disquieting aftereffects—practice only under the supervision of a professional autogenic training instructor.

BIOENERGETICS

★★★

Bioenergetics is a body-oriented form of psychotherapy. A direct descendent of Reichian therapy, it is sometimes grouped with radix and orgonomy under the heading of neo-Reichian therapies. It was founded by Alexander Lowen, a student of Reich's.

As it's practiced today, bioenergetics comes in two forms: private sessions, which combine bodywork with classical Freudian character analysis, and supplemental group sessions.

The group sessions are part of what makes bioenergetics different from Reichian therapy, which the late Dr. Wilhelm Reich developed in the 1930s. Reich, a one-time protégé of Freud's, came to discover that there was a relationship between tension and rigidity in the body, and rigidity—or psychological limitations—in the mind. In other words, when emotions are held in, rather than expressed, they begin to affect the musculature of the body. And when the body is tense, the mind itself is locked into the same set ways of perceiving things.

Emotions are a form of energy, Reich believed. If they overwhelm us, we may tense a muscle, or set of muscles, to stem the flow of feeling. The problem is that a one-time muscular defense can lead to chronic tension when we supress the emotion again and again.

Reich found that groups of muscles in the body tend to form protective "armor." Segments of the body prone to armoring are the oracular, or eye area, and the oral, cervical, thoraxic, diaphragmatic, abdominal, and pelvic areas. In therapy, he would gradually soften and remove armor, through physical manipulation and psychoanalysis. He preferred to work from the oracular segment on down.

Bioenergetics, conversely, works from the pelvis up. Ultimately, it seeks to help individuals learn how their emotions affect their bodies, and how their physical tension keeps them locked in the same self-defeating emotional responses to situations in their lives. Once rigidity is released from the mind and body, the individual is free to respond spontaneously and appropriately moment by moment.

Bioenergetic group sessions typically begin with strenuous yogalike poses and may end, sometime later, with the clients throwing temper tantrums on the floor. That's to bring about emotional release.

In private sessions, practitioners work to dissolve body armor through a combination of methods. In the more aggressive of these techniques, clients are encouraged to hit, cry, and scream. Other times, regulation of breath, pressure point massage, or stretching over a "breathing stool" are used. Clients roll backward over the 24-inch stool to help "open" the spine.

"When they stretch like that, it opens up breathing constrictions," says Dr. Robert Glazer, director of the Florida Society for Bioenergetic Analysis. "If someone is tight around the throat, the chest, or the diaphragm, this slowly but methodically stretches the body."

A typical session might begin with the client relating something of importance that's going on in his life—be it anxiety or depression, or happiness and well-being. If the feelings are negative, the therapist tries to discern how that emotion is being manifested in the body.

"You have to get to the fear or emotional pain that's keeping the body in its frozen pattern," says Dr. Glazer. "Then as you release the emotional energy, you can release the psychological component that put the body in that pattern to begin with."

Bioenergetics and Reichian therapy differ most in their end goals. Orthodox Reichians aim to help a client achieve "orgiastic potency," that state in which the individual is able to freely experience and express the full range of his sexuality and emotions. Reich saw sexual release as a key. Individuals who were capable of adequate sexual release, through orgasm, were not able to maintain neurosis, he believed.

Bioenergetics is more interested in helping clients attain a surer sense of self, an ease within which they can express their emotions honestly, and an awareness of an inner life. By integrating feelings with body awareness, it seeks to bring the body into a more vibrant state.

How well-trained are bioenergetic practitioners? Therapists undergo a four-year training course that consists of 160 hours of training therapy, a series of training workshops and another 12 hours of personal supervision under a qualified bioenergetic trainer. Would-be practioners need to possess or be working toward a graduate degree, preferably in the healing arts, in order to be accepted for training.

Prices for therapy vary according to your locale and the skill of the therapist. The price ranges from $70 to $100 an hour.

How much therapy you need to achieve results depends upon just what kind of results you're seeking. Dr. Glazer says that it "generally takes three to four months to deal with the 'presenting issue.' That's the depression, nightmares, or other problems that brought the person in. Once they get through that, I give my clients the option of going for broke—of going for character analysis." That can last two to three years.

To locate a practitioner in your area, contact the International Institute for Bioenergetic Analysis, 144 East 36th Street, New York, NY 10016, or call (212) 532-7742.

For further information on related therapies, see the entries on Radix, beginning on page 315, and Reichian Therapy, beginning on page 321.

BIOFEEDBACK

★★★★★

If you're like me, then you've probably flirted briefly with some sort of meditation or guided-imagery technique in an attempt to give stress the slip.

Unfortunately, I always ran into the same problem. After wrapping myself up into a reasonable facsimile of the lotus position, I'd close my eyes and set sail for inner peace. About 10 minutes into my journey, I'd start wondering if I was doing it right. "Am I relaxed now?" I'd ask myself. That little voice of doubt always managed to be just loud enough to disrupt any attempt at achieving relaxation.

The end result of all my endeavors was always the same: a sigh of defeat and a couple more instruction books relegated to the bottom of a closet.

But a couple of months ago, hope came to me through the mail in a package from a company called Thought Technology. Inside was a hand-size piece of machinery with the enigmatic label "GSR 2." It was a biofeedback unit. I vaguely recalled biofeedback as a sort of 1970s self-improvement fad that somewhere along the line was quietly forgotten. But since I

was about due for another adventure in stress control, it couldn't hurt to give biofeedback its turn.

Being inherently suspicious of anything I don't understand that promises to do me good, the first order of business was a call to Dr. John A. Corson, professor of psychiatry at Dartmouth Medical School and an expert in the field of biofeedback.

"Basically, what a biofeedback unit does is monitor a biological process that would be otherwise difficult or impossible for the subject to detect," Dr. Corson says. "Changes in body function are then transformed into an easily understood signal, such as a tone or meter reading, so that the subject can see exactly what a certain part of his body is doing from moment to moment."

"The Fire in the Boiler"

One reason for spying on your body's workings is that they oftentimes change as your emotional state changes. "The autonomic nervous system is a perfect exam-

253

ple of this," says Dr. Corson. "I call this system the emotional fire in the boiler because it initiates many physical and chemical changes as components of heightened emotional states, such as fear or excitement."

Perspiration is one of those functions controlled by the autonomic nervous system. You may have noticed yourself sweating a bit the last time you gave a recital at Carnegie Hall or were chased by a Siberian tiger. This is the autonomic system working at its best. On a subtler level, the size of your pores as well as the level of perspiration production are constantly changing in reaction to everyday stimuli and stress.

"These changes are very small and are measured in units called micro mhos," says Dr. Corson. "The GSR 2 biofeedback unit monitors the skin's micro-mho levels and emits a tone, which rises in pitch as more moisture is produced or drops as the skin becomes drier."

The end product is a direct line of communication with how you're really feeling. So it seemed as if biofeedback was the answer to my meditation struggles with the voice of doubt. Now I'd know for sure if I was relaxing correctly because the tone would tell me. It was time for some experimentation.

Mastering the Pitch

The actual unit fit easily in my hand and had a small elastic band that held my fingers snugly against two smooth metal plates. Upon contact, a small earphone began humming softly in my ear. I closed my eyes and started purposefully thinking about a stressful situation: my next

article deadline. Sure enough, within 3 seconds, the tone started climbing the scale until it resembled the high-pitched whine of a mosquito. No doubt about it, I was definitely worked up.

Bringing the tone back down took a little more work. Over the next two weeks, I practiced regularly with the unit while listening to a tape of relaxation exercises that came with the package. Soon I had the unit humming a low complacent tone that was a virtual one-note hymn to relaxation. If I heard the tone rise, I stopped and examined my thoughts to see what was bothering me. In this way, I not only learned correct relaxation techniques, I also dicovered hidden stressors that I never realized were upsetting me.

As I was lying on my living room floor totally calm after ½ hour of feedback, I wondered why such a great technique had been a mere fad 15 years ago. "The instrumentation and training techniques for clients were less sophisticated back then," says Dr. Corson. "People bought biofeedback units with the idea that they could just plug themselves in and rewire their emotions for relaxation."

That's not the case at all. If you're thinking of giving biofeedback a try, be prepared for some serious work. To start, you've got to find a good relaxation technique and really concentrate on making it work. "The unit itself only tells you how you're doing, not what to do," cautions Dr. Corson. A good analogy is that of a maze. At one end is you, at the other is relaxation. Biofeedback can tell you when you're on the right path and can also let you know when you're taking false turns.

I put in a good ½ hour a day at biofeedback. But Dr. Corson says even

10 to 20 minutes daily, done regularly, can have a beneficial effect. "Besides the promise of daily relaxation, I've found that biofeedback in conjunction with stress-management training often delivers other bonuses, such as better sleep and relief from stress-related high blood pressure," he says.

Eventually, when you've learned proper relaxation techniques, you can wean yourself from the biofeedback unit. But again, to make it work, you still must practice your exercises regularly. Otherwise your body will forget everything you taught it. "Occasionally it's a good idea to go back to the biofeedback unit to make sure your skills are in good order," says Dr. Corson.

If regeneration is high on your priority list, biofeedback may be just the ticket. It helps you gain control of your body and mind so that you can realize some of your latent potential. And it does this by rechanneling your own attention rather than by depending on external resources. If you just want to calm down a bit, biofeedback can show you how to do it faster and better.

M. G.

BODYWORK

Bodywork doesn't refer to any one technique, therefore it has no star rating. Rather it encompasses a virtual alphabet soup of methods, ranging from shiatsu, which has its roots in antiquity, to Hellerwork, launched in 1978. The idea that you can profoundly influence physical and emotional well-being, by using the hands to rid the body of chronic muscular tension, is at the core of the bodywork disciplines. The field is in such a state of expansion that new methods probably are under development as you read this.

Variety certainly isn't a problem. The real challenge is to separate what's half-baked from what's legitimate, and determine which of the reputable methods is most likely to offer you what you want. Once you select a method, you need to determine that the particular therapist you're considering is competent.

How do you do that? By researching carefully. Comparative reading is the cheapest way to begin. Some of the best-known methods are covered in greater detail in this chapter. One or two of them just might click with you.

You might also check the local listing section in your newspaper to see if bodyworkers in your area are planning an exchange weekend, or offering a workshop that will let you sample several styles.

To make a thorough comparison of the methods that interest you, determine for each one:

- Cost per session.

- Length of typical session.

- How many sessions you need to obtain the results you desire.

- Whether the touch involved is gentle, or forceful enough to cause pain.

- Whether the practitioners are well trained and who supervises the training.

- What the underlying premise is, and whether you are comfortable with it.

Don't feel shy about asking practitioners for a short demonstration, before you commit yourself.

Making sense of what's out there isn't easy. Here's a quick guide to what's what. Remember, though, that most of these definitions are basically *claims,* not facts.

Shiatsu and *acupressure* rely on manual stimulation of pressure points to bring the body's energy back into equilibrium.

Rolfing and *Hellerwork* use deep tissue massage and direct manipulation to restore the skeleton and joints to their intended alignment. Rolfing focuses just on the body. Hellerwork explores the psychological dimensions of posture and tension.

Trager psychophysical integration proceeds from the belief that pleasurable stimulation is the most effective teacher. It uses massage techniques and guided imagery to profoundly relax the body.

The Alexander Technique and *the Feldenkrais method* are more properly called movement reeducation techniques, rather than bodywork. They teach students to consciously replace poor movement habits with healthier, more efficient ones.

Only a few of these methods have been scrutinized by mainstream researchers. Rolfing got good grades from a study conducted by a UCLA professor and a research specialist with the California Department of Mental Health. Similiarly, a Tufts University professor found the Alexander Technique effective.

Despite the lack of formal study, some insurance companies will pay for bodywork sessions. The key, according to Chris Rosch, author of *Decoding the Insurance Puzzle,* is that (*a*) a licensed physician makes a diagnosis that you have a recognized health problem and (*b*) prescribes bodywork sessions as an adjunct to treatment. Typically, bodywork is described as "neuromuscular reeducation" on the insurance form, says Rosch.

The earliest forms of bodywork were very much part of the ancient medical traditions. The Egyptians, Greeks, and Romans relied on massage to relieve physical pain and keep the body supple. In China, acupuncture was considered the highest expression of medical care.

In modern times, bodywork takes its place among the alternative modalities that stand outside the boundaries of conventional medicine. Like other forms of alternative health care, the emphasis is on prevention rather than diagnosis and cure.

Another characteristic of bodywork is that it concerns itself as much with psychological issues as physical ones. The basic premise is that the physical body, intellect, and emotions are part of one dynamic, inseparable whole. If you create positive change at any one level, you bring improvement to every other level.

Much of the bodywork developed in the West shows the influence of the late Wilhelm Reich, an Austrian psychoanalyst who was a member of Freud's inner circle. For Reich, an intellectual understanding of one's neuroses wasn't enough: In order to end the offending behavior you had to effect a physical and emotional release. He was the first to show how personality shaped posture.

Reichian therapy, which continues to be in practice today, works to break down the "body armor," or chronic tension that individuals accumulate in their bodies when they hold their emotions in check, rather than expressing them.

Bodywork methods that build from this theory are gaining in popularity, even in some medical circles.

"The trend is slowly toward accepting more and more adjunctive therapies as a worthwhile part of patient care," says Dr. Susan Lark, author of *The Premenstrual Syndrome Self Help Book,* and a practicing physician who refers some of her patients to bodyworkers.

Dr. Lark has had Swedish massage, Trager psychophysical integration, shiatsu sessions, and some lessons in the Alexander Technique herself.

"I went for personal benefit, for relaxation," she says. "After a long day of seeing patients, my muscles tend to be tense and tight. I'm a believer in making time and space for oneself to receive care. Learning stress reduction also is important."

Certain techniques seem to work better for certain conditions, she believes. Musculoskeletal problems—like spasms, injuries, and arthritis—respond well to Trager and Swedish massage. Patients with internal problems, like asthma or digestive distress, might do better with acupressure or shiatsu, she says.

"In an ideal world, everyone would do some sort of self-nurturing bodywork," she says. "If you just go to the doctor's office to get a pill, you're not being made aware of how you can maintain your own health."

Are there times when people are better off avoiding bodywork?

Don't massage an open wound or a healing sore, says Dr. Lark. If you've just had a traumatic injury, wait until the swelling or inflammation goes down. Likewise, cancer patients are not to be massaged.

See the Contents for the list of entries on specific techniques in this section.

DREAM WORK

★★

You see the phrase "dream work" in articles and catalog descriptions, you hear it spoken by lecturers and talk show guests and you wonder: Is this some new, improved version of dream interpretation?

Nope. It's the very same thing.

That's not to take anything away from dream interpretation. In some self-growth and psychotherapeutic circles, dreams are the primary vehicle for self-understanding and healing. In other modalities, they're an important — if not central — therapeutic ingredient.

How much stock you want to put in your dreams is up to you. Sigmund Freud saw them as the "royal road" to the unconscious. The Talmud says a dream left uninterpreted is like an unopened letter. Carl Jung valued them as gateways to deeper and deeper levels of consciousness. That's why Jungian analysts spend so much time helping clients "translate" their dreams. But then again, there are scientists who see the whole process of dreaming as nothing but a nightly mental housecleaning.

If you have an area of your life you'd like to improve, dream teachers say you can look to your dreams for counsel. Maybe you'd like to know which approach would work best for a health problem...or how you might be getting in the way of your own success.

Practically, how do you do this? Dream experts like Henry Reed, psychologist, and Patricia Garfield recommend that you (a) find a quiet place, (b) deeply relax your body, (c) phrase the question as clearly as you can, (d) contemplate it, and (e) focus on the question again as you're falling asleep.

You may need to do this a couple of days in a row to let yourself know you're really serious.

You can even skip the questions altogether and let your dreams tell you what you ought to focus on. You'll find that what surfaces in your dreams is most relevant to what's currently going on in your life. You can use dreams to conquer old fears and point you in new directions.

And you can learn to translate your own dreams. If you lack confidence here, you might want to consult a book on the subject or take a workshop. But beware of becoming dependent on someone else's

259

260

interpretation of your dreams. Because dreams originate in your mind, you yourself are the most accurate interpreter of them.

That doesn't mean that a friend can't help you enlarge on the meaning you've gotten for yourself. Sometimes, when our dreams bring us thinly disguised versions of things we don't want to face, we may resist to the point where we misinterpret the dream.

The most important questions to ask yourself when you're interpreting your dreams are these:

1. What do I associate with the particular images in the dream?

2. How did the dream make me feel?

3. How do these images and feelings relate to what's going on in my life right now?

And keep at it. If you've been ignoring your dreams for years, it may take some persistence before you can catch even the last fleeting fragments of your dreams as you awaken in the morning.

For help in deciphering your dreams, you could check your library for books on the subject. Other resources include a newsletter called *Dream Network Bulletin,* 1083 Harvest Meadow Court, San Jose, CA 95136, and the *Dream Incubation Workbook,* a 25-page spiral-bound notebook that guides you through a four-week dream interpretation course. The book is available from Henry Reed, 503 Lake Drive, Virginia Beach, VA 23451.

Your community college or local bookstore may offer workshops on dream interpretation.

FELDENKRAIS

★★

Feldenkrais, the babe in the movement education playground, proceeds from the belief that your body can teach your brain new tricks. How? Through a series of intelligently conceived, deceptively simple movements.

The lessons are dispensed in two forms: private tablework sessions and group movement classes.

Both train you to use your muscles to "teach" the motor cortex that smarter options exist; that there are freer and more relaxed ways to walk, to sit, to carry yourself. Ways that make more efficient use of your body's structure that work with gravity instead of against it. With repetition and conscious attention, you forge the neural connections that make such sensible movement consistent.

If you choose "Functional Integration," you'll pay $30 to $70 for 40 minutes with a Feldenkrais instructor. You'll lie on a low, padded table, your awareness focused inward, while the instructor teaches you what it is to be relaxed right *there,* where his hands are at work, and to perceive the subtle differences in feeling that accompany slight alterations in movement. The manipulations are gentle.

Meanwhile, the movement keeps relaying a message to the motor cortex: "This body is capable of much more. You can drop the chronic tension and the inefficient patterns; the organism will survive." Gradually, you bring the posture back to the alignment nature intended it to have.

"Awareness through Movement" classes cost $10 to $20, and last 45 to 60 minutes. Typically, you'll do most of the movements while lying or sitting on the floor. That's to minimize gravity's impact on your exertions. The movements are simple and undemanding, making them ideal for the elderly or the physically challenged. They're also repetitive. Maybe you'll lift your hand just inches from the floor again and again and again, using a set of muscles you hardly knew you had. And then it's on to another tiny movement. Your muscle control becomes more refined.

The Feldenkrais repertoire includes over a thousand such movement sequences, designed to reeducate the skeletal, muscular, and nervous systems. The the-

262

ory is this: Teach the body to expand to its full range of motion, and you help the self reach toward the fullest expression of its potential.

The point of it all, to put it as simply as Feldenkrais Guild president Bonnie Humiston did, is to become "more alive, more alert, more awake, more out there."

Moshe Feldenkrais, the Israeli physicist who devised the method back in the 1940s to restore his knees, was certainly an out-there kind of guy. Physicist doesn't describe half of what he's about. A mechanical and electrical engineer who earned his doctorate in science at the Sorbonne, Feldenkrais was the first Caucasian to earn the sixth dan black belt in judo. He founded the Judo Club of Paris, wrote the manual on unarmed combat for the British army, and also worked on the French atomic research program. He's also the author of six books.

It seems entirely consistent with his character that he's not after "flexible bodies, but flexible minds," as he told one interviewer.

Feldenkrais, the method, owes a certain debt to soccer. It was the flaring up of an old knee injury from that sport that prompted Feldenkrais, the man, to search his knowledge of physics and engineering for a way to heal himself. He was in his thirties then, and unwilling to accept his doctor's advice that he have surgery, which only gave him a 50/50 chance of ever walking again.

Confined to bed, Feldenkrais devoured books on physiology and anatomy and thought hard about the body's relationship to gravity. Movement, he concluded, was the observable force for that relationship.

After restoring his knees to full functioning, Feldenkrais refined his ideas by working on family and friends. By the 1950s, friends were sending *their* friends to see him. A training session in San Francisco in 1975 led to the founding of the Feldenkrais Guild in San Francisco. Now there are over 400 trained instructors of Feldenkrais in the United States, and more on the way. (Teachers recognized by the guild have 800 hours of training, which they complete over a three-year period.)

To locate a trained Feldenkrais instructor in your area, contact the Feldenkrais Guild, P.O. Box 11145, San Francisco, CA 94101, or call (415) 550-8708.

Advocates of the method say it's well-suited to people with severe neuromuscular disturbances. One Feldenkrais book, a slim volume titled *The Case of Nora*, relates how he helped her regain her ability to read and write again, and move unassisted, after a stroke left her with limited muscle control.

No university studies exist to prove, or disprove, the effectiveness of the method. Guild members say that Feldenkrais is so new, it's probably only a matter of time until such a study is undertaken. (Rolfing and the Alexander Technique are among the bodywork disciplines that have been scrutinized by mainstream researchers.)

Still, Feldenkrais has attracted a number of well-known clients, including basketball star Julius Erving, violinst Yehudi Menuhin, and neurophysiologist Karl Pribam. The late Margaret Mead, an anthropologist, was also a fan.

Humiston describes "Functional Integration" as "a very inward experience. You get a very intimate physical acquaintance with yourself. What changes (in the process) is your physical image of yourself, your contact with the ground, and your relationship with gravity. At the end of a session, you're feeling very light, open, kind of floaty. You feel different and you don't know how to describe it. There's no language for it."

Like the movement theorists who preceeded him, Feldenkrais believes that a person's emotional history helps mold posture. In his view, emotions effect the body's flexor muscles to such an extent that the tightness of undischarged anger, sorrow, and fear remain locked in the muscles themselves. To release those tensions is to help cleanse the psyche, bringing about a greater clarity of emotions and thought processes.

"Feldenkrais teaches you how to organize yourself at every level," says Humiston. "Your movements reflect your entire neurological state of function. Your nervous system controls everything about you—your chemistry, digestive system, even how the brain works. When you begin to enhance the nervous system through movement, the whole physique, the whole spirit changes just by changing a little bit about the movement."

"The work is very subtle," she adds. "It's not typical to experience dramatic change. For learning, slow, continuous change is best."

How many sessions before you attain optimum results? That depends upon the condition of your body and what you're looking to achieve. Feldenkrais recommends that students in good health take 1 session for each year of their age. If you're 30, that's 30 sessions.

"Even a little bit can teach you something," Humiston says. "I compare it to learning French. It depends how fluent you want to be."

GESTALT THERAPY

★★★★

Gestalt therapy is a style of psycho-therapy that places more value on your honest expression of emotion than on your intellectual analysis of what happened to you. It aims to keep you focused on the present moment rather than mired in the past. In that sense, it's almost as if its founders turned classic psychoanalysis inside out.

Where does all this lead you? Toward wholeness, a fully alive state of being in which your thoughts, feelings, and actions concur.

This therapy can be quite intense at times. It is definitely confrontational. With its penchant for dramatic reenactments of inner conflict, it can also be a lot of fun.

What makes Gestalt therapy a mind/body therapy—even though it mostly involves sitting around and talking—is the primacy it gives to the emotions. Research into the causes of disease suggests that emotions held in check may be expressed through the body in the form of certain illnesses. Gestalt teaches you how to ver-balize those emotions and to clear out feelings you've locked inside.

"This type of therapy places the body, with its movements and sensations, on entirely the same level as the mind and its abstract thoughts and verbal symbols," explains Joe Kovel, in *A Complete Guide to Therapy.*

The term *Gestalt* comes from the Ger-man Gestalt psychology movement, which concerned itself with human perception and cognition. Yet this therapeutic ap-proach is wholly American, and positive, in that it operates from a belief in man's basic goodness.

Paul Hefferline and Ralph Goodman helped found this approach, but the late Fritz Perls is the person most associated with it. Perls, a German-born neuropsy-chiatrist, was at one time a practicing Freudian analyst.

Perls was influenced by Wilhelm Reich, who explored the connection between emotion and bodily posture; by neo-Freudian Karen Horney, with whom he underwent therapy; and by Carl Jung, whose system of dream translation he carried into Gestalt therapy.

The synthesis that resulted is organized around several key concepts. One key is: "Pay attention to the obvious, the utmost surface."

As Laura Perls, Fritz's wife, says in an essay for *Whole Dimensions in Healing*, "The past is present in the form of memory, with all its emotional ramifications, particularly in the futile repetitive attempts to resolve unfinished situations. It is present in the fixed attitudes and habit patterns originally developed as support that have now (like most Gestalt patterns) become blocks in the ongoing life process."

Gestaltists believe that needs can't be repressed, only re-directed. Denied needs are expressed in the voice, in one's movements or posture. Proponents of this theory also believe that verbal communication tends to be dishonest and protective.

Another key concept is that nature is always moving toward unity. In the human being, this occurs when thinking, feeling, and actions are integrated. When anxiety exists, it signals awareness that one part of the being has split off, and is struggling toward unification with the core self.

One goal of Gestalt therapy is to bring split-off projections back into the self, and to let the self identify with and accept all its sensations and urgings. Another goal is to get individuals to respond appropriately to the moment, instead of seeing it through the filter of the past.

For example, a woman who was constantly criticized by her parents may not hear a compliment when it is given to her by an authority figure. This decision to not hear what authority figures say arose from an initially positive instinct to ward off pain. But when this mode of operating becomes fixed, it prevents her from fully experiencing current reality.

What is a Gestalt session like?

That's a hard question to answer. In the first place, you can find Gestalt therapists in any number of settings offering individual sessions, group encounters, or intensive weekend workshops. Because Gestalt is opposed to closed systems of therapy, therapists may incorporate any number of modalities into their sessions, including movement, art therapy, and primal scream therapy. You may even find Gestalt techniques incorporated into hands-on healing systems, such as the Rubenfield Synergy Method. Purists prefer a hands-off approach however, because they feel Gestalt therapy is more empowering that way.

What will remain constant is that Gestalt is confrontational. You confront your feelings, your conflicts. You'll be expected to express them honestly; if you don't, cover-ups and evasions will be exposed for what they are. You may be asked to stay with a feeling and express it by screaming it, or you may be asked to dramatically reenact an inner struggle.

You'll do your reenactment using several chairs as props. While you're sitting in one chair, you'll take the part of the overbearing conscience who yells at the "self" to do better. When you shift to a new chair, you'll respond as the "underdog," that subversive, beaten-down part of you who wants to live fully but is constantly battling the conscience. From the dialogue, a sense of what's healthy for you as a whole being may emerge.

There are as many as 80 schools that teach Gestalt therapy around the country. Training standards vary widely, as do prices for the therapy.

With so much variety among Gestalt

therapists, how do you choose a competent one? Very carefully, says Lenore Hecht, director of the Gestalt Therapy Institute of New York. She suggests you visit a training institute in your area and determine whether you're comfortable with how they treat you and how much training they give their graduates. If you feel good about the school, ask them to match you with a graduate who practices in your area and has particular finesse with the issues you want to work on in therapy. Ask for a consultation with your proposed therapist before committing yourself. "Use your eyes and ears to see what you're buying," she suggests.

For reference, graduates of Hecht's school undergo three years of training after they are approved for the program. Potential trainees are typically required to have a graduate degree, or be working toward one. Personal readiness, as determined by an interview with the candidate, plays a big part in whether someone will be accepted into the training program.

HELLERWORK

★★

A lesser-known variant of Rolfing, after which it is patterned, Hellerwork also uses deep tissue massage and direct manipulation to bring the body's major segments back toward a more natural alignment. And like Rolfing, the work proceeds systematically over a number of sessions.

The main difference between them is that Hellerwork tries to be more inclusive. Unlike Rolfing, it doesn't begin and end on the massage table. If you're a Hellerwork client, you can expect to talk about the emotional issues that may be contributing to the tension that's pulled your body out of whack. You can also expect lessons in how to sit, stand, bend, walk, and balance yourself.

Hellerwork was developed by Joseph Heller, a Polish-born aerospace engineer who became a Rolfer around 1972, and then the International Rolf Institute's first president in 1975. In 1978, he branched out with his own method.

In a magazine interview ten years later, Heller explained the difference between his approach and Rolf's in this way:

"In Hellerwork, I create pressure by the weight of my body. In Rolfing, I create the same pressure through muscle tension . . . Same amount of pressure, but . . . your body reacts to it differently. As I worked with it more and more, I began to see it as a large philosophical difference that has to do with living what you're preaching. If I am trying to teach your body about relaxation, about flow, about alignment with gravity I'm much more likely to do it this way. You don't relax because your body can feel the tension in my body and it will respond automatically. When the touch is that hard, it is intrusive and your body will guard against it."

Adds Susan Belfiore, a Hellerworker in New Jersey, "If we come up against a place where there's tightness, it can be uncomfortable. What we don't do is barrel through it. I encourage the client to say stop, if it's just too much. But we will work on that edge so that they have the experience of letting go what's tight in their bodies."

Hellerwork costs about $75 to $100 for each 1½- to 2-hour session. Rolfing costs just about as much, although sessions may be as short as an hour. Hellerwork takes 11 sessions to complete; Rolfing takes 10.

During your first session, you'll do a

lot of talking. Your Hellerworker is interested in finding out about your body history: serious accidents, surgery, where you tend to hold tension. If you're under the care of a psychologist or physician, she'd like to know that also. "If so, we like to get permission and work hand in hand [with the doctor]," explains Belfiore.

Next, you'll be photographed standing in front of a wall chart with a plumb line. That's to help you and your Hellerworker monitor your results.

And then it's on to the massage table. You can expect a workout on the table, followed by movement instruction, for the first 10 sessions. The 11th session doesn't involve bodywork; it's more a graduation and a send-off.

Each session has a specific psychological theme, to be explored in discussion, and a specific physical goal. Ideally, sessions are spaced a week apart.

Session 1 is "Inspiration." The physical goal is to open up the breathing and align the rib cage over the pelvis.

Session 2 is "Standing On Your Own Two Feet." Its goal is to align the legs, create a horizontal positioning of the knee and ankle joints, and distribute the weight of the body over the arches of the feet.

Session 3 is "Reaching Out." Its goal is to release tension in the shoulders, arms and sides, and to bring vertical alignment to the sides of the torso.

Session 4 is "Control and Surrender." Its goal is to release the insides of the legs and the muscles of the pelvic floor and align the midlines of the inner thighs.

Session 5 is "Guts." Its goal is to lengthen the muscles of the front of the legs and release the deep muscles of the pelvis.

Session 6 is "Holding Back." Its goal is to lengthen the back.

Session 7 is "Losing Your Head." Its goal is to align the head over the torso and release tension in the head, face, and neck.

Session 8 is "The Feminine," and explores concepts like beauty, well-being, and receptivity. Anatomically, the focus is on the feet, legs, and pelvis.

Session 9 is "The Masculine," exploring such principles as "activity with purpose" and "movement with direction." Anatomically, the focus is on the upper half of the body.

Session 10, "Integration," attempts to establish the overall integrity of the body through working with the joints.

Session 11 "Coming Out," focuses on concepts like empowerment and self-expression. It's a time for review, both of results achieved and lessons learned. You'll get an "after" photo, to compare to the one taken your first session. "This is the session where we give it all back," says Belfiore. "You are the expert on your body. We use a lot of video in this session."

Hellerworkers recommend twice yearly "tune-ups."

Practitioners of the method are certified after completing 1,000 hours of training. Course work covers bodywork, psychology, movement awareness, and business practices. Students must complete a six-month internship after they finish training.

To locate a certified Hellerworker in your area, contact The Body of Knowledge, 147 Lomita Drive, Suite H, Mill Valley, CA 94941, or call (415) 383-4240.

See the entry on Rolfing, beginning on page 325.

HYPNOTHERAPY

★★★★★

Like alchemy and astrology, the practice of hypnosis once belonged to the world of the occult. But then, so did medicine.

Today, numerous medical schools teach hypnosis, and a handful of doctors, dentists, and psychologists are board-certified to practice it.

Although it's been successfully used to treat such things as phobias and bad habits, hypnosis's most significant role has been in the treatment of pain. Doctors first used it as an anesthetic in the 1840s and they still use it for that purpose today. In cases where chemical anesthesia is undesirable—in childbirth, or when the patient has an allergy to anesthesia—hypnosis has proved itself to be not only effective but also inexpensive, safe, and virtually side effect-free in patients able to enter profound hypnosis.

"Hypnosis is very, very good at pain control," says Dr. Eugene E. Levitt, secretary-treasurer of the American Board of Psychological Hypnosis and a professor at the Indiana University School of Medicine. "That is one of its outstanding applied uses, particularly in pain due to clear-cut bodily pathology [disease]," adds Dr. Mar-

tin Orne, director of the unit for experimental psychiatry at the Institute of Pennsylvania Hospital in Philadelphia. "For people who have the ability to respond well, hypnosis is one of the few effective ways for providing pain relief over a long period of time without risk."

Think Cool and Calm

Doctors have used hypnosis to treat many kinds of pain. In New Orleans, Dr. Dabney Ewin, a surgeon and psychiatrist who teaches hypnosis at Tulane University, uses it to treat patients with widespread third-degree burns. He's found that if he can hypnotize a burn victim within 2 hours after the accident, he can prevent much of the inflammation, pain, and skin damage that usually results.

"In a severe burn," Dr. Ewin explains, "two things happen. There is the heat damage to the outside of the skin, and there is the inflammatory reaction from the inside, which comes as a response to the patient's fear. If I can hypnotize him into believing that he is cool and comfort-

269

able, I can turn off that response and stop the inflammation."

Others have had similar positive results. Doctors from three Minnesota children's hospitals have taught a form of self-hypnosis called "relaxation-mental imagery" to children. Of headache patients, 70 percent got relief from pain. Of 36 children with other kinds of pain, 19 got complete relief and others got partial relief.

Obstetricians from Staten Island Hospital and Downstate Medical Center in New York have been teaching young mothers how to relax during delivery by repeating the thoughts, "You will be calm, confident, and brave. You will experience pressure and exertion but no pain. You will recover quickly and comfortably" and other suggestions.

Doctors now use hypnosis in cancer wards, according to Dr. Levitt, and there's evidence that it is effective. "The data are clear that when you introduce hypnosis techniques in a terminal-cancer ward, you will see the demand for painkillers such as Demerol go down."

Dentists often use hypnosis for patients who don't want procaine, usually with great success. Doctors have also used hypnosis to help people who suffer from migraine headaches, shingles, tinnitus, arthritis, and low back pain.

Before he can treat pain, a hypnotist has to put his patient into a relaxed state. He can use a variety of induction techniques. Typically, he will speak to the patient in a gentle, rhythmical voice. He might ask the patient to close his eyes. Then, using his voice and suggesting visual images, he will soothe the patient into a state of complete relaxation.

"I ask him to visualize a stairway," one hypnotist told us. "I ask him to walk down the stairs with me, one step at a time, while I count from 20 to 1. With each step, I tell the patient that he is becoming more and more relaxed, and that by the time we reach the bottom of the stairs, his conscious mind will be asleep."

If all goes well (and it may not on the first or even second session), the patient will have slipped into a hypnotic trance. Being under a trance, doctors say, is like being absorbed in a book or film, only more so. It is a state of focused awareness and of intense concentration. In a trance, the right hemisphere of the brain is thought to become dominant, says Dr. Helen Crawford, of the University of Wyoming, who chairs the American Psychological Association's division on psychological hypnosis. This is associated with the nonanalytical, imaginative side of the brain, and is the one more open to suggestion.

The trance is not, however, the "zombie state" that many people imagine. "People think that in a trance a person will do anything that the hypnotist wants him to do. None of that happens in real hypnosis," says Dr. Jeanine LaBaw, of Denver, who works with hypnosis and pain. "You totally maintain your own control. You won't do anything immoral. You won't take your clothes off and cluck like a chicken, unless you happen to like being the life of the party."

Once people enter a trance, a hypnotherapist enables them, in a sense, to imagine their pain away. By suggesting mental pictures at a time when the mind is especially receptive to them, the hypnotherapist can attach pain to an image and then move that image from one body part to another, or even push it out of the body. Says Dr. Daniel Kohen, associate director

IS HYPNOSIS A GOOD WAY TO LOSE WEIGHT?

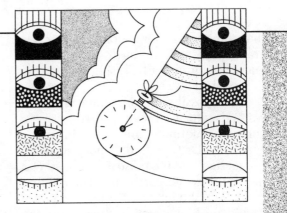

For years, you've been trying to shed those last 10 pounds, which stand between you and a terrific shape. You've tried several diets and nothing seems to help. Maybe you need more willpower. Maybe you need . . . hypnosis!

There's no shortage of hypnosis clinics that claim to help their clients lose weight. But will hypnosis really help trim those last inches? Actually, the experts give hypnosis about a C+ or B in the dieting category. "Hypnosis is no more or less effective than any other method used to help people curb their appetites and lose weight," says Dr. Thomas Wadden, a University of Pennsylvania psychologist who specializes in the treatment of obesity.

"When people go to a hypnotist and pay high fees and are told that it will help them, it may help and they may lose weight. But aside from offering a structure for change, hypnosis is generally no more helpful than other techniques," he says.

On the other hand, he says, "There are certain people for whom hypnosis works. In hypnosis, they learn to reinterpret the growling in their stomachs as a nice warm sensation rather than a signal to eat. Aside from that, the biggest plus for hypnosis is that the public has very high expectations for it. It gets them psyched up for change."

Others agree that hypnosis is not a magic cure. "The success rate of hypnosis for weight loss or smoking cessation is about 30 percent, which is not better than other methods," says Dr. Eugene E. Levitt, of the American Board of Psychological Hypnosis. "It's just that hypnosis might turn out to be the thing that works for you."

of behavior pediatrics at the Minneapolis Children's Medical Center, "The active ingredient in hypnosis is imagery."

Imagery helped one man overcome back pain, for example. "One of my patients, a 45-year-old executive named Henry, suffered from severe back pain," says David E. Bresler, author of *Free Yourself from Pain.* "But through symptom substitution (a mental technique for shifting pain from one place to another), he was able to move that pain from his back down to the bottoms of his feet." Eventu-

ally he was able to rid himself of his pain whenever it recurred by "walking it away." He imagined the pain leaving his body "and scattering on the ground as he walked along."

A very common technique called "glove anesthesia" has been used to reduce labor pains. An obstetrician might lead his patient to believe that her hand is numb by telling her under hypnosis that it's made of wood or stone or that it's a thick, woolly glove. He can then ask her, through symptom substitution, to transfer that numbness to her abdomen. After several sessions prior to birth, she will have learned to numb her belly simply by saying the word "belly."

The possibilities are endless. "I once worked with a woman with tinnitus [a chronic, sometimes painful, ringing in the ears]," says Dr. Crawford. "Under hypnosis, I suggested that the noise in her head was like the noise of a car. She was taught that every time she felt an attack coming, she should push that car farther down the road, away from her, until she couldn't see it anymore. The noise didn't go away completely, but she learned to make it more bearable."

"Fist therapy" also helps some people. Dr. Orne asks his patients to imagine capturing all of their pain in their fist. The tighter the fist, he says, the more pain it holds. When the pain is totally in that fist, they can throw it away and not have it come back for several hours.

The Ultimate Bedside Manner

While these techniques show *how* hypnosis works, they don't explain *why* it works. Assuming that there is no hocus-pocus involved, on what level of mind or body does hypnosis work?

One theory is that hypnosis, in a powerful way, distracts us from pain. "The explanation for suggested anesthesia," says Dr. Orne, "must probably be sought in the profound effect hypnosis may exert on selective attention." In other words, we can use the hypnotic state to focus all of our attention away from the pain.

"In experiments with cats," Dr. Orne relates, "it has been shown that the ani-mal won't hear a clicking noise, which it normally hears, if it's hungry and we put a mouse in front of it." People can "choose to see or not to see" their pain better, he says. He also thinks that hypnosis can work by relaxing those in pain, diminishing their fear of pain.

Another theory is that during hypnosis the brain releases natural opiatelike painkillers called endorphins. This theory is espoused by Dr. Paul Sacerdote, a New York psychiatrist and oncologist who has had great success treating cancer pain.

Others believe that hypnosis acts through the emotions. Dr. Theodore X. Barber, a Massachusetts psychologist and author, thinks the success of hypnosis depends on the rapport that the doctor establishes with the person whom he or she hypnotizes. Hypnosis, he suggests, is the ultimate bedside manner, one in which doctor/patient affection pushes aside the loneliness, anxiety, and tension that makes pain so much worse.

At the heart of hypnosis, says Dr. Barber, is the principle that pain fluctuates depending upon the way we perceive it. "Since the interpretation of pain sensations is such an important part of the total pain experience, hypnosuggestive procedures can play an important role in pain control," he writes in *Handbook of Clinical Health Psychology*.

Are You a Good Candidate?

But, supposing that hypnosis works, does that mean it will work for everyone? The question "Who is hypnotizable?" is very much debated among researchers. The consensus is that there are a few people who can be hypnotized so deeply that they could undergo open-heart surgery without chemical anesthesia. At the other extreme are people who can't be hypnotized. Most people, however, can be hypnotized to a certain degree.

"Almost anyone can get into a trance state," says Dr. LaBaw. "If you're motivated and work on it, then you can do it. I have been using hypnosis in my practice for 14 years. In that time, only one or two people weren't hypnotizable."

But not all are created equal. The better you are at letting your imagination run loose, it seems, the better your chances are of being hypnotized. "The main thing is the imagination," says Dr. Ernest Hilgard, a Stanford University professor and a pioneer in this field. "It means having the ability to believe that you are in a nice warm pool in the South Pacific instead of sitting in a dentist's chair having your teeth drilled."

Because imagination is so big a part of their lives, children have been found to be highly hypnotizable. "We know that children whose parents read them stories are likely to be good candidates for hypnosis. "By age 12, some people lose a lot of their ability to be hypnotized—a phenomenon not fully understood," says Dr. Crawford.

Dr. Barber suggests this instant "litmus test" to find out if a person is highly hypnotizable: "Ask someone to close her eyes and to imagine that she is holding a baby. Ask her to smell the baby, to feel the baby, to listen to the baby for a short while. Then tell her to open her eyes and *see* the baby. If she really sees the baby, she's a good candidate for hypnosis."

Then there are those for whom hypnosis represents the last resort for pain relief. The fact that they often focus all of their hope and attention on the doctor makes them more sensitive to trance induction. "Motivation is as important as hypnotic responsiveness in predicting the patient's ability to derive pain relief," says Dr. Orne.

But can people learn how to hypnotize themselves so that they can slip into a trance whenever pain occurs, without needing the reassuring presence of a hypnotherapist? Every doctor we spoke to said yes to this question.

Self-hypnosis, which calls on the patient to say the words of induction to himself, is effective against pain in part because it offers empowerment, doctors say. It gives patients a tool with which they can fight their pain actively. In doing so, self-hypnosis reduces the sense of helplessness that is known to make pain seem worse than it might necessarily be. "All good hypnotists teach self-hypnosis," says Dr. Hilgard.

In fact, some doctors don't even want their patients to listen to cassette tapes of their sessions when they get home, because it delays self-hypnosis. "We seldom use tapes," says Dr. LaBaw. "Using a tape is passive. People learn faster if they play an active role."

IMAGERY

★★★★

Long before the real race is run, world-class track star James Robinson is running it in his mind, rehearsing every second of the half-mile as surely as he practiced each day on the track. The image is so clear he can hear his heartbeat, feel the cinders crunching under his shoes, see himself surge ahead near the end, and feel the finish line snap across his chest.

When all the athletes in a race are in virtually the same tip-top shape, it's presence of mind that makes the difference.

Lester L., a Florida businessman, was running a different race—for his life. A tumor had invaded his throat. It was going to have to come out, and with it, possibly, his vocal cords.

A week before the operation, Lester started an imaginary attack on his tumor. His white blood cells became busy miners with pickaxes, hacking away at the mass. Once fearful of surgery, Lester now imagined that it would go well. He saw himself controlling his bleeding during surgery and recovering quickly. When the doctor did operate, the tumor was half its expected size. Lester awakened as he left the operating room, and was on the phone 2 hours later. He left the hospital in two days. Just a coincidence? Lester doesn't think so.

Sarah M., a Boston journalist, had embarked on a new career as a free-lance writer, something she'd always wanted to do. But she was having trouble writing. She couldn't take herself seriously. She was afraid she'd fail, and indeed, seemed to be setting herself up for just that.

Instead, she learned to imagine her new self—at parties, talking with confidence and self-respect about her career change. She also gained a strong new image of sitting down and writing for a full day without distractions. Pie-in-the-sky fantasies? Not for Sarah. She's already started doing the same things in real life, and her writing career has taken off.

So what's going on here? Are we to believe that if we think about something hard enough and long enough and in enough detail that it will become real?

Yes, to a large extent. We *can* maximize our potential, both in performance and in health, and within the realm of possibility. And there's good evidence to show that our potential goes far beyond what we think of as normal, everyday functioning.

Tricking the Subconscious

One widely held theory for imagery's powerful effect is that it fools the subconscious mind. The subconscious, it seems, cannot always tell the difference between an actual experience and a vivid image. And that's one reason researchers think imagery can so easily produce physical responses. Image a near miss in your car and your blood pressure, pulse rate, and adrenaline levels soar. See yourself on a sunny beach and watch them drop.

It was this sort of observation that convinced Dr. Jeanne Achterberg, a leading researcher and author in the field, that there was a definite link between the imagination and the body's healing process.

Dr. Achterberg states that in the medical literature on people who recovered from a diagnosis of terminal cancer, the only thing in common was a change of attitude. "Something happened to cause them to begin to have a different image of themselves—not of a dying person but of a well person," she says. In her clinical practice, Dr. Achterberg observes that, "Someone would come in with total liver failure, yellow as a pumpkin, and be up and walking around in two weeks. Another person would have a simple diagnosis of a small breast tumor and soon be dead.

"Now this goes beyond physiology. You cannot die from a small breast tumor.

It doesn't impinge on any vital organs. But you *can* die from giving up. You can die from the workings of the imagination. And from it you can also gain life."

The Imagery of Cancer

"See" yourself as a healthy, whole person despite what the doctors say, Dr. Achterberg says. Doing so actually beefs up the immune system, cuts down on stress, and may give you a new lease on life. "I am not saying this is for everyone, or that anyone can do it," she emphasizes. "It takes 100 percent commitment, and sometimes the body is just too worn out and tired for this sort of thing." And one of the prerequisites seems to be that you really have to believe that it will work for you for it actually to work.

Dr. Achterberg found that terminal cancer patients who went into remission or had experienced a shrinkage of their tumors not only had an incredible will to live, they imagined their cancers, their immune systems, and their treatments in a certain, positive way.

One man, for instance, saw his cancer as small, easily squashed creatures being lanced by white knights on horses—his own white blood cells. "Having images of goodness and purity of the immune system was important," she says. So was being able to see a treatment as effective and safe. One woman imaged her radiation as the healing rays of the sun; another, her chemotherapy as a powerful substance that exploded her cancer cells the instant it touched them.

Imagery can be a basis for diagnosis, Dr. Achterberg believes. "It could be that

276

those who saw white knights were simply getting in touch with the intuitive sense that tells us what's going on in the body. And that those whose cancers were imagined as ants or crabs—clinging, pinching images that meant a poor prognosis for recovery—somehow sensed that they weren't going to get well."

The question now is—can changing these images into a more positive form help to fight the disease? Preliminary research seems to indicate yes, Dr. Achterberg says, although she emphasizes that very few people have actually done so. "Only recently have we begun to get some work showing that if the images are changed, you actually get changes in the healing mechanism of the body itself."

In a classic study conducted at Penn State University, certain people (those who are younger or more susceptible to hypnosis) who twice each day for a week imagined their germ-killing white blood cells as sharks showed a significant increase in the numbers of white blood cells.

Several repeats of this and similar tests have shown the same results, Dr. Achterberg says.

And researchers at Michigan State University demonstrated that people could change the number and function of a specific white blood cell, called a neutrophil, by first seeing actual pictures of the blood cell and then, under induced relaxation, imaging the process by which the blood cells act. Bordering on science fiction? Perhaps. But Dr. Achterberg envisions a day when people will help themselves to heal with images of knitting bone tissue, dilated arteries, and an army of white blood cells coming to their defense.

Walking Tightropes and Chasing Butterflies

Dr. James Meade, Jr., a California psychologist, uses imagery to help brain-injured adults walk and talk again. A man who was having trouble with balance learned to see himself as a tightrope walker, an image that forced his brain to make subtle balance corrections. He also learned to no longer fear falling. If he imaged himself slipping off the rope, he'd then see himself catching the rope, pulling himself up and continuing along.

Another man, depressed and with many coordination problems, learned how to move his arms and walk again with the aid of a most pleasant scene. From his hospital bed, he would imagine himself in a field of wildflowers, catching beautiful butterflies in a net, examining them, and releasing them to fly again.

Drunk Self/Sober Self

Drug addicts and alcoholics who successfully kick the habit share a common image, says Dr. Lawrence Horberg, a Chicago psychologist specializing in drug addiction. "They can bring back quite strongly a picture of themselves doing something that can be humiliating and degrading or resulted in personal loss. This negative image can be a powerful source of motivation in the lifelong struggle to remain drug-free." One cocaine addict, for instance, could see himself combing his carpet for a trace of the spilled powder.

Typically, addicts *can't* remember such scenes. Drugs and alcohol and ordinary psychological defenses block their awareness. The details are stored in the brain, though, and can be retrieved in the form of imagery. Dr. Horberg provides a supportive environment and encourages the patient to listen to family, friends, and employers recount scenes of addiction or intoxication. Then, he uses a similar technique to help the addict create a healthy, happy image of his new sober self.

Image Your Best Self

You don't have to be an addict to benefit from developing a new self-image. Dr. Timothy Hodgens, a Massachusetts psychologist, uses imagery in perhaps its largest sense — to help people gain a sense of themselves, their goals, and their place in life.

"Many people who go through therapy and discover some of their problems get scared when they start trying to change," Dr. Hodgens says. "They don't want to continue as they are, but they have no idea who it is they eventually want to be, and how they are going to get there."

To help them tackle this problem, Dr. Hodgens asks them to image themselves during a time when they felt things were going well, when everything seemed to come together. For him, that time was when he had just finished giving a speech at a conference.

The next step, then, is to start talking with your ideal self, and to listen to what it has to say to you. "Everyone has to ask their own, very personal questions, but it's in this dialogue that new insights are uncovered."

The final step, a lifelong process really, is to project yourself into your image of your ideal self. "It becomes a transformation," Dr. Hodgens says. "Over a period of time you start to lose your old self in the process. You project yourself into that image, right now, and then begin to see yourself feeling, acting, behaving in that way and that context.

"There has to be a very serious intent of moving toward this best possible self. It's not easy, but it's possible."

277

INTEGRATIVE
BODY PSYCHOTHERAPY

★

Take a Jungian analyst, Gestalt therapist, Rolfer, acupuncturist, Reichian bodyworker, spiritual teacher, and Freudian psychotherapist and roll them into one.

What do you get?

Most likely, a practitioner of Integrative Body Psychotherapy (IBP).

This body-oriented style of psychotherapy, developed by Dr. Jack Lee Rosenberg, draws together the theories and tools of ancient and modern healing systems in a single coherent package. It grew out of Dr. Rosenberg's attempt to discover why existing therapies aren't consistently effective.

A synthesis itself, IBP seeks to bring about a "coming-together" in the individual, an experience of aliveness in which mind, emotions, body, and spirit interact as cooperative parts of a unified whole. That whole is "Self," and re-awakening this "Self" is the goal of therapy.

Much of the work is done on a massage table. That's because Dr. Rosenberg and collaborator, Dr. Marjorie Rand, believe that the surest route to this core self is through the body.

In their book, *Body, Self & Soul: Sustaining Integration*, they define the self as "that nonverbal sense of well-being, identity, and continuity that is felt in the body." This feeling of well-being should have been our natural condition as infants, they say. Whether it was or not depends upon how lovingly our needs were met during our preverbal years.

For most of us to return to that inherent state of well-being, we have to reopen our capacity to feel. Since feelings are a form of energy, this means increasing our ability to contain energy in our bodies.

Contain is the key word here. What makes IBP different from most other body-centered styles of psychotherapy is that it emphasizes building energy and spreading it through the body, rather than emotional or muscular release. Also, unlike the Reichian- or Rolfing-based therapies, IBP is noninvasive. The therapist may work the pressure points to get the energy moving again, but don't expect her to reconstruct your body the way a Rolfer would.

"We're not focused on release at all," says Dr. Rand. "We emphasize well-being and aliveness. We want people to get in touch with the energy that flows through them. When they feel good, they lose their fear of contacting their feelings."

The concept of energy is fundamental to Intergrative Body Psychotherapy. Dr. Rosenberg and Dr. Rand suggest in their book that a healthy person is a mass of free-flowing energy, which is "instantly accessible to the person whenever he needs it for any purpose." An unhealthy person, conversely "has blocks in his system and the flow of energy is impeded."

IBP's body focus reflects Dr. Rosenberg's eclectic background. A 20-year practitioner of yoga, and a Gestalt therapy trainer, both at Esalen Institute and in San Francisco, he also studied Reichian therapy.

"He thought it was ridiculous to do so many different kinds of therapies," says Dr. Rand. She met him in 1976, as a graduate student in his training class at the Center for the Healing Arts in Los Angeles. Together, they organized his methods and theories and wrote *Body, Self & Soul* to explain them. In 1982, they opened the Rosenberg-Rand Institute for Integrative Body Psychotherapy and began offering a five-year training program.

During training, IBP therapists learn to use a variety of diagnostic and therapeutic tools.

One tool used is the client journal. That's to show you, the client, you're in charge of your own healing. You record dreams, feelings, inner dialogues, and other therapy assignments.

Two other diagnostic tools IBP uses are an extensive physical history (it even asks about eating and exercise habits and drug consumption) and what Dr. Rosenberg and Dr. Rand call the primary scenario. This requires some sleuthing through the family history to put together a detailed look at your earliest relations with your parents, their relations with their parents, and anything else that may have influenced your earliest perceptions of the world and your response to it.

But the centerpiece of IBP is the energy-building exercises you'll do on the massage table. These Reichian-inspired exercises help show where tension blocks energy from moving freely through your body. Working with the tension will give you access to emotional situations that were never fully resolved, and which continue to influence your feelings and behavior, they say.

In session, you'll lie down on the table, bend your knees so that your feet rest flat on the table, about pelvic-width apart. You'll relax and breathe as instructed. This breathing will build up what Dr. Rosenberg and Dr. Rand call an energy charge, which intensifies what you're feeling so you can identify and work with it. Your therapist observes you closely while you're on the table. Subtle movements you make and color changes in your skin will indicate to her where constriction begins. Her careful observations give her clues about what's going on within you emotionally.

As you "charge" your body, memories may surface, memories of painful events and situations you never fully resolved.

"Breathing causes people to go into regression, and what they come up with is material from the first three years of life," Dr. Rand explains. "Since much of what's in the body is precognitive and preverbal, you have to get at it through the body."

279

With your therapist, you'll reframe that early situation by applying your adult logic to the emotions and perceptions that overwhelmed you at the time.

If you're so tense you have difficulty moving energy through your body, your therapist may work your pressure points or guide you through an appropriate stress-building exercise that will work the tight muscles until they give up and let go.

Throughout, she'll work to keep you focused on the feelings and sensations in your body. Her goal is to teach you where you cut your feelings off, where you shut your energy down, and what it would feel like to take yourself one step further. IBP theorists believe that when you work your feelings through, a palpable sense of well-being results.

As a variation, you may build up "charge" and then share a recent dream in a Gestalt type of way, reenacting the dream by playing each of the characters in it. Together, you'll explore the dream for ideas about areas in your life that need healing.

Information that these exercises yield about you will help your therapists determine whether you've successfully completed each of early childhood developmental stages needed to build a secure sense of self.

"The therapist works to heal those early injuries by using certain reparenting techniques," Dr. Rand says. "The more that happens, the more the client expands and relaxes, and the more willing he is to have his own energy."

At this point, you may work with imagery, develop a sense of your own energy boundaries, or experiment with other techniques designed to reinforce the self. Throughout, you'll be taught to give yourself the acceptance, love, and permission to be yourself that you might not have gotten as a child.

What's happening in your current relationships will also provide material to work with. Dr. Rosenberg and Dr. Rand believe that a person's relationship patterns as an adult reflect his childhood experiences.

Dr. Rand and Dr. Rosenberg say their therapy is a transpersonal approach. They believe that when you systematically rid the body of physical tension, work through unfinished emotions, and broaden your self-concept, you pave the way for the transformation of being.

The goal, says Dr. Rand, is to guide the client toward a "feeling of openness and love that is transcendent of emotional and muscular blocks. It leads to a shift in consciousness. It's a way that you live."

The process can take two to three years.

Because the therapy is so new, the great majority of practitioners are located on the West Coast or in Canada. That's slowly changing, however. Dr. Rand has been conducting training workshops throughout the country, and will offer workshops wherever there's interest. Applicants must be either licensed or certified health professionals.

She says the cost of therapy is competitive with most other forms of psychotherapy in the surrounding community.

For information about the training, or referral to a practitioner, contact The Rosenberg-Rand Institute, 1551 Ocean Avenue, Suite 230, Santa Monica, CA 90401, or call (213) 394-0147.

JIN SHIN DO
BODYMIND ACUPRESSURE

★

Imagine talking to your psychotherapist while she presses her fingertips into specific points along your body. And imagine that her firm touch helps you sink deeply into your psyche, where you find the long-buried memories and hurts that help you make sense of your current situation.

This is a snapshot of Jin Shin Do Bodymind Acupressure, a relative newcomer to the field of body-oriented psychotherapies. As in other forms of bodywork, the therapy is done on a massage table, with the client fully clothed. And, like the others, it is presented as a tool for transforming painful feelings into pleasurable ones. Its Asian flavor is what sets it apart.

Iona Marsaa Teeguarden, who developed this system, drew from traditional acupressure theory and technique, ancient Taoist philosophy, and contemporary Western psychology, particularly Wilhelm Reich's theories about muscular tension and psychological limitations.

What she came up with is a systematic therapy with its own scheme for understanding the connection between the various muscle groups, the body's internal energy channels and the emotions that influence both.

Emotions are of primary importance in Jin Shin Do. In her book *The Joy of Feeling Body-Mind: Acupressure*, Teeguarden asserts that feelings are "the *driving energy* of the body," and are what keeps you in touch with the changing needs of your inner self. One goal of her therapy is to get clients to accept and allow each of their feelings. Resolution of a feeling brings peace and a sense of well-being. But when feelings are ignored, or prematurely shut down because they're just too painful, physical problems arise. And the good feelings are blocked off.

During Jin Shin Do sessions, therapists "read" these physical problems (the muscular tension, the tenderness at pressure points) as if they were a road map pointing to ongoing difficulties in the psyche. "Freeing the body helps free the psyche, and psychological growth is accompanied by the release of physical tensions," Teeguarden asserts in *The Joy of Feeling*.

East Meets West

Jin Shin Do (literally, the "way of the compassionate spirit") traces its roots back to the 1970s, when an interest in macrobiotics and Asian philosophy drew Teeguarden, a University of Michigan music major, to Los Angeles.

Eventually, she sought out acupressure for treatment of a physical problem and was so impressed by the results she decided to study it. Around the same time, she was introduced to the theoretical work of Reich. "Instinctively, I knew that acupressure and Reichian therapy should be together," she says.

She studied acupressure first, intent on understanding what the "strange flows" of Chinese medicine were all about. (These 12 energy channels are believed by the Chinese to regulate the internal balance of energy in the body, by continually modulating and adjusting the flow of energy to the body's major organs.) In time, she came to view the "strange flows" as the body's most primary means for maintaining homeostasis. So she made the pressure points that relate to these flows a key part of her Jin Shin Do system.

Teeguarden's interest in acupressure led her to Japan. In 1976, after returning from a three-month visit to the East, she became director of the Acupressure Workshop in Los Angeles. In her work with clients, she began noticing things. They felt a need to talk as the acupressure helped release tension. And their physical ills,

she claims, virtually disappeared as they developed the self-confidence to do what they wanted.

In 1978, Teeguarden published *The Acupressure Way of Health: Jin Shin Do.* But she felt she hadn't taken her method far enough. A year later, interested in exploring the correlation between the Eastern and Taoist view of the psyche, and Western psychological theory, she applied to the graduate psychology program at Antioch University in Ohio. In 1982, she began the Jin Shin Do Foundation for Bodymind Acupressure, where she continued to refine her methods. Her *The Joy of Feeling*, published in 1987, adds Western psychology and insights from her clinical experience to the synthesis.

Teacher training is ongoing at the foundation. Currently, practitioners trained in her methods are working in 18 states, three Canadian provinces and several European countries. Among those who have practitioner certification are licensed massage therapists, physical therapists, nurses, doctors, and psychotherapists, she says.

She also offers "Joy of Feeling" workshops around the country to teach people a simplified version of Jin Shin Do they can use at home.

"This is ideal for couples to learn to do for each other," she asserts. "I've never met a person who doesn't build up a little bit of stress. Sometimes we really need the release valve of a session like this."

■ Softening Away
■ Your Tensions

When the session begins, the therapist checks the major points to see what's sore, and asks the client what he wants to work on. Information gained here tells the therapist which acu-points to employ. (Most of the points are found within the muscles, although some are located on the joints.)

Firm but gentle finger pressure is applied to the points until the therapist feels a softening of the tension. Usually, she'll press several points at once — a main point and some distal points, which are related to the problem area but distant from it.

In the tradition of Reich, the Jin Shin Do therapist begins at the top of the body and works down, easing the kinks out of the scalp, neck, and shoulders first. That's because Teeguarden believes that relaxation in these areas is crucial to self-expression and free circulation of feelings. Then the therapist's attention continues to move down the body.

As the acu-points are worked, clients are asked to "feel into" the tension and discover what the body is trying to tell them. Verbal counseling continues throughout.

"It's a back-and-forth process," says Teeguarden. "Physical tension reflects psychological stress level and anxiety. Working the spots brings up emotional material. The release allows for resolution and replacement with more pleasant feelings.

"Acupressure is just a tool," she adds. "The thing that does the work is the person's own mind and spirit. But when the body and mind are uncomfortable, people are not able to access those inner resources."

How Often? Only You Know

How often clients go for a Jin Shin Do session depends upon what they're after.

"I like, personally, to work in a way that leaves up to the client how often, how many sessions," says Teeguarden. "Ultimately, I want to get the person in touch with the core self, which is wise, capable, lovable, and loving. That self knows the answer to a whole lot of things, including what kind of therapy is going to be most useful and how often."

Sessions tend to cost anywhere from $30 to $75 each, depending upon the going rate in the locale and the experience of the practitioner. Some practitioners have sliding scale fees to make the therapy more accessible.

Teeguarden's training institute offers three levels of mastery: basic, intermediate, and advanced. Registered practitioners who complete the basic course must have undertaken 125 hours or more of training and experience and must have undergone ten sessions themselves.

For more information, contact the Jin Shin Do Foundation for Bodymind Acupressure, P.O. Box 1097, Felton, CA 95018, or call (408) 338-9454.

For information on related therapies, see the entries on Acupressure, beginning on page 243, and Reichian Therapy, beginning on page 321.

MUSIC

★★★★★

Patients at the Kaiser Permanente Medical Center in Los Angeles have a choice. When in pain, they can either turn to prescriptions or turn on their portable tape players for 20 minutes of soothing harp music and guided relaxation. Some of the center's doctors even "prescribe" the music tape instead of painkillers and tranquilizers. It is being used before cardiac surgery, during chemotherapy, and for patients with chronic back pain and crippling spinal injuries. In the hospital's outpatient stress-management center, the same music and relaxation training is used to treat many stress-related illnesses—including high blood pressure, migraine headaches, and ulcers.

"Difficulty in relaxing is a common problem in many illnesses," says Dr. David Walker, one of Kaiser Permanente's psychiatrists, specializing in behavioral medicine. "It's not unusual at all for people who are having surgery, or who have been told they have cancer, to stay awake late into the night, obsessed with what is happening to them. Relaxation is universally therapeutic, and people who can learn to relax deeply can create a better state of mind for getting well.

"Just knowing they have a way to reduce the anxiety helps. We tell them to use this any time they need it—just before they are wheeled into the operating room, or even as the doctors are talking to them. They can replay the tape in their minds, even if they can't listen to it, and get the same results."

Kaiser Permanente is one of several facilities across the United States using music as a way to reduce stress, relieve pain, and personalize the often anxious, sterile hospital environment. Others include the University of Massachusetts Medical Center in Worcester, Beth Israel Hospital in Boston, and Hahnemann University Hospital in Philadelphia.

These hospitals are using music for everything from helping couples celebrate the birth of a baby to aiding a child prepare for heart catheterization, from enabling a stroke victim to learn to speak again to evoking the memories of a lifetime as someone prepares for death.

"Music is a marvelous and extremely powerful tool," says Nancy Hunt, a St. Louis music therapist who works in both a childbirth center and a hospice. "Music has a direct physiological effect on people.

It increases blood volume, decreases and helps stabilize heart rate, and lowers blood pressure. And psychologically, it does a whole lot. It can make us relax, or remember, or to have all sorts of feelings. It all depends on what we project onto the music."

Perhaps this is the biggest part of music's magic—that it can transform an environment by changing our own state of mind.

"We get a lot of patients here who have been through a number of different referrals," says Dr. Stephen Kibrick, the clinical psychologist who directs Kaiser Permanente's stress-management program and who developed the tapes.

"We have cancer patients and other patients with chronic pain who are going through a lot of distressing treatments. We give them a tape and a little player and a set of headphones and they find that it not only relieves the intensity of the pain, it helps them to calm their minds and relax their bodies."

Burn patients, in the hospital for weeks or months, have a difficult time because they are often in pain as their burns heal. "These people often can't be kept on drugs all the time," Dr. Kibrick says. "This kind of music and relaxation instruction has proven very effective in helping them stay in a relatively calm, relaxed state while undergoing treatment."

A 57-minute-long University of Massachusetts Medical Center television program take its viewers through what is called mindfulness meditation, says Dr. Jon Kabat-Zinn, director of the hospital's stress-reduction and relaxation department. "The tape teaches people to pay attention to their bodies, the quality of their breathing, the sensations in their bodies, the music, and their thoughts as the thoughts move through their minds."

The end result, he says, is a state of detachment from, and relaxed observation of, the body—a state particularly useful if one is experiencing pain. He chose to have musical accompaniment for this tape, he says, because he theorizes that the meditation instructions would be more accessible to the patients within the flow established by the music. And he chose harp music, he says, because "the harp has traditionally been an instrument for healing and calming the mind."

Dr. Kabat-Zinn's intent was to make available to all the hospital's patients (and its doctors) a relaxation program based on his eight-week outpatient training at the hospital's stress-reduction center. Of the 20 percent of the hospital's patients who have already used the relaxation tape, 80 percent have found it beneficial.

Dr. Kabat-Zinn plans to begin formal controlled studies of kidney-dialysis and cardiac-care patients to determine exact physical and psychological responses to the tape.

A Long Tradition

These contemporary uses of music may be new, but traditionally music has had a long and strong connection with medicine. The philosopher Pythagoras prescribed a daily regimen of music to wake up by, to work by, and to relax and sleep by. Ancient physicians used music to regulate the heartbeat, and from the Renaissance through the nineteenth century, music and singing were used as a cure for "melancholy" and to bring the body's mysterious "vapours" into balance.

In the nineteenth and twentieth centuries, medical "progress" in anesthetics and painkillers left music far behind. It wasn't until the late 1950s that it started to be used again in the form of "dentist office music"—bland, mindless tunes that attempted to camouflage the nerve-racking whine of the dentist's drill and distract the distraught patient.

Since then, however, the medical use of music has grown steadily, often in conjunction with other alternative medical practices like biofeedback and hypnosis.

Just how music works its wonders is something researchers are only beginning to understand. Both its physical and psychological responses involve complex brain chemistry changes, not only in the "thinking" part of our brain, but in our "emotional" brain, the limbic system, and the "primitive" brain, the brain stem, which controls heartbeat, respiration, and muscle tension.

Therapists like Janalea Hoffman of Kansas City, Missouri, say you need to combine the music "with the mental awareness of what is going on in your body" and that most people must be trained to do that.

In her graduate study at the University of Kansas, she used visual imagery and music to teach 60 people to lower their blood pressures an average of 10 to 20 points. She uses the same techniques to help people with heart arrhythmias and migraine headaches, using music with a 60-beats-per-minute tempo, which is the ideal, or relaxed, heart rate.

How does music work to help reduce the perception of pain and to create a positive state of mind?

One theory is that some kinds of music can produce in the brain the same "feel good" chemicals that running and meditation produce. These are called endorphins, natural opiates secreted by the hypothalamus, which can reduce the intensity with which we feel pain.

The one thing music therapists do agree on is that more research must be done. Because music does work, even if many of its effects have yet to be documented.

Georgia Kelly, whose lilting, free-flowing harp music has been used in several medical tapes, including the University of Massachusetts's and Kaiser Permanente's, says she didn't realize the potential of her music until people began to write to her that they were playing it during childbirth, in the operating room, and to relax and fall asleep.

"A Place without Pain"

"I feel my music takes the mind to another place," she says. "It helps you to move away from identifying with your body, and in doing that it is calming. It reduces your awareness of pain. It puts your mind someplace else for a while, in a place where there is no pain—psychic or physical."

At Hahnemann University Hospital, Cynthia Briggs, director of music therapy, helps young patients to choose music that will be played for them while they undergo heart catheterization. "We use everything from Sesame Street to Neil Diamond." she says. "It's a way to personalize the experience, and, hopefully, to make things more pleasant." Although the children's physical responses have not been monitored, Briggs says the surgeons performing the procedure have been extremely happy with the children's reactions.

At the Charing Cross Hospital in London, patients who opt for spinal rather than general anesthesia for certain kinds of surgery, like hip replacement, are given headphones and music to block out the noises of drilling and sawing.

Perhaps one of the more joyful ways music has been used in medicine is in childbirth and delivery. Music therapist Hunt uses musical cues as part of her program to teach couples relaxation methods during childbirth.

For a child's birth, she prepares an 8- to 21-hour tape that includes some of the songs the couple has learned to relax to, along with others of their choice. She says the theme from *Chariots of Fire* is particularly popular during the pushing stages of the delivery, and that for the celebration of the birth she has been asked to include everything from "Isn't She Lovely?" by Stevie Wonder to "For unto Us a Child Is Born" from Handel's *Messiah.*

Hunt also works in a hospice, where she uses music to help terminally ill patients resolve their feelings toward death and talk with their family members. In what she calls life review, she will play songs that were popular during the time the patient was most active—during courtship and early marriage, perhaps during a war.

"I use songs that are like mileposts in their lives," she says. Such music often evokes strong memories and facilitates heartfelt communication between loved ones. Many times, too, she will do something as simple and effective as sitting at someone's bedside and singing with them the old favorite church hymns they may

have learned as children. "Amazing Grace," "The Old Rugged Cross," and "In the Garden" are songs requested over and over again, she says. "They give real comfort."

And therapist Hoffman uses music to help people express their grief over a death. "Music elicits imagery in people," she says. "The best way to say how it works is that you are helping someone to have a dream in a waking state. And dreams help to work out subconscious things, so it is very useful."

Some music seems to induce the same kinds of images in many people, she says. For instance, she often uses Richard Strauss's "Death and Transfiguration," with its plaintive oboes, bassoons, flutes, and harps, to help people feel their buried grief.

Finding the Right Music

Both Georgia Kelly and Dr. Steve Halpern, a California composer and music-therapy researcher, say a personal library of music can enhance your environment and your health. They suggest you use your public library and local record stores to experiment with different kinds of music, old and new.

If you are looking for music to relax by, Dr. Halpern suggests you watch your breathing. If the music helps you to breathe slower and deeper, it is relaxing you. If you find yourself experiencing pain, particularly in your chest area, neck, or shoulders, it could be the music, he contends. He says bad rock music is the usual culprit, but also suggests you watch out for some classical music such as Tchaikovsky's "Pathetique."

288

"Just watch your body and see how you feel," he says. "Allow the music to be your center of attention. Try to sit down or lie down, but even if you can't, do notice how you are feeling. The bottom line with any music is your personal response.

"Get music you can pick and choose according to your mood, so when you want some rousing music or dance music or emotionally uplifting music, you have it right there. So you don't have to play what is called radio roulette, which is just turning on the radio and hoping you'll hear a good song."

Kelly suggests the usually slow, second movement of some classical pieces. Many baroque pieces—by composers such as Bach, Handel, Telemann—have parts with 60-beats-per-minute tempos. And she suggests you avoid music where the musical phrasing is forced to follow a mechanically produced beat, as it is in much popular dance music. "Unless you are moving with the music, it can be very disturbing," she says. And for any piece of music, she says, "the individual performance can make all the difference."

Don't think that only classical music is beneficial. Both also suggest jazz, blues, some popular music, electronic synthesizer, even rock 'n' roll, as long as you know your body is responding the way you want it to, by being relaxed, or energized, or whatever.

For starters among the classics, they suggest: Beethoven's "Fifth Symphony," anything by Bach, but particularly his "Mass in B Minor," Mozart's "The Vespers," Schubert's "Ave Maria," Schumann's "E-Flat Major Symphony," and Dvořák's "New World Symphony."

And don't forget that memories associated with music can be powerful mood setters. If "Begin the Beguine" still knocks your socks off, or if Wayne Newton makes you drool, why not have them there any time you want them? Music is energy, just like food, Dr. Halpern says. "Having the right music around the house is as important as having the right food and the right vitamins."

Sources of Soothing Sound

Most music therapists recommend that people with medical problems like high blood pressure who want to use music to relax, first train with a therapist. For information on music-based relaxation programs near you, contact the National Association for Music Therapy, 1001 Connecticut Avenue NW, Suite 800, Washington, DC 20036.

The University of Massachusetts Medical Center has an eight-week stress-management program for patients referred by their doctors. Its videotape is for rent or sale to other hospitals. Contact William Stickley, Center for Educational Resources, University of Massachusetts Medical Center, 55 Lake Avenue N, Worcester, MA 01605.

Kaiser Permanente Medical Center's tapes are available to its health-plan members in Southern California, but other tapes by Dr. Kibrick are available through Self-Health Cassettes, 16661 Ventura Boulevard, Suite 822, Encino, CA 91436.

For more information on Kelly's music, write to Heru Records, Box 954, Topanga, CA 92090.

For a catalog of Dr. Halpern's music, write to Halpern Sounds, 1775 Old Country Road, Suite 9, Belmont, CA 94002.

Heaven on Earth, 803 Fourth Street, San Raphael, CA 94901, is a recording company for a number of West Coast artists involved in therapeutic music. Write for a free catalog and sample tape (there's a fee for the tape).

The Institute for Consciousness and Music offers a Music Rx package of five cassettes. Their address is ICM West, Box 173, Port Townsend, WA 98368.

Hoffman has put together a tape of 60-beats-per-minute baroque piano music of her own composition. These are available through Mellow Minds, Box 6431, Shawnee Mission, KS 66206.

For information on behavior-change, stress-management, and optimal-performance tapes, contact Dr. Emmett Miller, c/o Source, Box W, Stanford, CA 94305.

NAPRAPATHY

★ ★

After the long car drive, the slight, dull pain that's almost always present in your back is feeling particularly troublesome. You sit stiffly on the chair in Dr. Robert Burg's Pennsylvania office. A doctor of naprapathy, he begins by asking you a series of pointed questions. Many are similar to those you'd be asked in any doctor's office, but others seem to be much more to the point. "Exactly where is the pain?" "When did the pain first start?" "Does your mother remember you having it when you were very young?" "What kind of pain is it: Does it ache or radiate? Is it sore or sharp?"

Next, he asks you to bend in all directions as he watches your spine and your hips. How flexible are you? Does each vertebra move on its own, or do a few move as a unit? Are your legs the same length? He gathers more data.

There's no sense of hurry or judgment as Dr. Burg, who asks you to call him Bob, questions you. Moments later, however, you are lying face down on a massage table wearing a green cotton robe that's open in back.

Hands That See, Hands That Heal

As he begins to touch your back, encouraging you to relax completely and let him move your body, you realize that this is not to be your typical massage. He's still gathering data.

You provide the feedback as he asks, "Does it hurt when I touch here?" "Tell me if anything feels particularly good or relieving." "Try to pull your arm down toward the table while I hold it back."

"I see with my hands," says Dr. Burg, explaining his technique. "I start working the tissues with my hands and when I feel limitations, I try to increase the range of motion in those areas."

Dr. Burg watches your muscles as you pull against his hold, and tests each of your joints with his hands. He reaches under your leg and lifts it back. He pulls back on your right arm and shoulder until you are nearly lying on your back. Whenever he finds a joint that isn't as flexible in one direction as the other, or is less flexible than the same joint on your other side, he gently stretches it, coaxing it to relax and release its tension.

"Stretching is the most important thing you can do structurally," he comments. "Building up muscle mass is less important. Very few people need a whole lot of muscle in their lives, but they do need structural integrity."

Nothing he does is really painful— every stretch, push, and pull is gentle. The only discomfort is at places where your muscles or tissues are already sensitive or sore. Once you stop worrying about *how* he's going to touch you, you begin to become concerned about *where* he's going to touch. But soon you relax, realizing that his treatment will be confined to your back and shoulders, legs, arms and hands, and neck and face.

He touches all the vertebrae on your back, pausing to massage the ones that hurt. It's sore under your shoulder blade, and so he spends a long time working there.

The data gathering, the massage of sore points, and what naprapaths call stretchment of inflexible areas, extends down your arms and legs and on to your hands and feet.

A Balanced Body Is a Healthy Body

Naprapaths believe that tensions in the connective tissues of the body, triggered by stress or trauma, cause the tissues to contract and move out of balance. This imbalance gets in the way of good circulation, nerve conduction, and lymphatic drainage, explains Dr. Burg, who is a former member of the board of trustees and former naprapathic department chairman at the Chicago National College of Naprapathy, the only school of naprapathy in the United States.

"Connective tissue is everywhere, and if it is out of balance, you'll have sickness," he says. "If, on the other hand, the body is structurally healthy, it will be able to take care of itself."

Later, you lie on your back, while Dr. Burg checks how flexible your neck is, lifts your arms, and massages your shoulders.

After 2 hours, the session is over. "I always spend 1½ or 2 hours the first time someone visits me," he explains. "After that, sessions cost $50 instead of the first-visit charge of $60, and they tend to be shorter." Other naprapaths often charge about half what he does, and spend about half the time with each client, he points out.

Once you're dressed again, Dr. Burg returns to the small, plant-decorated office, and explains what went on. "Your right shoulder is pulled forward for some reason. That's why I worked your right shoulder back so far; I was trying to stretch the connective tissue holding your shoulder blade.

"Also, your right side needs stretching in comparison to your left. The left side is more flexible and stretched out." You feel a sudden flash of recognition and intuitive agreement. Had he said your left side needed stretching you know you would have disagreed.

Dr. Burg recommends some stretching exercises, expecially tailored to your body, and explains that he doesn't know how much effect one treatment will have. Most people feel relief from back or neck

291

292

pain with three or four treatments, he says. Others prefer to maintain their health by seeing a naprapath regularly—once a month or less frequently—over a period of years.

What Is Naprapathy?

The word *naprapathy* (nuh-PRAH-pathy) comes from the Czechoslovakian word *napravit,* which means "to correct or fix," combined with the Greek word *pathos,* which means "suffering." So naprapathy means "to correct suffering." Practitioners of this hands-on healing system manipulate the muscles, tendons, and ligaments of the body in order to alleviate tension and promote fluidity of motion, according to Dr. Burg. Many naprapaths also make dietary recommendations because they believe that the chemistry of the body must, like its connective tissues, be in balance.

Developed by a chiropractor named Oakley Smith in 1905, naprapathy bears a great resemblance to chiropractic. But chiropractors do *bone* alignment, explains Chicago naprapath Jacquelin S. McCord. "The advantage of naprapathy is that we do connective tissue manipulation. So while chiropractors just promote nerve conduction, we promote nerve conduction *and* improved circulation."

In 1905, Smith founded the Chicago College of Naprapathy. The school has since separated into two schools, reunited itself back into one school called the Chicago National College of Naprapathy, and is now approved by the Illinois Board of Higher Education to grant a Doctor of Naprapathy degree.

All naprapaths are trained in Chicago,

at the School of Naprapathy in Sweden, where the field is widely accepted and popular, or at a new college in Spain. During the four-year academic program, students learn naprapathic theory and technique, a full range of biological sciences, and nutrition. The final year they work in a supervised clinic.

Because the field is relatively small, the practice of naprapathy is still flexible. In fact, it has changed considerably over the past 50 years. About 40 years ago dietary recommendations were added to the practice, and neuromuscular methods picked up from other types of body therapists followed in recent years. As a result, each naprapath you visit could have a slightly different focus or way of treating you.

Some naprapaths do "mono-treatments," focusing on just one part of the body or a particular problem. Others, like Dr. Burg, do whole-body treatments, either to correct problems, or for prevention. It's important to ask a naprapath which approach he or she follows before making an appointment.

"I do a whole-body treatment," Dr. Burg explains, "because I've never found where a particular problem ends. If you have a cervical problem, for example, I could just treat your neck. But if I don't also change the balance in the rest of your body, the connective tissues in your neck will just go back to the way they were before."

The large majority of naprapaths work in the Chicago area. But to find a naprapath in your area, you can contact the Chicago National College of Naprapathy, 3330 North Milwaukee Avenue, Chicago, IL 60641, or call (312) 282-2686.

The Healing Power of Naprapathy

Most naprapaths maintain that their method of healing may be helpful for all physical problems. The theory is that a body with unobstructed nerve conduction, lymphatic drainage, and blood circulation will be healthier. If you aren't healthy, then the physical structure will also reflect this. Just as obstructions and tension in the connective tissues could cause back or neck pain, they could also contribute to liver disorders or a weak heart, say naprapaths.

"You could have an infected kidney, for instance," says Dr. Burg. "An M.D. would kill the germ in the kidney that is infecting it. We ask, 'Why did the germ get in there in the first place?' If the kidney tissues were truly healthy, the germ couldn't infect it.

"Or maybe you have an ulcer," he continues. "You could take medicine to coat the ulcerated lining of your stomach. But we think that you'll be better off if you correct the problem that led to the stomach lining losing its natural protection. To do that, we determine if contracted muscles and ligaments are irritating nerves that lead to the area, or are blocking good circulation somehow. When we reduce the structural pressure and get the body back into balance, it will often heal itself."

Most people see naprapaths to alleviate body pain—usually back or neck pain, and Dr. Burg says he is most successful treating those problems. But sometimes there are happy surprises, as well. "I get lots of patients with sports injuries, or knee or neck pain, and I help them, usually quickly and easily," he says. "Some of them, though, find that the treatments have relieved their allergies or asthma, too."

NEUROLINGUISTIC PROGRAMMING

★

Neurolinguistic Programming (NLP) is attracting much attention as a method that promises lasting cures in very little time, sometimes just a session or two. People who teach the method claim it can cure phobias in an hour, eliminate unwanted habits, change the dynamics of relationships, and relieve physical problems.

But it's incorrect to call NLP a therapy. Its creators see it as a model for understanding how human beings communicate and learn. As such, it has "tremendous implications" for business, sales training, educational institutions, and clinical practice, claims Dot Feldman, counselor, consultant, and former president of the national NLP organization.

No two therapists use NLP in exactly the same way. But they follow a basic framework. For instance, NLP teaches therapists to match their speech patterns — the words, rhythm, intonation, and metaphor — to the client's. If a client's dominant sense is visual, the therapist may suggest she "reframe that image" or "see the big picture." But if the client is kinestheti-

cally oriented, he may be asked his "gut reaction" to something or directed to get "a full grasp" of the problem.

Or, the therapist may pace her speech so that her rhythm follows a client's absentminded opening and closing of his fist. NLP teaches therapists to use the available clues to enter the client's world as completely as possible.

The other thing therapists can do, once they determine a client's dominant sense, is to refine their understanding of precisely how that sense colors the client's experience. "You find other useful distinctions, for example, by asking 'how do you visualize?,' " says Steven Leeds, a New York area therapist who has masters level NLP training. "Let's say the problem is that someone intimidates you. Well, how do you picture them? How close are they? How big? Is your picture light or dark?

"You can teach someone to have control over how they visualize. They can make the person smaller or move them away, or make the image still and put it in a frame," he says. "This takes out the intensity and discomfort and teaches people to use their own brains, to be active in their perceptions."

NLP's tactics are derived from several fundamental assumptions.

1. Each one of us has the resources inside to get what we want and need.

2. The mind and body is one cybernetic system.

3. Every behavior originates because of a positive intention. (The way to loosen the hold destructive behaviors have on you is to recognize what the original, positive intention was and find other more positive ways to achieve the same result.)

4. There is no such thing as failure, only feedback. Every experience offers information about how you can develop and grow.

5. People are responsible for the results of their communication. If your communication style isn't producing the desired result, how can you adjust it to be more effective?

6. All of the above presuppositions are true only to the extent that they're useful.

"NLP isn't just about becoming aware, but once you become aware, how to change," says Leeds.

He used NLP with a couple who came to see him because they weren't getting anywhere when they talked. He watched closely and saw that when the man leaned forward and pointed his finger, the woman got really upset. Her breathing changed, her face flushed with anger, and her voice got progressively louder. That made the man so angry he jabbed his finger even more.

"I asked them if that was the response they wanted," says Leeds. "It wasn't. I pointed out to them that they were more aware of their feelings than their behavior. And it was their behavior that was triggering the other person."

Leeds knew the man practiced T'ai Chi, so he asked the man to take a T'ai Chi stance as he talked to the woman. "She calmed down, although the content of their conversation was the same," says Leeds. "NLP explores the form, as opposed to the content. It's looking at how to change the form of the communication. The form is powerful. Usually, what we're not paying attention to is what's messing us up."

With another client, a woman who realized she was excessively jealous and insecure around her boyfriend, Leed used her current feelings to take her back to the source of the problem.

He directed "Cindy" to let herself really feel the jealousy and insecurity she often experiences. Then he suggested that she use those feelings like a thread to take her back to another time she felt that way. Cindy remembered what it was like for her as a child, when her parents' marriage broke up and her father left.

Leeds told Cindy her feelings were an appropriate response to that situation. He asked her what the younger Cindy needed at the time. "A sense of security," she told him.

"I had her give that sense of security to herself, by getting in touch with her adult feelings of self-confidence. We created a multi-sensory experience where she could see the younger self, talk to and touch the child. I had her tell that younger self, 'I'm from your future. You're going to be okay.' "

Leeds did the work in a 1½-hour session. One regression proved to be effective in this case, Leeds says, although the process "often needs to be done with a number of experiences until the younger self really feels secure."

Leeds checks his work by taking the client forward into a similiar future situation. He had Cindy visualize herself at a party, where her boyfriend had wandered away from her. Leeds had her describe what she was experiencing.

"The therapist makes sure the person is feeling secure and comfortable," he says. "If not, more work is needed."

NLP was devised in the early 1970s by a group of people, including John Grinder, a well-known linguist, and Richard Bandler, a mathematician who became interested in psychotherapy.

Grinder's understanding of linguistics formed the core of NLP. Around this core, the group added techniques based on what they observed in other successful therapists. They were most influenced by Virginia Satir, a well-respected family therapist; Milton Erickson, an unconventional hypnotherapist; and Fritz Perls, the founder of Gestalt therapy.

What emerged was not a therapy but a model for studying the structure of subjective experience, says Feldman. From this model, the founders developed several therapeutic techniques. But NLP does not consist of therapeutic techniques above.

"The most remarkable thing for me about NLP is the hopeful, positive way it thinks about human beings," she adds. "There's a belief that people really can change. The second thing I can say,

although I do not subscribe to the idea of the 5-minute cure, is that I haven't found anything in my mind that approaches the speed NLP does.

"I've spent about 20 minutes on certain clients' phobias. Literally, that's been the end," she says. "In a single session, where you're building someone a resource state, I've seen incredible changes across context. Yes, there have been clients I've worked with for several months, but very few I work with for years."

These days, NLP has its own national organization, which is based in Indianapolis. There's an effort underway to standardize the training.

Three levels of training are offered: practitioner, master, and trainer, but course requirements differ from school to school. Leeds say that the course usually takes up to 25 days to complete. There are NLP practitioners in most major cities. How much they charge per session depends partly upon their background, and the cost of competitive therapies in the region.

If you're looking for an NLP practitioner, Feldman cautions that you choose someone with a clinicial license. While "there are some competent practitioners who are not clinicians, I'd choose someone with a clinical degree," she says.

Leeds advises people to interview their proposed therapist. "Ask yourself: Do I feel like this person is respecting my model of the world? Is the way I perceive things respected by this person?"

For more information or a referral, contact the National Association for Neurolinguistic Programming, 310 North Alabama Street, Suite A100, Indianapolis, IN 46204, or call (317) 636-6059.

PET THERAPY

★★★★

It's exercise hour at the Tacoma Lutheran Home in the state of Washington and P. T., an exotic yellow-crested bird called a cockatiel, is having the time of his life. He's sitting on the foot of 81-year-old Ben Ereth, riding in circles while Ereth pedals vigorously on an exercise bicycle. The bird likes it so much that if Ereth stops too soon, he'll squawk at him.

A bizarre sort of activity to find in a nursing home? Not at Tacoma Lutheran. Three years ago, the nursing home adopted an angora rabbit. Then a puppy. Then tropical birds. The home's elderly residents have taken to these animals with a passion. And, says Virginia Davis, director of resident services, the animals have breathed enthusiasm into what otherwise might have been a listless nursing-home atmosphere.

"The animals help in several ways," says Davis. "One of the cockatiels gives a wolf whistle whenever anyone passes its cage. That gives them an unexpected boost in morale. And the birds seem to alleviate the tension associated with exercise. They make exercise more acceptable and relaxing."

What's happening at Tacoma Lutheran is just one example of an increasingly popular phenomenon called pet therapy. Although humans have adopted pets for thousands of years, only recently have social scientists taken a close look at the nature of the relationships that people form with dogs, cats, and other companion animals.

At places like the Center for the Interaction of Animals and Society, in Philadelphia, and the Center for the Study of Human Animal Relationships and Environments (CENSHARE), in Minneapolis, they've discovered that there is something mutually therapeutic about those relationships. They say that pets relax us, help us communicate with each other, build our self-esteem, and comfort us when we're feeling down.

In fact, many now believe that pets play a small but very significant role in determining how well, for example, a heart-attack survivor recuperates, how a family

298

handles domestic strife, whether a disturbed teenager grows up straight, or even whether a nursing-home resident like Ben Ereth enjoys and sticks to his daily exercycle program.

Pets, in short, may affect our health.

The modern history of pet therapy began in the late 1950s and can be traced through three landmark events.

The first occurred in 1959, when Dr. Boris M. Levinson, the late New York child psychiatrist, happened to have his pet dog, Jingles, with him when a patient paid an unexpected visit. Before anyone knew it, the dog ran up to the patient, a young boy, and licked his face. At that instant, the boy broke out of his usually impregnable withdrawal and started playing with the dog. Eventually the boy warmed up to Dr. Levinson, who went on to use pets as icebreakers in his practice and to publish a book, *Pet-Oriented Child Psychotherapy*, in 1969.

The next major event in the field was also serendipitous. In the mid-1970s at Ohio State University, Dr. Samuel A. Corson, psychologist, kept a kennel for the dogs he was using for behavioral studies. Mental patients in the adjoining hospital heard the dogs barking and insisted on seeing them. Visits were arranged, and the trust and affection that developed between the patients and the dogs enabled some of the patients to trust their doctors.

Then, in 1980, the third and possibly the most influential discovery took place. While interviewing a group of heart-attack survivors, University of Pennsylvania researchers Dr. Aaron Katcher, Dr. Erika Friedmann, and others unexpectedly found that people with pets lived longer after their attacks than those without pets. Soon after, they discovered a link between pet ownership and blood pressure.

The lessons of these discoveries, according to those who made them, were that, in simplest terms, companion animals have two powerful assets—they help people communicate with each other and they help people relax.

Animal Magnetism at Work

Pet therapists have put these capacities to work in a variety of ways. Pet therapy is very often used, for example, to combat the isolation and loneliness so common in nursing homes. At the Tacoma Lutheran Home, Davis has found that the pets help many residents break their customary silence.

"Animals are a catalyst for conversation," she says. "Most people can remember a story from their past about a pet animal. And people are more comfortable talking to animals than they are to people. Sometimes a person who hasn't spoken for a long time, or who has had a stroke and doesn't talk, will talk to an animal."

Animals also seem to draw everyone into the conversation. "Even in a nursing home there are some people who are more attractive or responsive than others," says Phil Arkow, of the Humane Society of the Pike's Peak Region in Colorado, who drives a "Petmobile" to local nursing homes. "Human visitors try not to do it, but they inevitably focus on those who are most attractive. But animals don't make those distinctions. They focus on everyone equally."

A person doesn't have to live in a nursing home, however, in order to reap the benefits of a pet. Pets typically influence the communication that goes on between family members in a normal household. During a research project a few years ago, Dr. Ann Cain, University of Maryland professor, discovered that pets help spouses and siblings express highly charged feelings.

"When family members want to say something to each other that they can't say directly," Dr. Cain says, "they might say it to the pet and let the other person overhear it. That also lets the listener off the hook, because he doesn't have to respond directly."

She also found that many people talk to and even confide in their pets. "I would ask people who they felt closest to in the family. Very often they said that it was the pet. One woman told me that her pet is like a psychiatrist she doesn't have to pay." Pets can even stop quarrels. "During family arguments, one woman used to say, 'Stop fighting, you're upsetting the dog.'"

Though it's still in the experimental stage, researchers are discovering that watching or petting friendly animals—not only dogs and cats but almost any pet— can produce the kind of deep relaxation usually associated with meditation, biofeedback, and hypnosis. Pets are apparently so good at this that they can actually lower blood pressure.

At the Center for the Interaction of Animals and Society, for instance, researchers Katcher and Friedmann monitored the blood pressures of healthy children while the children were sitting quietly or reading aloud either with or without a dog in the room. Their blood pressures were always lower when the dog was in the room.

The researchers went on to discover, remarkably, that looking at fish could temporarily reduce blood pressures of patients with hypertension. In one widely reported study, they found that the systolic and diastolic pressure of people with high blood pressures dipped into the normal range when they gazed at an aquarium full of colorful tropical fish, green plants, and rocks for 20 minutes.

This calming power of pets has found at least a few noteworthy applications. In Chicago, one volunteer from the Anti-Cruelty Society took an animal to a hospital and arranged for a surgical patient to be greeted by it when he awoke from anesthesia. "It's a comforting way to come back to reality," says one volunteer. "For children, pets can make a hospital seem safer. It's a reminder of home."

Animals may also have the power to soften the aggressive tendencies of disturbed adolescents. At Winslow Therapeutic Riding Unlimited, in Warwick, New York, where horseback riding is used to help handicapped children of all kinds, problem teenagers seem to behave differently when they're put on a horse.

"These are the kids who fight in school. Some of their fathers are alcoholics," says Mickey Pulis of the nonprofit facility. "But when they come here they're different. When they groom and tack the horses, they learn about the gentle and caring side of life.

"The horse seems to act like an equalizer," she says. "It doesn't care what reading levels these kids are at. It accepts them as they are."

Ultimately, researchers like Dr.

Friedmann believe that the companionship of pets can reduce a person's risk of dying from stress-related illnesses, such as heart disease.

"The leading causes of mortality and morbidity in the United States are stress-related or lifestyle-related," she says. "Pets, by decreasing the level of arousal and moderating the stress response, can help slow the progression of those diseases or even prevent them."

Pets Are Touching

But what is it about pets that makes them capable of all this? And why do millions of people go to the trouble and expense of keeping them? Pet therapists offer several answers.

For one thing, animals don't talk back to us. Researchers have discovered that a person's blood pressure goes up whenever he talks to another person. But we talk to animals in a different way, often touching them at the same time, which minimizes stress.

Another theory holds that pets remind us of our ancestral link with other animals. "By domesticating an animal, man demonstrates his kinship to nature," Dr. Levinson wrote. "A human being has to remain in contact with all of nature throughout his lifetime if he is to maintain good mental health."

Dr. Corson, on the other hand, says that we love pets because they are perpetual infants. Human infants charm us but they eventually grow up. Pets never do. They never stop being cuddly and dependent. Likewise, pets are faithful. "Pets can offer a relationship that is more con-stant than relationships with people," says Dr. Cain. "You can count on them."

Some argue that the most important ingredient in our relationships with animals is that we can touch them whenever we want to. "Having access to affectionate touch that is not related to sex is important," says Dr. Katcher. "If you want to touch another person, you can't always do it immediately. But with pets you can."

Most advocates of pet therapy are quick to admit that it has limitations. Dr. Friedmann points out that interaction with pets only reduces blood pressure temporarily, and that it is not meant to replace exercise, diet therapy, or medication. "Pets are just one component of care," agrees Dr. Corson. "They're never a substitute for other therapies."

Nor is pet therapy for everyone. "We want to protect the rights of people who don't want contact with animals," says Linda Hines, executive director of the Delta Society, a pet-therapy information clearinghouse in the Seattle area. "And we caution people against choosing inappropriate animals."

The safety of having animals in nursing homes is also being questioned. "We're looking at the incidence of allergies, infections, and injuries associated with having pets in nursing homes," says Dr. R. K. Anderson, director of CENSHARE. "So far, pets appear to be one of the safest things you can do for a nursing-home population."

In other ways, however, the field of pet therapy seems to have very few limits at all. It is expanding rapidly. Chicago's Anti-Cruelty Society, for instance, which takes pets to 22 area hospitals, has a waiting list of 17 more. Meanwhile, at CEN-

SHARE, Dr. Anderson and others are about to distribute a videotape that demonstrates how to initiate pet-therapy programs at a nursing home.

Then there's the research front. The Delta Society, for its part, has been awarding research grants to answer questions like, Do people's attitudes affect their response to animals? And does raising a pet make people good at raising children? At the University of Pennsylvania, research-

ers are studying the expressions on people's faces when they greet animals. And in Washington, D.C., friends of pet therapy are trying to make sure that the government enforces a 1983 law mandating that the elderly residents of an estimated 900,000 federally funded housing units can't be barred from owning pets.

"There's a lot of ferment," says Linda Hines at Delta Society. "It's amazing how many things are happening at once."

301

PLANT THERAPY

★★★

The first thing you see when visiting Jenny's is the plants. A potted Norwegian pine races the spindly avocado to the ceiling. Spider plants dangle a plush yellow-green web over the apartment's picture window.

You'll find Jenny here most days after work, watering or carefully pruning the African violets on the end table, recharging herself after a stress-filled day as a medical social worker. Sometimes she just relaxes on the couch and gazes absent-mindedly at her plants.

But whether diligent or daydreaming, chances are Jenny is forgetting about the patient whose file was lost in the computer and the disagreement she had with her boss. She is letting worries slip away and thinking about how her children like to hike in the woods behind the house, or about the vacation she is planning.

Jenny's plants, like the ones you grow out back or see on your way to work, are a fitting antidote for the high-tech, high-stress rat race. Potted on the windowsill, landscaped around the house, or planted in a city park, trees, flowers, and other vegetation can fascinate us, soften the environment, and subtly remind us of life's natural rhythms.

Dr. Rachel Kaplan, a University of Michigan pyschologist, says that people "resonate to plants." Research by Dr. Kaplan, as well as horticultural therapists, city planners, and others, indicates that plants are excellent tools for helping people focus their lives, become more attuned to natural cycles, and more aware of themselves.

Patrick Horsbrugh, an architect and city planner from Notre Dame, Indiana, calls it phyto-psychotherapy, or "distracting people from whatever their worries and illnesses may be through cultivation of plants.

"There is something marvelous about looking at a plant every morning and seeing it grow," he says.

While many people get into gardening thinking they'll supplement their food supply, the intangible benefits gardening produces are, for many, more worthwhile, according to Dr. Kaplan.

▪ Pruning Away Frustrations

It may feel as though the exercise you are getting planting and weeding the garden or mowing the lawn is breaking your back. But it is also therapeutic, breaking down any frustrations or tension you may be feeling, says Dr. Diane Relf, extension services specialist in home horticulture at Virginia Polytechnic Institute and State University, and one of the founders of the National Council for Therapy and Rehabilitation through Horticulture.

"I remember as a kid I practiced 'horticultural therapy' on myself," says Dr. Relf. "I had a kid brother, and I would get so mad at him. I'd go out into the yard and get the hedge pruners and prune the hedge. Now I've never told anybody what I pretended the hedge was, but by the time I got through pruning the hedge, I wasn't going to hurt my brother anymore. Working with plants, you can do something good, something positive, with the anger and hostility. You are turning it outside instead of turning it in on yourself."

Hard physiological data on horticulture's benefits (such as slowed pulse rate) that would confirm this calming effect are just now beginning to appear, according to Dr. Richard Mattson, horticultural therapist at Kansas State University. "Of course," he says, "anytime you garden, there is a release of nervous tension and rechanneling of anxiety and factors related to stress. There should be some kind of calming process going on mentally, and physically as well."

Lynn Doxon, a master's candidate at Kansas State University, recently studied pulse rate, blood pressure, skin temperature, and other indicators in a group of retarded individuals in horticultural and more traditional rehabilitation workshops.

Doxon says that final analyses show that the subjects were more relaxed in the greenhouse than in the other programs.

Meditating on Greenery

303

The mental pleasures we derive from plants seem to be based in the fascination that they engender, according to Dr. Stephen Kaplan, Dr. Rachel Kaplan's husband and, for more than a decade, her research partner at the University of Michigan.

If you have spent hours happily hypnotizing yourself while raking leaves, or just minutes staring at the cluster of trees below your office window, you know this fascination.

"The basic idea is that there are two kinds of attention," Dr. Stephen Kaplan says, "one that takes effort and one that doesn't. We tend to use the kind that takes effort much of the time," and this may be the cause of much mental fatigue.

"We are eager to rest that effort and attend to things that are inherently interesting, such as plants," he says.

Charles Lewis, horticulturist and administrator of the collections program at the Morton Arboretum in Lisle, Illinois, believes that plants' growth cycles reveal an innate intelligence, a larger force that is controlling them. "In our world, modern, man-made things just happen out of the blue. There is a lack of order. That's why it's nice to work with plants, because it is a situation where there is order, where things are nice and predictable."

Plants are also nonthreatening, according to Lewis. "they can't talk back, they can't bite you, but they *will* respond to what you do for them. A dog can get mad at you and growl, but a plant can't do that. It is totally benign. It doesn't care who you are or what you are. A plant is not interested in human values. You have to work with it according to *nature's* rules."

Roots That Bind

This makes gardens and other plant-scapes great social levelers. "If you go to a community garden you will find working right next to each other all classes of society, and they are getting to know each other," Lewis says. "In the garden it doesn't matter who you are if you grow the best tomato."

Beautification programs sponsored by housing authorities in cities such as Chicago and New York have prompted residents to take more control over their environments, planting in open and unused areas and policing the shared ground, according to Lewis, who first became interested in people's relationships to plants when he was asked to judge a New York Housing Authority contest in 1961.

Lewis was struck by the creative, nurturing effort put into the inner-city gardens. "As a judge, I would come back so full emotionally . . . I was just soaking it up. I realized that emotional gratification was an important part of these gardens," he says.

One plot struck him in particular, a Japanese garden created by the members of a street gang.

"They found out they could change their environment, physically change it, and not only so they would know it, but so everybody who passed would know it," Lewis says.

Gardening is an example of an "active" nature experience, according to Dr. Rachel Kaplan. But getting dirty isn't necessary in order to enjoy plants; "observing" and "conceptual" experiences may prove as beneficial, she says.

Just viewing scenes of vegetation can "significantly improve" emotional states, according to studies recently completed at the University of Delaware. That work shows that people have a consistent preference for views including nature rather than those showing only man-made elements.

POETRY

★★★★

In 1882, a young British physician named Robert Seymour Bridges shocked his London colleagues when he gave up medicine to practice poetry. "I will be what God made me," he explained in a poem he penned at the time, "The Growth of Love." "My toil is for man's joy, his joy my own."

If Dr. Bridges's career change was a gamble, he won. He was appointed poet laureate of England in 1913. More people were touched by his poems than might ever have felt the touch of his stethoscope. Today, his poems still bring people joy — and health. Poetry is one of the latest tools of the health professions. Dr. Bridges was simply a specialist ahead of his time.

Nowadays, poetry is used in fields as diverse as mental health and dentistry. Poetry is helping the stressed to relax, the stricken to recover, and the psychotic to relate. A new breed of psychotherapist, the poetry therapist, is dispensing verses that may work better than Valium. Whether a person is mildly depressed by everyday cares or traumatized by rape or cancer, help is available through the poetic prescription.

And nationwide, in mental hospitals, drug-abuse clinics, and prisons, poetry is helping the severely disturbed to face reality. This application seems ironic, because people have an initial tendency to look at a poem as a thing apart from reality. "The truth is that poetry is, in fact, one of the most effective 'grounding' mechanisms that exists," according to Dr. Jack J. Leedy, psychiatrist and author. Working with numerous agencies in New York City, Dr. Leedy has seen "addicts go from being hooked on heroin to being hooked on Hopkins, Herrick, and Homer." In responding to the words of a poem, the patient learns his problems are universal; that somebody — even a long-dead English poet — understands. Fear and rage no longer loom as monsters about to engulf him, but may be seen for what they are: all-too-human emotions.

"Poetry may be utilized in reflecting the inner turbulent mental state experienced by the patient. Thus the inner becomes the outer, or the conscious, making it tangible and workable," explains W. Douglas Hitchings, therapist and contributor to Dr. Leedy's books *Poetry Therapy*

305

and *Poetry the Healer.* When depressed patients are given poems to read, they will often "open up" and start talking about their own emotions while they are talking about a poem.

The Road Not Taken

Two roads diverged in a yellow wood,
And sorry I could not travel both
And be one traveler, long I stood
And looked down one as far as I could
To where it bent in the undergrowth;

Then took the other, as just as fair,
And having perhaps the better claim,
Because it was grassy and wanted wear;
Though as for that the passing there
Had worn them really about the same,

And both that morning equally lay
In leaves no step had trodden black.
Oh, I kept the first for another day!
Yet knowing how way leads on to way,
I doubted if I should ever come back.

I shall be telling this with a sigh
Somewhere ages and ages hence:
Two roads diverged in a wood, and I—
I took the one less traveled by,
And that has made all the difference.

—Robert Frost

Warming Up to Frost

"Something there is that doesn't love a wall," wrote poet Robert Frost. And, says certified poetry therapist Joy Shieman, poetry is one such thing. "Poetry tears down walls, whether they exist between people or within ourselves."

Shieman is director of the poetry ther-apy program at El Camino Hospital, in Mountain View, California. One of the most useful poems in her work is Robert Frost's classic "The Road Not Taken." It is a poem about indecision, an affliction that all of us have experienced at some point in our lives. One depressed woman, after reading it, was able to face the conflicting demands of her husband and job. Another poet prominent in Shieman's work is the late Loren Eiseley, who was also respected as an anthropologist. One of Eiseley's poems, "The Face of the Lion," has been especially useful.

"It is a poem about a stuffed toy that Eiseley held as a child, in the dark when no help ever came," Shieman explains. "In the poem, he confesses how he, grown to be a great man of science, is humble enough to keep the toy, is human enough to still find comfort in its shoe-button eyes, which stare at him from the bookshelf over his desk."

Reading this poem often leads into a discussion of strength, for which the lion provides an excellent metaphor. Sheiman, whose list of clients has even included truck drivers, says, "Men respond to this poem because it builds their self-esteem and allows them to accept a part of them-selves that may have made them feel embar-rassed or guilty. But they learn that true strength is revealed in admitting one's weakness."

Metaphor is unbeatable for project-ing a holistic grasp of a situation, agrees Dr. Michael Shiryon, chief psychologist in the Department of Psychiatry at Kaiser Medical Center and Hospital in Oakland, California. In truckers' jargon, a name is a handle. A metaphor is a name that gives you something to hold on to. Metaphors also give you the opportunity to hold your affliction at arm's length and look at it from a more objective perspective.

"It's a matter of distancing," Dr. Shiryon explains. "Art, the metaphor, takes your feelings and puts them outside so you can review them. Poetry enables us to take a second look to reframe something in our experience."

Poetry helps foster the proverbial courage to change the things we can, serenity to accept what we can't change, and wisdom to know the difference. One of Dr. Shiryon's patients was profoundly affected upon reading William Blake's poem "The Poison Tree."

The Poison Tree

I was angry with my friend:
I told my wrath, my wrath did end.
I was angry with my foe:
I told it not, my wrath did grow.

And I watered it in fears,
Night and morning with my tears;
And I sunned it with smiles,
And with soft deceitful wiles.

And it grew both day and night
till it bore an apple bright;
And my foe beheld it shine,
And he knew that it was mine,

And into my garden stole
When the night had veiled the pole:
In the morning glad I see
My foe outstretch'd beneath the tree.

— *William Blake*

The patient was moved to express the anger that was poisoning her relationship with her family. "She felt guilt over her feelings of anger, and so she was keeping it inside, breeding resentment and more guilt. The poem helped her to realize that while she had no control over her feelings, she did have control over what she did about them. And that is what counts," Dr. Shiryon says.

A Kentucky social worker learned a similar lesson when poetry helped her to battle breast cancer.

Margaret Massie Simpson discovered she had breast cancer in 1959. After two radical mastectomies, she was moved to chronicle her experience in a book, *Coping with Cancer.* Poetry enabled her to cope.

In the hospital for her first operation, Simpson started reading poetry to take her mind off her pain. Within two years, she was writing verses of her own, dwelling heavily on images of water and the sea. She wrote a poem called "Devil Fish," and seemed fixated on a waterskiing trip she had taken shortly before surgery. Later, she told Dr. Leedy she understood the full meaning of her metaphor: She had been drowning in self-pity.

"A few months after surgery, I recognized that my main problem was emotional, not physical," she wrote to Dr. Leedy. "I had thought I was running from death and fear. My problem was that I was afraid of life."

In the meantime, she discovered that the physical benefits of poetry were also very real. "Under cobalt, linear acceleration, and during chemotherapy treatments, I have found that recitation of remembered poetry and the writing of my own poetry have been powerful anesthetizers," she wrote in 1974. "During each crisis or period of pain over the past 15 years, I have found the writing of poetry a trance-

A POETIC PRESCRIPTION

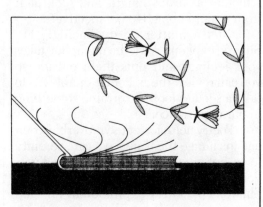

"Instead of one aspirin, take two poems," says Dr. Jack J. Leedy, psychiatrist from New York City. When his patients have trouble getting to sleep, are anxious or depressed, he has found that the following poems work wonders.

For Insomnia

"Hymn to the Night," by Henry Wadsworth Longfellow

"A Ballad of Dreamland," by Algernon Charles Swinburne

"To Sleep," by William Wordsworth

"Oft, in the Stilly Night," by Thomas Moore

"Night," by John Whitaker

"To Sleep," by John Keats

"La Belle Dame Sans Merci," by John Keats

"Annabel Lee," by Edgar Allan Poe

"Tintern Abbey," by William Wordsworth

For Anxiety

"Anxiety," by Paul F. Whitaker

"I'm Nobody! Who Are You?," by Emily Dickinson

"The Road Not Taken," by Robert Frost

"Time, You Old Gypsy Man," by Ralph Hodgson

"Ode on a Grecian Urn," by John Keats

"The Day Is Done," by Henry Wadsworth Longfellow

"Song of Myself," by Walt Whitman

"She Dwelt Among the Untrodden Ways," by William Wordsworth

"The Lake Isle of Innisfree," by William Butler Yeats

For Depression

"Today," by Thomas Carlyle

"Light Shining Out of Darkness," by William Cowper

"The Chambered Nautilus," by Oliver Wendell Holmes

"The Day Is Done," by Henry Wadsworth Longfellow

"On His Blindness," by John Milton

"Ode to the West Wind," by Percy Bysshe Shelley

"The Celestial Surgeon," by Robert Louis Stevenson

"In No Strange Land," by Francis Thompson

"The Eternal Goodness," by John Greenleaf Whittier

like anesthesia, relieving me from fear and confusion. There was no fear and confusion. There was no fear of the operation. There was only anticipation of removing the lump, one barrier between me and health. Without fear, I did not develop many of the side difficulties experienced by many other cancer patients, such as the nausea and the pain produced by fear."

Pain induced by the fear of pain is a factor in many types of surgery, not just mastectomies. In Brooklyn, an oral surgeon has found that "poetry could be considered a good substitute for tranquilizing drugs, narcotics, and sedatives in producing preoperative relaxation." Dr. Mort Malkin has an assistant read poems to the patients in his waiting room. "My own judgment was that fear and anxiety were diminished noticeably during the poetry sessions," says Dr. Malkin. "Most patients felt that doctors who were concerned enough about their patients to present poetry in the waiting room would necessarily be more gentle and compassionate. This reduced apprehension even further.

"And poetry can also help members of the patient's family, who are often just as nervous as the patient.

Dr. Malkin's patients are partial to the poems of Emily Dickinson, Robert Frost, and William Carlos Williams.

Body Rhythms and Rhyme

Poetry doesn't always rhyme, but it does have a rhythm structure that is sometimes unsophisticated, sometimes quite profound, according to Dr. Joost A. M. Meerloo, a psychiatrist and communication researcher. There is rhythm even in free verse. Verses tend to be clocked to a poet's body rhythms, Dr. Meerloo says, and the poets we like best tend to be those whose body rhythms match our own. Rhythm is what gives poetry its "balancing" effect. Poet Allen Ginsberg links poetry to measured breathing and meditation.

Some people retain their metaphoric capacity; others recover it in old age. Among the elderly, "everyone is a poet, didn't you know?" says Sylvia Baron, editor of *Expanding Horizons,* a literary magazine of poetry and prose that specializes in publishing the works of the elderly. She calls it a forum for "voices of the third age." Some of the most powerful verses of our day are being written by hands so stiff they can barely hold a pen. Older people have the experience and insight that gives them a lot to say, and they have need to say it. Poetry gives them a way to say it; *Expanding Horizons* gives them a means to be heard.

"Writing poetry helps fulfill the will to live on, to continue engaging in worthwhile and satisfying endeavors of an artistic nature or a service nature, and these factors should not be overlooked when we want to consider preventive 'medicine' as one of the goals in life," Baron says. "Writing poetry motivates us to go on living. There is also much pleasure in being published in a worthwhile literary magazine."

Dr. Leedy agrees, adding that there is much pleasure to be gained by subscribing to one—or in keeping a collection of poetry in your medicine chest. Dr. Leedy quotes literary giant Robert Graves, who said that "a well-chosen anthology is a complete dispensary of medicine for the more common mental disorders and may be used as much for prevention as cure."

POLARITY THERAPY

★

Polarity therapy, an American-styled variation of pressure-point massage, is said to balance the flow of vital energy in the body through strategic use of the positive and negative energy currents the body is supposed to contain.

Practitioners claim this mind/body healing technique can recharge the nervous system, normalize the major organs, and restore mental and emotional balance.

What can you expect from a session? You're likely to start by telling the practitioner a little something about your lifestyle—your eating and exersise habits, your health history, and current complaints, the nature of your relationships and even your general outlook on life.

Then you'll be asked to lie on a massage table. The therapist will press his fingertips or palms at strategic points to increase the energy flow throughout your body. Then he'll test your reflexes to determine where energy might be blocked.

"What people experience during their sessions varies greatly," says Howard Moskow, founder of the Polarity Wellness Center, New York. "Most will feel the electrical charge moving through them. For some, emotions will come up. Others may feel a deep sense of relaxation; maybe they'll see colors and lights. What happens depends upon how much the person is willing to let go. It's like riding a surf board."

Moskow says the method is especially valuable for stress-related conditions, digestive disturbances, and neck and lower back problems. He also finds it helps therapy patients achieve a more successful outcome. The work can help them remove the physical tension that helps keep their thinking fixed, he says.

"One of the primary things that causes energy blockages are stuck emotions," says Moskow. "The nature of emotions is to move. There are several ways to deal with emotions. One way is suppression. When that happens, the emotional energy gets compressed into the body and causes a blockage.

"When you find the energy blockage and work to release it, emotion and memory of the incident will come up," he says. "All healing, I think, is primarily emotional."

Moskow says that many of his clients are referred by psychologists.

"A psychologist may help persuade a client to make a much-needed change, but as soon as the client walks out of the room, the physiology reimposes itself. But when the person comes in for a session, we go right to the body and release the energy structure involved. The physiolgy returns to balance. Now the client is in an extremely receptive state to make changes. At this point, visualization and affirmations can be extremely effective."

In addition to the bodywork component, polarity therapy stresses correct diet, regular exercise, and clear thinking. Dietary recommendations are based on an analysis of the five elements that proponents of polarity therapy believe are basic to all of life: earth, air, fire, water, and ether.

Sessions average about $50 each, depending upon the skill of the practitioner and the going rate in the area. Moskow says it usually takes about three sessions to really make a significant change.

How does polarity therapy work?

The system is called polarity because it is based on the idea that all of nature—the atom, the cell, the organism, the planet—is structured to reflect the forces of positive and negative energy. In the human body, polarity expresses itself in a "positive pole" in the head, and a "negative pole" in the feet. Similiarly, the right hand is said to give off positive energy and the left hand, negative energy.

According to this theory, electromagnetic energy circulates through invisible channels connected to these poles. That energy helps keep the body's major systems working optimally. If stress or toxins create a short circuit in the system, disease can occur.

"When energy is stuck, the secret is to reestablish polarity," says Moskow. "Since the head is the positive pole, you can increase the charge over the head and get energy to move rapidly over the poles. It will sweep through any neutral stuck areas in the body."

Polarity also proceeds from the belief that the body is holographic, meaning that every region of the body contains reference points to every other part of the body. Reflexologists, for instance, believe that specific points on the feet correspond to all of the major organs of the body. Iridologists look for their "body map" in the eyes. Moskow says that such maps also exist on the ears and abdomen. Polarity therapy makes use of all of them.

How, specifically?

"Let's say the neck is tender," Moskow begins. "I'd press the neck reflex on the big toe, with one hand. Then I'll find a neck reflex on another pole—maybe the hand, the ear, or the neck itself. Using my right and left hand, just like they were wires connecting the poles, I increase the charge by connecting that circuit. The charge goes to the sore neck, clears the blockage and the body establishes improved circulation."

The system was devised by Randolph Stone, a chiropractor and osteopath who spent years exploring other health systems, such as homeopathy and naturopathy in the West, and acupuncture and reflexology in the East. Moskow says Stone refined the system through trials on "hundreds of thousands of patients" in his Chicago clinic.

312

"He was known for working with people who were considered incurable," Moskow adds.

In the late 1940s, Stone began publishing reports of his work but he didn't attract much attention until years later, when the Esalen Institute, a California support center for the human potential movement, invited him to demonstrate his work.

Practitioners of Stone's method are trying to establish standardized requirements for training. Graduates of polarity therapy schools typically complete 100 to 300 hours of classwork, 20 to 50 hours of counseling, 25 to 50 hours of nutritional work plus an internship.

To determine whether the practitioner you're considering is competent, ask about their training and how long they've been practicing.

For more information, contact the Polarity Wellness Center, 145 West 28th Street, 9th Floor, New York, NY 10001, or call (212) 465-8062.

PROGRESSIVE RELAXATION

★★★★★

At its most basic, Progressive Relaxation involves tensing your muscles, holding the tension for a certain period of time, and then relaxing the muscles. You work one muscle group at a time, typically starting with your feet and working your way up to your facial muscles.

You may need to do this several times to feel profoundly relaxed, but that is the end goal of this simple technique. Coordinating your breathing with your tense-it/relax-it rythmn will enhance its effectiveness.

The technique was developed in the 1930s by Edmund Jacobson, a University of Chicago researcher. That's why you'll sometimes hear people refer to it as Jacobson's technique after him. These days, Progressive Relaxation is a staple in stress management programs.

Practiced often enough, Progressive Relaxation can help you develop a very heightened awareness of your body and its particular tension zones. Expect to get better with practice. You may find that the level of relaxation it took you 20 minutes to achieve when you first started can,

after several weeks of practice, take you only 5 minutes. And that's sure to come in handy next time you find yourself in a pressure-cooker situation you can't avoid.

Sometimes, Progressive Relaxation is just a single ingredient in a larger therapeutic package. You may learn to combine it with self-hypnosis, peaceful music, imagery or movement exercises.

Be aware, however, that if you add visualization techniques to your Progressive Relaxation effort, you may retain a measurable amount of tension around your face and eyes. The alternative is to keep your mind clear and focus on your breath.

Progressive Relaxation can be used as a prelude to other work, such as visualization techniques to heal an affected area of the body, or positive self-talk to improve your self-image. Researchers have found that the subconscious mind is most receptive to change when its owner is deeply relaxed.

You can do Progressive Relaxation lying down, or sitting up straight in a comfortable chair. Until you get used to the exercise sequence, it may be helpful

313

314

to make yourself a tape. (See the entry on how to Make Your Own Relaxation Tape, beginning on page 200.)

Be sure to focus on how wonderful your muscles feel when they unclench. Savor that feeling; try to hold it in your memory so you can refer back to it when you feel yourself tighten up.

If you don't want to make your own tape, there are plenty of commercially available relaxation tapes for you to explore. Look for a music store or boutique that will let you sample tapes, on an in-store cassette player, before you purchase.

See also the entries on Autogenic Training, beginning on page 249, Imagery, beginning on page 274, and Relaxation Response, beginning on page 323.

RADIX

★★

Radix is an offshoot of Reichian therapy, the body-oriented psychotherapy Wilhelm Reich developed in the 1930s. Radix differs from its prototype and other neo-Reichian therapies in that it places greater emphasis on group work than private work, and sees itself as educational rather than medical in nature.

Reichian therapy, conversely, grows out of the one-to-one relationship between therapist and patient.

What radix shares with Reichian therapy is Reich's belief that body posture perfectly reflects a person's emotional state. In other words, when emotions are suppressed, rather than expressed, muscles tense in the body to diminish the flow of painful feelings. Over time, an often-used muscular defense can turn into habitual tension, or what Reich termed "body armor." The armor then blocks bodily energy, which Reich called orgone, from circulating throughout the body. Proper circulation of that energy is what keeps the body systems functioning optimally.

Reich identified seven muscle groups in which the muscles work in unison to create segments of body armor. The muscle group near the eyes, he calls the oracular segment. Below that are the oral, cervical, thoraxic, diaphragmatic, and pelvic segments. Radix teachers, like Reichian therapists, work to release blocks from the oracular segment on down.

Radix, in fact, is noted for its usefulness in helping correct visual disorders. People familiar with the technique say it emphasizes the improvement of visual awareness and eye contact as precursors to a more general sense of well-being.

Reichian therapy and radix differ most in terms of the psychoanalytic theory used to determine a client's level of emotional maturity. Reich, a one-time protégé of Freud, paired his notions of body-armoring with classical Freudian psychoanalysis, which classifies emotional maturity according to certain psychosexual stages of development.

But Charles Kelly, the experimental psychologist who created radix in the 1960s, prefers clients to see where they are with regard to their feelings. Are they blocked by fear? anger? pain? Or some combination of all three?

Radix does its teaching through body and voice. You can expect to engage in bioenergetics exercises that will help you raise the energy level in your body, by gradually stressing the armored muscles until exhaustion causes them to let go. You and your teacher may engage in one-on-one counseling. You'll also be shown how to work with your breath to aid the process. You may also be asked to engage in cathartic types of movement: kicking and screaming, or hitting a tennis racket against a mattress.

Individual sessions are offered, as well as group work and workshop intensives.

The core of radix is a technique called the radix intensive, which stresses deep emotional release. In a group setting, members of the group get their turn to do the intensive, and are supported through it by every member of the group.

The intent of all of this is to teach you to use your body, mind, and mouth to honestly express your feelings so you can experience a deeper satisfaction with life.

Radix also makes use of various "paired feeling" exercises, in which participants pair off and aid in each other's therapeutic work. Tools used include guided fantasy and direct body contact between the client partners, as ways to help each other release body armoring.

But since Kelly believes that a certain amount of character armoring has a valuable psychological focus, radix doesn't concern itself with eliminating all armoring, the way Reichian therapy does.

Another significant difference between radix and other Reichian therapies is the focus, prerequisites, and intensity of its training program. Kelly insists that potential trainers complete about 50 radix sessions before they begin the training, and another 100 before they finish. Kelly believes that psychological readiness, rather than academic training, is more important if a teacher is to be effective.

Radix instructors spend three weeks in an intensive program at the Radix Institute in Texas, then complete two to three years of training with regional instructors. There are some 200 radix practitioners in the country today.

Individual sessions range from $40 to $90. Prices for groups and workshops vary, depending upon the scope.

For more information, contact the Radix Institute, Route 2, Box 89A, Granbury, TX 76048, or call (817) 326-5670.

REBIRTHING

★

Imagine putting on a mask and snorkel, submerging yourself in a tub of water and letting your breath carry you back in time to that difficult, perplexing journey through the birth canal.

How did the world seem to you then — the bright lights, the noise, the large alien beings? Did you find it scary, inhospitable, harsh?

Examining your initial impressions is what rebirthing is about. Theorists of this method believe that the attitudes you developed during your first few minutes of exposure to the outside world still color the way you see it.

The practice was developed by Leonard Orr in the 1970s and has generated a lot of interest in New Age circles. In one sense, rebirthing is a new take on the ancient practice of using the breath to purify and energize the body, and bring the mind to greater awareness of the inner self. Like many modern therapies, it aims to help you unburden yourself of past emotional trauma.

How does rebirthing work?

A technique called connected breathing is central to the process. You inhale-exhale-inhale-exhale, without taking the customary pause between breaths. By doing this, rebirthers say, you bring more oxygen to your blood, rev up your circulation, and throw off toxins more quickly.

Over time, say rebirthers, this deep and energetic style of breathing will leave you feeling profoundly relaxed. Chronic tension will melt away. As the tension dissipates, the new energy you bring into your body enters areas where tension normally blocks it off. Bringing sensation to these normally shut-down areas may trigger certain feelings for you.

Meanwhile, your relaxed state allows unconscious thoughts to surface in your conscious awareness. There you can examine your thoughts and consciously choose to change the ones that get in the way of your happiness.

Michael Adamedes and Alia Paulusz, authors of an article on rebirthing in *The Bodywork Book,* say that it typically takes three to eight weeks just to get clear of the emotional issues the breathing is likely to bring to the fore.

In the article, they explain that rebirthing proceeds from the premise that

317

318

our innate nature is perfection, and that if we were in our natural state, we'd have abundant energy and happiness.

"It is the conditioning from the environment that makes us believe we are not happy with ourselves and tends to make us lose confidence in ourselves," they write. "By relaxing, a person lets go of the conditioning and reconnects with this innate perfect Self. . . . Once a person relaxes and stops 'avoiding,' then whatever is in the unconscious will spontaneously come to the surface, enabling it to be integrated and released by the breathing process."

Getting Wet Is Optional

Rebirthing can be done dry or wet. Wet rebirthing simply means that you are rebirthed in a bath tub, hot tub, or other body of water. Even among wet rebirthers there are lots of variations. You could lie face down in the water and breath through a snorkel, with your rebirther holding you. You could lie on your back, supported by your rebirther. Or you could simply sit in the water, with your head above the water.

You could choose between warm water, with the temperature between 98° and 102°F, or cold water. The warm water helps simulate conditions in the womb.

But beginners to rebirthing can usually expect a dry rebirthing, which means that you practice the breath work someplace dry, like on a mattress or bed. You can choose an introductory "group rebirth" or opt for a solo consultation.

Sessions usually last 1 to 2 hours. The first one is typically preceded by an hour-long counseling session. You'll then lie on something soft, be guided through a deep relaxation exercise and be given breath work instructions.

How long does it take to see results? Rebirthers say it's best to do the first 10 to 20 sessions with a qualified rebirther and then continue the work on your own. They say the process helps peel back ever deeper layers of conditioning.

Philadelphia rebirther Tony LoMastro claims that the technique has helped his clients relieve arthritic pain, narcolepsy, nerve conditions, and "a wide range of symptoms." The more people experience mental well-being, the more they experience physical well-being.

Individual sessions cost $40 to $100 depending upon locale. LoMastro says $75 to $100 is average.

Rebirther trainees attend three weekend "Loving Relationships Training (LRT)" seminars and assist at a fourth one. They are also asked to go through ten rebirthing sessions with a qualified rebirther, and to continue their training with ongoing seminars sponsored by the LRT foundation, founded by Sondra Rey, a colleague of Leonard Orr's. But there is no system for determining whether the people who call themselves rebirthers are qualified to do it.

For more information, write to the International Office of the Loving Relationships Training, P.O. Box 1465, Washington, CT 06793, or call 1-800-INTL-LRT. This organization can put you in touch with rebirthers in your area.

REFLEXOLOGY

★ ★

Reflexology is a pressure-point style of massage for the feet. Practitioners claim its effects can be felt throughout the body, in the form of relaxation and increased vitality.

This specialized foot massage also functions as an early-detection system. Tender areas on the feet may signal that something's amiss in a particular organ or body system. That's because the points your reflexologist digs into with her fingers, or knuckles, correspond to the major organs and systems in your body.

According to reflexology theory, the feet contain "maps" of the entire body. (Other alternative healing systems say that the hands, ears, face, and eyes also contain such maps.) Moreover, there is a direct connection between a particular organ and its corresponding reference points. For instance, if you have kidney problems, you may also find a blemish on the forehead, between the eyebrows; a tenderness on the liver "points" on the ears and feet, and some discoloration along a tiny band below the pupil of the eye and toward the outer corner.

If the reflexologist finds that the kidney "point" on your foot is extremely tender, she'll probably advise you to have your kidneys checked by a doctor. If you can tolerate pressure on that area of the foot, she'll work with it. As she does so, practitioners claim, the warmth from her fingers gives off a tiny electrical charge, which helps get energy moving again along the body channel that feeds your kidney and related organs.

This theory of "body energy channels" is the same one underlying acupuncture. The concepts were in place in China more than 2,000 years ago, and introduced to Japan around the sixth century. The central notion is that *chi,* or life energy, flows through the body along a series of pathways known as meridians. The meridians are named for the vital organ whose function they help facilitate.

According to this view, the central source and reservoir for body energy is the hara, the soft area between the rib cage and the pelvic bone. In a healthy body, energy flows from the hara, through the meridians, circulating freely among

319

320

the vital organs. Tsubos, points just under the skin that connect to form the meridians, serve as energy conductors. (These are the same points as those on an acupuncture chart.)

But sometimes, the tsubos don't do their job, and the energy stagnates. Any number of factors can contribute to blockages along the way: stress, injury, trauma, poor posture, or diet. Pressing on the tsubos is said to release the trapped energy so it can circulate, bringing about the internal balance needed to activate the body's own healing mechanisms.

Reflexologists say that by massaging these reference points, they help the corresponding body parts heal themselves through improved circulation, elimination of toxic by-products of metabolism, and overall reduction of stress.

Massaging the feet also helps break up calcium deposits and the crystals that form from excess uric acid, says reflexologist Ki Tomlinson.

"It's just a gateway into the energy and organ systems of the body," says Dr. Ronald Hoffman, medical director of the Whole Life Medical Center in Manhattan.

He says there is "definitely documentation suggesting that if you press certain points on the outer ear, you have a concrete effect on the vagus nerve regulating digestion, heartbeat, and appetite." He thinks "reflexology has scientific validity that hasn't been discovered yet. It's an empirical science—it's been researched in the clinic, not the laboratory."

Reflexology is said to help everything from acne to wrist pain, though no reflexologist will promise a cure.

Sessions range from $25 to $100 per hour, depending on locale.

For preventive health care, one session every two weeks is considered optimum. For treatment of a particular condition, one to three sessions a week may be needed.

You can probably find a reflexologist in your area through a physician who practices holistic medicine. Others likely to know of reflexologists are osteopaths, chiropractors, and massage therapists.

Another good source of information is the International Institute of Reflexology, which has trained about 12,000 reflexologists in the last 30 years. It presents seminars and workshops around the country. Write to the Institute of Reflexology, P.O. Box 12642, St. Petersburg, FL 33733-2642.

REICHIAN THERAPY

★★

Reichian therapy is the model for a number of body-oriented forms of psychoanalysis in vogue today. It was developed in the 1930s by Dr. Wilhelm Reich, a brilliant and controversial theoretician who was at one time a member of Freud's inner circle.

There is no one today who duplicates Reich's therapeutic approach exactly. Orgonomy comes closest. It was developed by Dr. Elsworth Baker, who studied with Reich for 11 years.

What follows, then, is a not a description of an available therapy, but a summary of the key Reichian concepts that have powerfully influenced modern mind/body therapies. These concepts helped generate orgonomy, bioenergetics, and radix, all of which are considered neo-Reichian therapies. They have also influenced Gestalt therapy, actualism, primal therapy, the Rubenfield Synergy Method, Integrative Body Psychotherapy, and prefigure psychoneuroimmunology.

For this reason, Reichian therapy can be considered the great-granddaddy of many modern bodywork approaches. For it was Reich who, as Joseph Heller so succinctly puts it, "was the first Westerner to concentrate attention on the relationship between body tensions and rigidity, and psychological limitations to a person's well-being."

Reich's contribution was his emphasis on the importance of heightened body awareness, and on releasing emotions. Those two routes, he said, were more essential to an effective cure than intellectual analysis.

Exactly how did he do this in practice?

Reich observed his patients standing, or had them lie on his table, and he instructed them to breathe in specific ways. He would then monitor the body for changes in skin temperature and color, and attempt to detect just where the bodily energy was blocked.

He saw these energy blocks as the protective "armor" that developed in reaction to some physical or emotional injury. To him, structural disorders in the body were physical manifestations of blocked emotional energy.

Reich used physical manipulation and psychoanalyis to gradually dissolve blockages. He began at the most superficial

322

level and cleared away until he reached the deepest defenses of the individual. To his way of thinking, an individual could never fully rid himself of psychological trauma without relieving the physical tension that accompanied it.

Reich found that certain groups of muscles work together as a unit to create armor, and that there were seven such units in the body. These he labeled the oracular (eye area), oral, cervical, thoraxic, diaphragmatic, abdominal, and pelvic. Reich always began at the top, with the oracular segment, and worked his way down.

When the stressed muscles brought memories to the surface, he'd work with them psychoanalytically.

His goal was to guide the patient toward a full release of blocked emotional energy and corresponding physical tension. After that occurred, the patient would be free to experience and express the full range of his or her sexuality and emotions, and live a freer, healthier life.

Like Freud, Reich believed that emotional, physical, and mental disorders were caused by sexual repression. He theorized that human character was ultimately based upon the movement and blocking of sexual energy. In this view, sex becomes the body's primary method for discharging excess energy and maintaining equilibrium. Consequently, Reich believed that an indi-

vidual is healthy only to the degree in which he or she can experience a full sexual orgasm, which is felt as pleasure throughout the body.

And, as early as the 1940s, Reich advanced ideas about the connection between personality traits and specific diseases; a question now being explored in mainstream medical universities. He came to believe that the particular disease a person develops relates very much to his or her personality traits.

Reich himself died in a federal prison in 1957, where he was jailed after a colleague of his ignored a federal injunction and shipped a truckload of "orgone energy accumulators" across interstate lines. Reich served six months of his two-year sentence, and many of his books were burned during that period. The "orgone energy accumulator" was a device he had invented to help collect the life energy, or orgone, he claimed every individual possesses. The government—and most other people—regarded the device as quackery.

Interest in Reich's work revived again in the 1970s, spawning societies, pro-Reichian journals and books and influencing new forms of therapy. For specific information on the neo-Reichian therapies that grew out of his work, see the entries on Bioenergetics, beginning on page 251, and Radix, beginning on 315.

RELAXATION RESPONSE

★★★★★

The relaxation response isn't a therapy. It is a bodily state you can elicit by practicing certain techniques. In this state, specific and desirable physiological changes occur.

The process is analogous to shifting gears in your mind. You downshift, and your body responds by slowing its metabolism, blood pressure, breathing, and heart rate. The other important change occurs in your brain, which begins to produce the larger, slower alpha and theta brainwave frequencies. Communication between the right and left cortical hemispheres of the brain becomes more coherent.

Why is this good for you? What's the big deal about alpha and theta waves?

In your normal state of consciousness, your brain typically emits small and rapid beta rhythm waves. When this rhythm predominates, you're more conscious of what's going on around you than inside you. But when you shift to the alpha and theta rhythms, the waves become larger — large enough to disturb old patterns of thinking. This altered state of consciousness opens the door for significant change

to occur, to a higher level of brain organization.

In his book *Your Maximum Mind,* Dr. Herbert Benson, the Harvard Medical School professor credited with popularizing the relaxation response, explains the phenomena this way:

"When we change our patterns of thinking and acting, the brain cells begin to establish additional connections or new 'wirings.' These new connections then communicate in fresh ways with other cells and before long, the pathways or wirings that kept the phobia or other habit alive are replaced or altered."

The improved communication between brain hemispheres also opens the door to new insights, says Dr. Benson. What this means, in simple terms, is that the nonverbal, intuitive part of your mind is able to communicate with the rational, verbal part about what kind of care you need.

Dr. Benson views the relaxation response as the counterpart of the body's "fight-or-flight" mechanism, which kicks in when you experience lots of stress. Excess

323

stress may make you feel nauseous, tense, short-tempered, or make you have difficulty sleeping.

Over time, a body too prone to "fight-or-flight" gear is liable to develop hypertension, cardiac arrythmias, digestive problems, various pains, and a chronic depression of the immune system.

Dr. Benson says that regular use of the relaxation response will bring about relief to the same degree that the fight-or-flight syndrome makes a disease worse.

Several different techniques will bring on the relaxation response. To work, they must provide you with some mechanism for arresting the flow of thoughts that disturb you and some way to detach yourself from these thoughts.

You could meditate, for instance; practice T'ai Chi or Chi Gong, or progressively relax your muscles. The more you are able to absorb yourself in your practice and clear your mind, the better. Dr. Benson believes that all of these techniques will bring about the same physiological changes.

Or you could follow Dr. Benson's formula and experiment with the following sequence. The important thing is to be open-minded about what you expect from the process. Don't try to change yourself. If you try to affect change, you'll lose the passive, receptive attitude essential to coaxing in the relaxation response.

Let's begin:

1. Pick out a word, a short phrase, or brief prayer that has a lot of meaning for you. Maybe there's a biblical phrase that sustains you. If you're not religious, a word like "one," "peace," or "calm" will do it.

But be sure to keep your phrase or prayer passive and undirected. Don't let your rational, logical self function like a drill sergeant that says "you must" to the body. Instead, allow your body wisdom to surface in the silence. Make the space for insight.

2. Sit in a comfortable position in a quiet room. If you keep your spine straight, it will help.

3. Close your eyes.

4. Relax your muscles.

5. Breathe slowly and naturally. As you do, focus on your word, phrase, or short prayer. Repeat it each time you exhale.

6. Don't worry about whether you're doing it right. As distracting thoughts come to mind, let them float away gently without following them. Return your focus to the word or phrase you've chosen.

7. Continue the technique for 10 to 20 minutes. Do this twice daily for optimum results.

The beauty of this sequence is that you can practice it at home without getting any outside instruction.

Dr. Benson and his colleagues observed the relaxation response when they were studying practitioners of transcendental meditation in the late 1960s and early 1970s. In 1975, Dr. Benson published *The Relaxation Response.*

For more information, consult either of Dr. Benson's books or see the entries on Autogenic Training, beginning on page 249, and Progressive Relaxation, beginning on page 313.

ROLFING

★★★

How'd you like to rewrite the history of your body? Get "Rolfed" and you can finally erase the ankle sprain you had at age 6, the ski accident that put you in a cast at 14, the break-up with the "love of your life" that leveled you at 22.

"Wait a minute," you're saying. "I've long since healed." But have you . . . totally? Or are you still out of joint, so to speak, because of the way your body recorded the trauma?

Rolfers believe the latter. Their mission is nothing short of restructuring your body in ten sessions, lasting 1 to 1½ hours each.

Focusing on specific groups of muscles each session, the Rolfer massages deeply into the connective tissue, working out tension until the tissue regains its resiliency. That allows the bones to move back into a more natural alignment with each other.

By the final session, they claim, the body is longer, the posture straighter and the joints restored to their normal position. Movement requires far less energy, Rolfers say, a statement corroborated by academic research. A study by Dr. Valerie Hunt,

director of the Movement Behavior Lab at UCLA, and Dr. Julian Silverman, a research specialist with the California Department of Mental Hygiene, found that subjects who completed the ten sessions showed specific improvements in neurological control over their muscles. Muscles were used more efficiently, conserving energy, and response to stimuli was more refined, the research showed.

What will the whole process cost you? $600 to $1,000 for all ten sessions, which translates to $60 to $100 a pop. Sessions work best when they're scheduled seven to ten days apart.

The system was devised by the late Dr. Ida Rolf, a Columbia University-trained biochemist who worked for the Rockefeller Institute as an organic chemist. After treatment by an osteopath, she was inspired to create a system of bodily manipulations that would, in her words "realign the random body into an orderly, balanced energy system that can operate in the field of gravity." She called the work Structural Integration.

Not much is known about how she developed her ideas. What motivated her,

325

326

she has said, was that she was prediabetic then, and suffering from curvature of the spine.

Rolf originally viewed her system as an adjunct to osteopathy. Then in the 1960s, she came to the Esalen Institute, in California, to work with Fritz Perls, the founder of Gestalt therapy. Stimulated by conversations with him, she came to appreciate more fully the profound connection between emotion and muscular tone.

Together, Dr. Rolf and Perls explored the idea of "Gestalt of character, balance of stucture." In that view, the radiantly healthy individual was one whose feet solidly touched the ground, whose bearing was erect, whose body was free from any habitual tension. This ideal person's psyche carried no extra baggage, and so was able to respond appropriately to each new experience, instead of perceiving it through the framework of issues left unresolved in the past.

That's the ideal. What Dr. Rolf found more typical was the individual who became "stuck" in certain patterns of behavior that felt safe.

Consider the child whose father bullies him. Provoked enough, the child feels an urge to strike back. But he stifles it, and that unfulfilled impulse is stored as tension in his arm. If the child doesn't acquire the skills to fully express his anger, he may find himself unconsciously tensing his arm in each new situation where he feels bullied. The muscular tension and emotion become two aspects of the same organic pattern. If the tension becomes chronic, the connective tissue may harden, pulling the surrounding body parts out of alignment.

That's precisely the kind of tension Rolfing works to eliminate. Rolfers say

that it's not uncommon for clients to recall a specific traumatic episode as the therapist makes headway on a particularly troublesome spot. Pain, they say, frequently marks an emotional release.

And Rolfing can be painful.

"Rolfing is a process of change," explains Don Hazen, a director for the International Rolf Institute. "The way that your body lets you know the status quo is being interrupted is that it gives you pain. Sometimes, in the course of a session, as things change, it is going to be intense. It can be a burning kind of sensation that leaves as soon as the Rolfer removes his hands from the client's body."

If a specific emotional issue surfaces during the work, be aware that the best a Rolfer can do is refer you to a psychotherapist. Rolfers do not have the training to offer psychological counseling.

What's nice about Rolfing is that you will know what to expect from week to week. The work is sequential. On the other hand, numerous clients tell us they found the experience startlingly painful.

During your first session, the Rolfer will concentrate on the outer layer of connective tissue, working the shoulder girdle, rib cage, legs, hips, and lower back. The front of the body should lengthen as a result.

After session two, your feet may finally feel like they really touch ground. Your back may appear to be longer.

During session three, the Rolfer will try to organize your major body segments around a 'center line.'

Session four works with the abductor muscles and the pelvic floor.

The next one focuses on the muscles of the pelvis, abdomen, and front of the thigh.

Session six works the muscles of the hip and gluteal structure, the hamstrings, sacrum, and lower back.

Session seven focuses on getting the jaw, neck, and head to line up neatly with the overall structure of the body.

During sessions eight and nine, the Rolfer works with the lower or upper half of the body, making sure that everything is centered and symmetrical. One session works with the arms and shoulder girdle, the other with the legs.

Session ten, says Hazen "puts it all together." The Rolfer makes sure that the joints are horizontal and that the planes of fascia are as smooth as possible.

"The thing that struck me about Rolfing is how simple it is," says Hazen, who has been doing the work himself for more than a decade. "It's a simplicity that speaks to me about what's possible when the aches and pains and energy blocks that are normally in the system get freed up. When I can turn my energy toward what I'm doing rather than hold it in my body."

What kind of training can you expect from the Rolfer who's about to rearrange your body? The actual course work used to take two eight-week periods to complete. That's being extended to one year, Hazen says, to make sure everyone has a similiar background.

To qualify for training, candidates must be versed in anatomy, physiology, and kinesiology and have hands-on health-care experience, such as a registered nurse, chiropractor, or massage practitioner might have. Additionally, says Hazen, candidates must have an adequate psychological background "to deal with the things that happen in a session." Finally, the institute must find them emotionally and physically capable of doing the work.

There are about 600 trained Rolfers located throughout the world, and more in training. For a referral to a qualified practitioner in your area, write the International Rolf Institute, P.O. Box 1868, Boulder, CO 80306, or call (303) 449-5903.

See also the entry on Hellerwork, beginning on page 267.

SHIATSU

★★★

Shiatsu, a Japanese word meaning "finger" *(shi)* "pressure" *(atsu),* is a relatively recent coinage for a style of bodywork based on the same ancient oriental theories of health as acupressure.

In practice, the method is relatively simple and straightforward. You, the client, recline on a mat on the floor while the practitioner applies steady pressure to a series of points on your body. More often than not, the therapist will work with her hands, but some also use knees, elbows, and feet. Your muscles will be gently stretched in the process.

A full massage lasts 45 minutes or longer. The focus throughout is on helping you restore the energy equilibrium in your body. Results may not be immediately apparent, but within hours, you may feel a difference. Maybe the minor aches you brought to the session will be gone, or noticeably diminished. Maybe you'll feel more energetic and clear-headed.

How does it work?

The concepts that shiatsu draws from were in place in China more than 2,000 years ago and introduced to Japan around the sixth century. Central is the notion that *chi,* or life energy, flows through the body along a series of pathways known as meridians. Shiatsu concerns itself with 14 major meridians, most of which are named for the vital organ whose function they help aid, such as the lung or liver.

According to this view, the central storehouse for body energy is the hara, the soft area between the rib cage and the pelvic bone. When we're healthy, energy flows from the hara, through the meridians, circulating freely among the vital organs. Tsubos, points just under the skin that connect to form the meridians, serve as energy conduits. (These are the same points as those on an acupuncture chart.)

Sometimes, however, the tsubos don't do their job, and the energy backs up. Stress, injury, trauma, poor posture, or diet can all contribute to such blockages. Pressing on the tsubos is said to release the trapped energy so it can circulate, bringing about the internal balance needed to restore the body's own healing mechanisms.

Oriental theorists have found 361 such pressure points, although shiatsu generally concerns itself with only 92 of them.

Western medicine does not recognize the tsubos and meridians at all, because they do not correspond to any anatomical structure. Recently, however, American osteopath Robert Becker, author of *The Body Electric,* was able to show that if you measure the electrical current along the skin, you will be able to pinpoint the location of about half the acupuncture points, through changes in the current. Becker found the same points on every body he tested and theorized that a more sophisticated measuring device might enable him to locate other points.

Shiatsu differs from acupressure (acupuncture without needles) only in that practitioners of this Japanese art also manipulate parts of the body. (Acupressure refers strictly to the application of pressure.)

Many different schools have grown up around the practice of shiatsu, making for many variations in approach. Practitioners are not licensed, and the degree of training schools require to grant certificates varies according to the school.

It pays to ask the shiatsu therapist you're considering whether she favors firm, sometimes painful pressure or a much lighter touch. And don't feel funny about asking to see credentials or a short demonstration or to be given the names of other clients you can talk to.

One man credited with helping to popularize shiatsu in the United States is Wataru Ohashi, a Hiroshima-born dynamo who lists Henry Kissinger, Martha Graham, Gay Talese, and Mohammed Ali among his clients.

Ohashi, who studied American literature at a Tokyo university before he entered the Nippon Shiatsu School, came to the United States in 1969. He worked as chief shiatsu therapist at the Watergate Health Club and created Ohashiatsu™, his trademarked blend of shiatsu, Zen philosophy, and exercise. The author of six books, he also produced the videotape "Ohashiatsu for a Healthy and Happy Pregnancy."

In 1976, Ohashi established a nonprofit institute in New York to spread his method. The institute offers courses throughout the United States and Europe. Students advance through six levels of training. Some complete only the first levels, learning just enough to give shiatsu massages to friends and family. But those who complete Advanced Ohashiatsu, Part II, have 540 hours of training under their belts.

Graduates of Ohashiatsu favor a firm but gentle touch. "They are putting their hands on to balance the energy flow," says Ohashi. "There is no painful finger pressure. That's one of the big differences."

Ohashiatsu sessions last about an hour, and include instruction in meditation and exercise. The cost ranges from about $45 to $85 a session, depending upon how much training the therapist has, and what the going rate is in your area.

Is Ohashiatsu successful for certain conditions? Ohashi says he isn't comfortable talking about that; he'd rather focus on prevention. "When you maintain a good, balanced lifestyle, you can prevent any abnormality," he says.

To locate a shiatsu practitioner in your area, you might try checking the bulletin boards of health food stores and alternative bookstores, or ask around at the yoga school or yoga-style retreat center in your area. If you're interested in Ohashiatsu or need a referral, write the Ohashi Institute, 12 West 27th Street, New York, NY 10001, or call (212) 684-4190.

See also the entry on Acupressure, beginning on page 243.

THERAPEUTIC TOUCH

★

Therapeutic touch looks much like faith healing, that ancient art of the laying on of hands. You sit in a chair while the therapist sweeps her hands along the contour of your body, keeping the palms a few inches out from the body itself. You may even feel warmth emanating from her hands, as some clients report; or a tingling sensation in the area she's working on.

But, unlike faith healing, therapeutic touch has gained a measure of respect in medical quarters. It was a registered nurse, Dolores Krieger, professor of nursing at New York University, who brought the practice into vogue in this country. These days, leading university nursing and medical schools across the country teach the technique.

And in hospitals around the world, nurses use therapeutic touch daily to relieve pain, reduce swelling, help bones knit, and enable patients to sleep more comfortably.

The technique has been defined, and its effects documented since the 1970s. Studies suggest there is something to it,

whether it's used on its own or paired with conventional medical care.

One series of experiments showed that wounded mice who received the laying on of hands healed much faster than mice who didn't. Those results were interpreted to mean that therapeutic touch is effective whether or not the patient believes it will work.

A 1975 clinical study, later published by the *Journal of Nursing,* showed that hemoglobin levels rose significantly higher in patients after a session of therapeutic touch, than they did in a control group. Hemoglobin, of course, is the component of the red blood corpuscle that carries oxygen to the cells.

Another study, done by the University of Missouri in Columbia, found that therapeutic touch reduced headache pain by up to 70 percent in most of the subjects tested. Four hours after the treatment, pain diminished even more.

How does therapeutic touch work?

Practitioners of this discipline, like those who practice shiatsu and other forms of massage, believe in the existence of a life energy that permeates every cell. This energy extends out beyond the body, they claim, creating "a bioelectric field." Therapeutic touch practitioners attempt to influence this field when they work. They use their intention to heal, to direct "life energy" to flow through them to the ailing patient.

Practitioners follow a standard process. First they establish their intent to heal, perhaps by saying a prayer. Then they use their hands to scan the body's "energy field" to see where the problems lie. Next they use the hands to clear away any "congestion" or to bring more energy to places where it seems to be depleted. What they're after is a feeling that the body's energy is evenly distributed, or balanced.

In *Therapeutic Touch: A Practical Guide*, author and registered nurse Janet McCrae theorizes that the process works like this: "In a state of health, the life energy flows freely in, through and out of the organism in a balanced manner, nourishing all the organs of the body. In disease, the flow of energy is obstructed, disordered, and/or depleted. Therapeutic touch practitioners, having learned to attune to the Universal [energy] Field through conscious intent, direct the life energy into the patients to enhance their vitality."

Practitioners of the method say that someone who is suffering from acute illness will respond more quickly than someone with a chronic illness. They claim the method can relieve discomfort and speed healing for people suffering from infections, wounds, burns, and operations. Therapeutic touch has also been used to aid arthritis sufferers.

To find a trained practitioner, or classes in the method, write to the Nurse Healers and Professional Associates Cooperative, Inc., 175 Fifth Avenue, Suite 3399, New York, NY 10010.

TRAGER APPROACH

★★

The full name for the method is a mouthful—Trager® Psychophysical Integration and Mentastics℠ Movement Education. Sounds harsh, but the method is anything but. If you can get past the formidable name, odds are you'll enjoy the experience.

Like Rolfing and Hellerwork, Trager includes a workout on the massage table and some movement instruction afterward. But it is unlike the other two in very distinct ways. While Rolfing and Hellerwork take a systematic approach to the body, working the muscle groups in a specific order, Trager is much more free form. Your body's responses will guide the practitioner. As she works with you, using a grab bag of massage techniques, you'll find she's much more concerned with getting your mind to register a certain quality of feeling, a pleasant sensation of lightness and flexibility, than with kneading the tension out of your flesh.

Among the most intuitive of the bodywork styles, "Tragering" is gentle, and yet it can be very effective. A skilled practitioner can help return to you that loose-limbed sense of well-being that was

yours as a child. A series of sessions may help induce more lasting changes.

An emphasis on things mental is what accounts for the strange-sounding name. Mentastics, playful, dancelike exercises, blends the word "mental" with "gymnastics." Psychophysical integration, the name for the tablework, speaks to the reuniting of the psyche with the physique.

The emphasis is where it is because Dr. Milton Trager, the Chicago-born originator of the technique, believes that patterns of tension are held in the mind.

He first hit upon his technique as an 18-year-old professional boxer in Miami. Mickey Martin, his trainer, used to give the young boxer rubdowns after every fight. One day, Trager returned the favor. Martin, according to an often-told story, was so stunned he asked Trager where he had learned to do that.

"You taught me," said Trager.

"I never taught you this, kid," Martin shot back. "But I don't care. Let me tell you, you got hands."

Elated, Trager went home and worked on his father, who was suffering from acute sciatica. Three sessions later, the legend goes, his father's symptoms disappeared. Success with a polio victim spurred Trager to explore his neighborhood for others to work on. Eventually, he quit boxing so he could take care of his hands.

In 1941, Trager received his Doctorate of Physical Medicine from the Los Angeles College of Drugless Physicians and certification from the state of California to practice in the field of neuromuscular disorders. Later, he sought more formal academic credentials and was accepted at a Mexican medical university. There he organized a polio clinic, completed his medical studies, and graduated with an M.D. in 1955. In 1959, he began a private practice in medicine and physical rehabilitation in Hawaii.

Throughout that time, Trager never had much success teaching his techniques to others. The central aim of his approach has been to reach "toward the unconscious mind of the patient, [so that] every thought, every move, communicates how the tissue should feel when everything is right."

In Trager lingo, that's called the hook-up. It's supposed to work like this: At the beginning of the session, the therapist enters a meditative state and empties his mind of all thoughts and feelings except for a sense of how light and free the body can feel. The therapist uses his hands to communicate that thought to the client's tissue. That positive, pleasant sensation is then supposed to "enter the central nervous system and begin to trigger tissue changes by means of the many sensory-motor feedback loops between the mind and the muscles," says Deane Juhan, author of *Job's Body: A Handbook for Bodywork.*

The breakthrough came in 1974, when Trager was called in to help provide rehabilitation therapy for a muscular dys-trophy sufferer. The patient asked Trager to teach his methods to his regular therapist, but Trager had little hope. Finally, Trager asked the therapist to place his hands on the patient while Trager worked on top of the therapist's hands. The therapist "got it" and a teaching method was born.

A year later, Trager met Betty Fuller at California's Esalen Institute and found he could teach her in the same fashion. She persuaded him to let her start an organization that would spread his methods. The result: The Trager Institute, 10 Old Mill Street, Mill Valley, CA 94941-1891. The phone number is (415) 388-2688.

The current training program takes a minimum of six months. Just to get accepted for study requires that a student experience the therapy himself, in two private sessions or a weekend workshop, and get a written recommendation from the Trager practitioner.

The easiest way to locate a Trager therapist in good standing in your area is to call the institute and ask for a referral. Sessions cost anywhere from $25 to $65, depending upon your locale. The tablework takes 1 to 1½ hours, and that's followed by instructions in Mentastics, simple movement sequences supposed to help you maintain the feeling of lightness and freedom.

The trick with Trager is to remember how you feel on the table while doing Mentastics and as you go about your daily affairs. How many sessions you need for optimum results may depend upon just how good your memory is. Trager practitioners say that if you can stamp indelibly in your memory the way your body feels after a Trager session, you can induce the same level of relaxation just by thinking about it. That, in fact, is the point.

RAISE YOUR INTIMACY INDEX

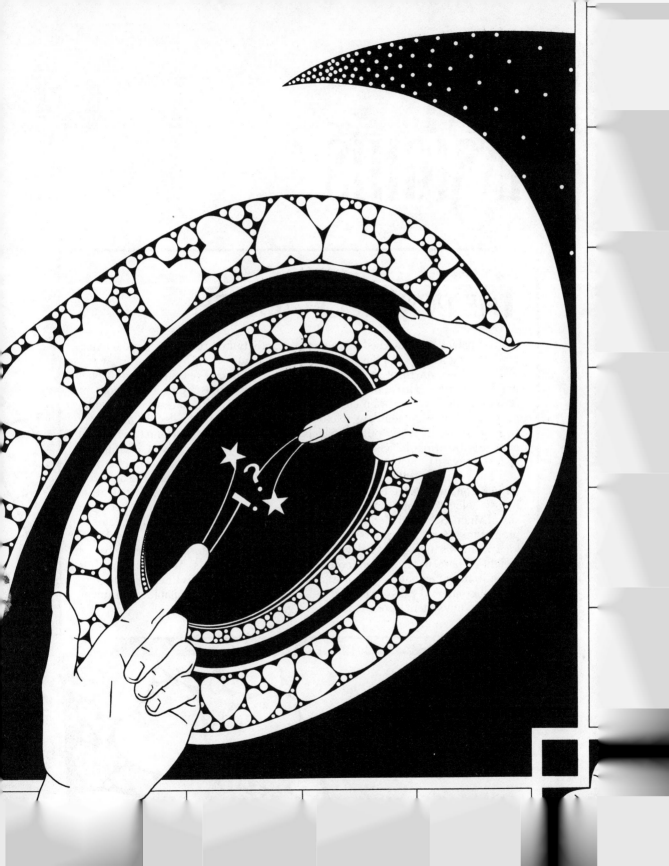

INSTANT INSIGHTS

THE POWER OF TOUCH

For babies, being touched is as important as being fed and can have a crucial effect on the growth of the body and mind. New research is pointing to the possibility that certain brain chemicals needed for development are released strictly by touch, while others, which impede growth, may be released because the infant wasn't touched.

Most of the speculation in this area is hinged on an unusual study conducted by psychologist Tiffany Field at University of Miami School of Medicine. Those premature infants who were massaged for 15 minutes three times a day gained weight 47 percent faster than those left alone in their incubator. The massaged babies also showed signs of a faster developing nervous system through their level of activity and responsiveness to external stimuli.

One line of reasoning for this phenomenon comes from observations of the animal world. Rats, when licked by their mother, show a decline in the production of beta-endorphin, a chemical that inhibits the levels of insulin and growth hormone production. But the beta-endorphin level rose when the baby rats were taken from their mother. Scientists are hypothesizing that this effect is a survival mechanism in all mammals. When the mother is away, heightened levels of beta-endorphin lower the baby's nutritional needs. When the mother returns and caresses the infant, its body knows that food is available and resumes growth.

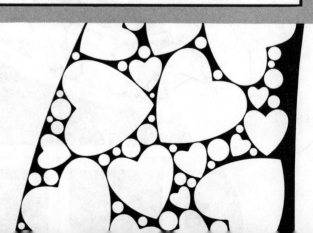

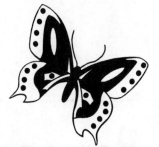

To AVOID CANCER, SAY "I DO!"

Want to reduce your risks of getting cancer, and increase your chances of beating it should you get it? Get married, says James Goodwin of the Medical College of Wisconsin.

Husbands and wives have better chances of living through a bout with cancer, Goodwin claims. Given similar treatments, he reports, married people pull through more often than singles. More emotional support from a spouse or better financial conditions could explain the differences in survival rates, Goodwin speculates. His findings also suggest that increased counseling for single people with cancer could save lives.

What GARBO KNEW

Maybe Greta Garbo was on to something. If you "vant to be alone" by all means, carve out some time in your schedule for it. It's good for you — and for your family.

Mental health experts have become increasingly aware of how important time spent alone is to personal well-being and healthy family relationships. Therapists find that when people regularly take time for themselves, they shed stress easily, deepen their creativity, and emerge from their solitude better able to handle the demands of others.

Laugh TOGETHER, LOVE TOGETHER

Falling in love? Check out each other's choice in comedy before thinking about tying that knot. According to the *Journal of Personality Assessment*, couples who share a similar sense of humor stay together longer and are more interested in getting married than those who don't laugh at the same things.

How does your marriage measure up?

If it seems that you and your spouse aren't as close as you were once upon a time, you may be right. The years may have put a little distance between you. Just to be certain, get out the yardstick and take a few measurements.

The emotional closeness of husbands and wives can be translated to inches, claims family therapist D. Russell Crane of Brigham Young University. Crane and his colleagues tested 108 couples to see how close they really were. Crane had the couples stand opposite, then walk toward each other. He instructed them to stop when they were at a "comfortable conversation distance." Crane measured this distance, then questioned the couples on marriage intimacy and divorce potential. He says that compared with happily married men, husbands unhappy with their marriages tended to stop a further distance away from their wives.

Crane says his test determined how strong the couples' bonding really was. The happy couples, he says, stopped an average of 11.4 inches apart; the unhappy, 14.8 inches apart.

Recognize the friend or foe behind a smile

Did you ever wonder if someone is truly enjoying your company or just trying to be polite? It may be difficult to tell, if their emotions are masked by a smile.

The trick to deciding is to check the skinfold of the eyes, says psychologist Paul Ekman of the University of California, San Francisco. True smiles of enjoyment can be detected by a characteristic wrinkling of the skin around the eyes, Ekman claims. He says lying smiles often can be detected by a tightening of the muscles around the mouth and narrowing of the lips.

In a study, Ekman and his colleagues had 31 students watch a pleasant film, then describe their feelings to an interviewer. Next they watched a gory tape showing amputations and burns; they were told to lie and tell the interviewer they enjoyed it. Ekman says those telltale signs of deceit showed up to a much greater degree during the deceptive interview.

THE LOVE THEORY WE HOPE IS WRONG

The Worst Idea of All Time Award from the Romeo and Juliet Society has to go to this one: Love may be just a chemical addiction to another person and not really "love" at all.

Kissing transfers an "addictive" substance, sebum, which chemically bonds two people, claims Bubba Nicholson, State University of New York graduate student of animal behavior. He says sebum is secreted by the sebaceous skin glands located all over the body, including the inside of the lips, scalp, face, neck, nipples, and outside surfaces of the sex organs. When kissing, Nicholson says, the lips' sucking action is perfect for extracting the sebum of another person.

Nicholson bases his theories on Chinese research involving the sebaceous exchanges of birds. He says when the sebaceous glands were removed and no sebum could be exchanged, the birds' interest in each other seemed to dwindle.

To us, the human connection seems like a long flight of fancy.

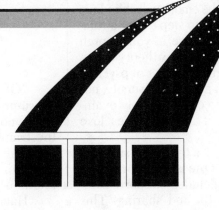

A LOVE TRIANGLE
MADE FOR TWO

"Love is good for anything that ails you," promises a popular song from the 1930s. "Love makes the world go round," says a more recent tune. "Love makes my head spin," complained a friend of mine the other day. With all this healing and spinning going on, love seems to be a rather potent form of energy.

In regenerative terms, love is a powerful resource that can and should be used to positively influence your life. The problem is that love can be emotionally blinding. Many times it's hard to step out of a relationship and be objective in your search for improvement. But a new theory by Dr. Robert J. Sternberg, professor of psychology and education at Yale University, not only offers a way to constructively examine relationships, it actually gives love a shape.

"Picture love as a triangle," suggests Dr. Sternberg. "One side represents *intimacy*, which includes support, communication, warmth, and sharing. This provides the emotional content of a relationship. Another side stands for *passion*. Passion is a motivational force that

leads to arousal, physical excitement, and a desire to be united with the loved one. *Commitment* makes up the final side. This is where a decision to love another person and maintain that love is made."

Putting the three sides together, Dr. Sternberg's portrait of love looks like this:

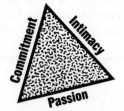

"Of course what you have here is *consummate love*, or the perfect relationship," notes Dr. Sternberg. "Not only is the triangle complete, but as shown by the length of its sides, passion, commitment, and intimacy all play equal roles in the relationship it represents."

Having looked at first prize, perfect love, let's get back down to earth a moment and build a triangle from scratch. After all, true love isn't created in a day. It's a process in which a couple begins with a particular component and then adds on.

"Many times, the way a relationship begins will set the tone for the love that ensues," says Dr. Sternberg. "If I had to pick the best way to build a strong triangle, I would start with the intimacy side. Communication and understanding are very important for a healthy and meaningful love."

At this point, a diagram of your feelings toward the object of affection looks like this:

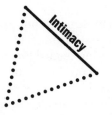

You like the person and feel closeness, but right now it's more of a high-grade friendship than a love affair.

After getting to know and like another person, *passion* may be the next thing to develop:

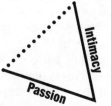

"When physical attraction is added to emotional involvement, the result is *romantic love,*" says Dr. Sternberg. "This is a Romeo-and-Juliet type of relationship —strong while it lasts but probably short-lived without a decision toward commitment.

"Sometimes, instead of passion, commitment will come after intimacy," notes Dr. Sternberg. "Known as *companionate love,* this type of relationship is more of a long-term relationship. You also see companionate love in many marriages where passion has faded away."

Using Dr. Sternberg's three love components, there are eight possible relationships that can be formed, ranging from *infatuation,* where only the passion side of the triangle exists, to *empty love,* a relationship relying completely on commitment for its survival.

But suppose you and your significant other have assembled all three sides of the triangle and love smiles upon you. What next? Is your triangle stabilized?

"I'm afraid not," answers Dr. Sternberg. "Over the course of a relationship, all three components fluctuate at different rates, some increasing in strength while others gradually fade. And of course there is the ever-present possibility that one or more of the components may disappear altogether should the relationship start to falter."

The dimensions of the triangle, meaning the length of the sides, represent the amounts of passion, commitment, and intimacy present in a relationship. The area of the triangle portrays the overall amount of love. As such, over a ten-year period a typical marriage might look like this:

YEAR 1

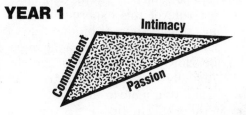

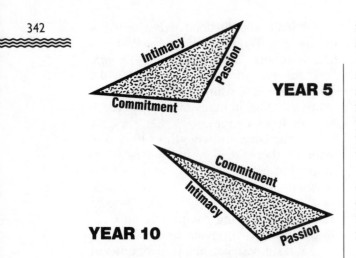

Year one shows a high degree of passion in the relationship. By year five, intimacy has become the dominant theme of the marriage, with passion fading. By the tenth year, commitment is the strongest bond in the relationship. In this case, although the priorities have changed, the area of the triangle (and the total amount of love) has remained the same.

How to Apply the Theory

Now that you've mastered the basic mechanics of the theory, it's time to apply it to your own relationship. The next quiet evening you have, round up the object of your affection, two pencils, and a couple pads of paper, and head for the den. Since the first rule of this experiment is no peeking, situate yourself on one side of the room and assign your mate the opposite side. Now you're ready to triangulate.

"Actually, there are several triangles for you and your mate to each draw," says Dr. Sternberg. "The first one is your *real* triangle. This is how you feel right now about your mate."

Before drawing your commitment line, ask yourself a couple of questions. Do you still hold firm to your decision to love your mate? Is this love still a long-term prospect? Take into account fidelity as well as the amount of energy you expend to keep the relationship on its feet.

Passion. How's your sex life? How excited or aroused do you feel about the other person? What amount of daily touching, holding, and kissing do you initiate?

Intimacy. Are you happy and having fun in the relationship? Have you been gaining or losing regard for the other person? Can you count on your loved one in times of need? Is there mutual understanding? Do you give emotional support to your loved one? Do you receive it? Are you or your partner starting to close up when it comes to intimate communication?

Of course there are no quantitive measurements on which to base your triangle. But after honestly thinking over the above questions, just draw the lines as large or small as your overall answers seem to warrant. You'll get a fair enough approximation of how you feel.

Next, each of you should draw your *ideal* triangle. This is how you would like to feel about the relationship. According to Dr. Sternberg, your ideal triangle will be developed in part from the best that previous relationships offered you as well as expectations of how good the present relationship could really be.

"The third triangle to draw is your *perceived* triangle," says Dr. Sternberg. "This is how *you* think your partner feels about you."

Now it's time for show-and-tell. First compare your *real* triangle with your partner's. Where are the differences? Was yours long on intimacy where his was short? It may be time for some discussion. Compare your ideal triangles and see if both of you have the same amount of desire for intimacy. If you do, then it could be time for you to spend a little more time together, share a few secrets, and start working toward that ideal you both have. It may even be a little easier to do when you know you have the same thing in mind.

Many times there is a gap between feeling and action in a relationship that can cause misunderstandings. Suppose your perceived triangle (how you think your mate feels about you) shows a short passion side, for example, but your mate's real triangle shows a long-sided passion. Obviously, your mate is big on romance but doesn't seem to show it as far as you're concerned. Now you know how she really feels, and perhaps the two of you can spend a little extra time bringing that passion to the surface.

Perceived triangles can work the opposite way also. You may find that while you think you're extremely intimate, your partner's perceived triangle is saying that he's not receiving that message. Or you both might think of yourselves as intimate, but neither one thinks the other feels that way.

In a case like this it could be time to go digging for buried treasure. "*Expressed intimacy,* or the intimacy that is exhibited in everyday behavior, often declines over the years," says Dr. Sternberg. "But underneath there is another thing known as *latent intimacy,* in which a couple becomes so attuned that they don't notice how much they rely on one another."

It sometimes takes a shock or disruption of daily events to bring latent intimacy to the surface. A death in the family may suddenly bring people closer together just as a temporary separation can uncover a sense of need and interdependence. But you can also manufacture disruptions of a more positive nature. Take an unusual trip together, dare to do something out of the ordinary.

"The triangle theory is a place to start rather than the answer," says Dr. Sternberg. "It's a way of straightening out the lines of communication between you and your significant other. Once you've done that, it's really up to you whether you work to improve. But at least now you have a direction and goal to move toward."

Start drawing.

M. G.

LISTENING AND OTHER INTIMATE ACTS

Cupid's arrow whizzed, bells rang, and angels sang. You found your one and only, and the best part of your life was about to begin. So, what happened? You know you still love each other (or at least you're almost positive you do), but you don't seem as close as you once dreamed you could be.

Don't worry—here comes that arrow again. If you've got just two simple things, you can bring lost zing back to your relationship and even supplement it with some desirable qualities it never had, says counselor Stuart R. Johnson, a clinical faculty member of the Yale University Department of Psychiatry.

The necessary base: a mature love and 60 percent compatibility, says Johnson. "Mature love means you and your partner can recognize and appreciate the good and the bad in each other. You see more in each other than just what you want to see, and you've gotten beyond infatuation," he explains. Sixty percent compatibility isn't all that much of the stuff. All it means is that you and your partner want to do the same things and agree on ideas a little more than half the time.

But even if you have those crucial ingredients, it doesn't mean everything is as rosy as it could be. One thing even the best-adjusted couples want more of is intimacy. It comes up again and again in surveys. After interviewing hundreds of women and men, Dr. Michael McGill, author of *The McGill Report on Male Intimacy,* reports that virtually every woman he spoke to wanted to improve the level of intimacy in her love relationship. Men often *appear* to want emotional closeness less than women, but Dr. Dan McAdams, a psychologist of Loyola University of Chicago, says that they like it when they get it. Dr. McAdams learned from his own survey that the greater a man's need for intimacy, the greater his sense of security and certainty in life.

Emotional closeness (and the exciting lovemaking it usually leads to) may be a popular goal, but it's hardly the Holy Grail. That is, it isn't impossible to find. Therapists say a few exercises, a little effort, and a bit of self-understanding can go a long way toward improving even the best of relationships.

The Rhythms of Your Intimacy

How will you maximize the emotional closeness in your relationship? Start by pinpointing those times when the potential for intimacy is *naturally* at its peak—then you can take advantage of those "intimate instants" by being sure to spend them together. "Couples who do not have children living at home usually feel closest late at night or very early in the morning," says therapist Olga Silverstein, senior faculty member at the Ackerman Institute for Family Therapy in New York City. "Even when it's not sexual, their most intimate time together centers around bed, because going to bed is a ritual that leads to talking and closeness.

"Recognize the importance of this rhythm and take advantage of it," suggests Silverstein. "Go to bed at the same time. One of you should not stay downstairs watching TV."

As parents well know, children in the home change the rhythms of a relationship. "With children, there are no more uninterrupted morning hours together, nor do the children always sleep through the night," says Silverstein. "Couples with children must work out a whole new arrangement to have intimacy. Rather than one partner becoming absorbed in work and the other in the children, both people have to make intimacy with each other a priority. They have to grab it when they can."

When there *is* intimacy, it often seems that everything else in the relationship clicks into place. And for most couples, there are times like that, when it's working perfectly. But what about those other times, when one or both partners feel dissatisfied?

It's important to realize that, while everyone wants those good times to exist all the time, they just can't. Even the best of relationships will only be harmonious about 60 percent of the time, experts say. So the goal is not to get rid of all the conflicts in your relationship, but rather to work out the disputes in a way that doesn't cause you both a lot of pain, says Johnson.

The conflicts in your relationship could be about almost anything on which you and your partner can take opposite sides: you're too emotional and he's not emotional enough, you're very social and she's not social at all, you're physically demonstrative and he won't touch you in public, you're passive while she's assertive . . . the list goes on.

The core struggle, though, says Johnson—the one the conflicts are really about—is almost always the pull between autonomy and intimacy. How often do you want to go for a long walk together while your partner wants to finish a book? What happens when your partner wants to make love while you'd rather visit with friends? "Being out of sync about these desires does not indicate that there is anything wrong with the relationship," says Johnson. "It is perfectly normal that there will be many times when you won't both want to be together at the same moment.

"For most couples, the problem is not that, over the long run, one person wants

345

How to Recover from an Extramarital Affair

If your partner doesn't know, the main question on your mind is probably "Should I tell?"

The answer: Not if you want the relationship to continue. "If you've learned from the affair and don't intend to have another, there is no reason to tell," says Dr. Lonnie Barbach, clinical faculty member at the University of California, San Francisco, and author of *For Each Other: Sharing Sexual Intimacy.* "If you tell, then your partner will just have to work through everything you've already finished with. Your main reason for telling would probably be to relieve your own guilt." Not the most commendable justification for honesty above and beyond the call of duty.

If your spouse has found out, then all you can do is help your spouse learn to trust you again. "Your spouse wants a guarantee that you will never do it again," says Dr. Barbach. It takes time to rebuild trust, but you can help it along by acting particularly trustworthy. Reassure her that you still love her. Call him from work to say you're on your way home—and then go home right away. "If your spouse feels violated, you both might feel better seeking help from a counselor," says Dr. Barbach.

One step on the road to recovery is understanding why you or your spouse had the affair. Extramarital affairs usually occur, not because one spouse loves the other less than before, but rather as a reaction to loss or stress, says sex therapist Dr. Avodah K. Offit, clinical assistant professor at Cornell University Medical College and author of *Night Thoughts: Reflections of a Sex Therapist.* "The course of married life provides at least fourteen predictable times for sexual infidelity to occur," she says. "All have to do with loss or stress, and represent attempts to cope or adapt." These include any point when a man or woman is:

- Deciding on or beginning a career.
- Heavily involved in expansion or success.
- Changing jobs.
- Traveling extensively alone.
- Depressed by failure.
- Bored by monotony or fatigued by dull overwork.
- Retiring.

Other times when extramarital affairs may occur have less to do with work and more to do with life events and family crises. These include:

- Pregnancy and childbirth.
- The period when small children require a great deal of attention.
- Times of bereavement, such as the death of a parent.
- Periods of other emotional crisis—a child's accident or a mate's illness.
- When children leave the home for work, school, or college.
- Any time in a person's life when she or he confronts the process of physical aging, an awareness that occurs at least in every decade of life.
- Major changes in style of life, such as moving or buying a home.

more or less intimacy than his or her partner," says Johnson. "People tend to choose partners who want about the same level of intimacy as they do." The real problem is finding a satisfactory method you can use to decide how much intimacy to have at *this moment.*

One method many couples use, says Johnson, is to unconsciously make up rules about the relationship. These rules usually say that one person will initiate all the intimacy while the other will make sure both partners get enough time alone, enough "space." The way it works is that the intimacy partner chases after the autonomy partner who always runs away.

Think, for instance, of the wife who's always complaining that her husband goes out with "the boys" when she wants them to spend time together. When they do spend time together, the husband feels resentful; he's only there to appease his wife. He may actually want to be close to his wife just as much as she wants to be close to him—at least sometimes. And she would really like to be alone, or away from him, some of the time—probably the same amount of time he wants to be away from her. But instead of each of them deciding, whether they want to be intimate with their partner at a particular moment, they find it easier to fit into their assigned roles.

This method of one partner chasing and the other running away *can* work well, according to Johnson. Since the chaser occasionally catches up with the one running away, "in the long run, a couple like this will probably end up getting enough time together to be close and enough time apart to be separate individuals," he says.

"The problem with the technique, though, is that it's so painful and unpleasant."

How do you and your partner solve your conflicts? Does one of you run while the other chases? How well do you tolerate your differences? Does one of you believe the old fantasy that "If you really loved me, we would always want to do the same thing at the same time?"

Exercises for Increasing Intimacy

No matter what the state of your relationship, you can improve it by doing these four exercises developed by Stuart Johnson, and outlined by Maggie Scarf in her book, *Intimate Partners: Patterns in Love and Marriage.* They may seem like a strange way to improve your relationship, but, according to Johnson, they can be remarkably effective tools to help you change the unspoken rules of your relationship. Want further proof they can work? Their creator met his wife in college and today, more than 31 years later, they are still happily married.

Exercise 1: Talking and Listening

Mutually select 1 hour a week and agree that this time will be spent together with no interruptions allowed. Flip a coin to see who will go first. Then, the first person talks to the other for half an hour. She (or he) can talk only about herself. She is not to say anything about the partner or the relationship.

The other partner will listen attentively but make no verbal response at all.

How to Stop an Argument

One of the main reasons an argument escalates into a screaming fight is because the yeller is never sure that the yellee has understood the reason for the anger. Not necessarily believed or agreed with—just understood, says Dr. Shirley Zussman, a sex and marital therapist in New York City. If the angry one isn't sure the other person got it, he or she is likely to repeat the point, at a higher decibel level, in different words, again and again.

To stop an argument before it escalates, often all you need to do is make sure that your points are getting across and that you understand your partner's points, says Dr. Zussman. She suggests that you repeat back, in your own words, what your partner is saying. For example, "Let me get this straight. You're saying that you're angry because you always have to walk the dog and today the dog pooped on the rug. So you feel I should have walked the dog today since I never do it. I can see why you would feel that way."

If you've got it, then you can go on and present your side of the dispute, which your partner can then paraphrase back to you. If you don't have it—well, now your partner has a reason to repeat what he or she is angry about. Maybe once you understand, you'll even agree. Then the fight will really be over.

After the half hour is over, the speaker and listener switch positions. The second partner talks and the first pays attention. Again, no discussion of the mate or the relationship is allowed.

At the end of the hour, each partner will go about his or her business. No discussion of the exercise is allowed for at least three days.

This task forces the partners to face each other as separate, autonomous beings; to act autonomously themselves, taking responsibility for their own feelings; and to pay attention to and value the other, in an intimate way.

Repeat this exercise as often as you like, even as you begin to do exercise 2.

Exercise 2:
Odd Day, Even Day

Divide up the days of the week between you. One may take Tuesday, Thursday, and Saturday, for instance, while the other takes Wednesday, Friday, and Sunday. Each partner, on his or her days, must make an intimacy request of the other. The mate has agreed ahead of time to meet it. Other needs can be expressed during the day, but the mate is only under obligation to meet the one need that is presented as part of the exercise.

It is important that the needs be realistic and specific. Do not ask for an hour of time when your partner is on the way to the dentist. Do not ask your partner to love you forever, or even to express his or her love. Most couples also agree in advance that the most volatile issues—usually sex and money—will not be approached in this exercise.

Good requests might include a 10-minute back rub, a walk together in the park, or ½ hour to discuss a problem at work.

This task helps couples resolve power struggles by giving each one power over the relationship on alternating days. It also helps partners identify what their own needs really are.

Exercise 3:
Adding Requests

Take your time before you embark on this exercise; you should be thoroughly comfortable with exercise 2 before going on. When you are ready, very slowly increase the number of intimacy requests that must be made on the alternating days. There is no prescribed upper level, nor does it matter how quickly you increase the number—do whatever is comfortable for you both. Other than the higher number of requests made, exercise 3 is identical to exercise 2.

Exercise 4:
Control and Meta-Control

When you are satisfied that you have gotten all you can out of exercise 3, move on to this one. The overall schedule for each partner stays the same as in the last two exercises—you each have control on alternating days. Now, however, you will be allowed to make as many requests as you like during your assigned days. All intimacy requests made at this point may be considered automatically part of the game (though certain off-limit requests, such as those dealing with sex and money, can still be considered separate from the exercise, if desired).

But while one partner is allowed to have control of the day by making as many intimacy requests as she likes, the other partner is now given a control of another sort—a *meta-control*. The other partner must respond positively to all requests made *until he decides that his limit has been met, at which time he can call off the game for the day.* After that, he is under no obligation to meet any more requests made that day.

In other words, the second partner can not respond selectively—he must say yes to all requests in the order they are made, but can end the exercise for the day whenever he wants.

The next day, the partners switch positions.

Thus, both partners are in control *at the same time.* And, each person's control does not compete directly with that of the other. Scarf writes, "Both spouses can negotiate intimate needs from a position of strength and entitlement, because each maintains control of a different yet important domain.

"When this small set of new rules is introduced . . . interesting things usually begin to happen in the relationship. As might be readily imagined, each partner is a bit reluctant to refuse one of the other's requests (thereby canceling the game for the rest of the day), because it is so

350

clear that the other partner can, on the following day, retaliate in precisely the same manner. And what has been learned about the partner in the course of carrying out the preceding assignments is now very handy information to have," continues Scarf.

"Each person knows (from the Talking and Listening task) what matters are foremost on the partner's mind. Each person knows also (from the Odd Day, Even Day exercise) which particular intimate needs and desires are of critical importance to the mate. Negotiations with the partner are, as a result, far more easily manageable—because such information makes it easier to trim the sails of one's own intimate needs to the winds of the relationship's reality."

By this time, your relationship is probably getting really enjoyable. Just doing the exercises above has given you more intimacy and a better understanding of each other. You're probably arguing less and doing more together. Most likely, you're having a pretty good time.

So, how will you react the next time a conflict comes up? Remember, since you only need 60 percent compatibility to have a good relationship, conflicts are bound to come up. Since you are having such fun with each other, you won't want to fight about the conflict. But what if you don't know any other way to settle the dispute? Really, a "good fight" isn't so good. Fortunately there's a much better way.

The Fine Art of Negotiating with Your Partner

"Even if you do have an egalitarian relationship, where neither partner can veto the other one, you may not know how to negotiate in an egalitarian way," says Johnson.

The first step, he says, is for both of you to state your needs or desires clearly. The key to this step is making sure you don't prenegotiate. Prenegotiating is when you want to do something—say, to go on an all-day picnic. But you think your partner won't want to. So, rather than suggesting an all-day picnic, you suggest going out for a couple of hours. When your partner still turns you down, you get angry and think, "Boy, am I mad. He didn't even appreciate that I already scaled down my plans. I give up so much, and get so little!"

Obviously, your partner doesn't know how much you have already given up, because you lied about what you wanted in the first place.

So, suppose you state your needs clearly. It might go like this:

TERRY: "Let's go see a movie."
JIM: 'I'm tired, and I wanted you to make us dinner so I could take a nap."

Next, check out your needs and see if they are compatible. If Jim had said, "Yeah, let's go," there would have been no conflict. Terry and Jim would be in the car by now. But there was a conflict.

Now comes a danger point, says Johnson. What could happen next is that both Terry and Jim will feel that they had better protect their positions because the other one is about to launch an attack. Each one will then start explaining why their need is the better one.

TERRY: "The movie is only going to be around for another few days and there are leftovers in the fridge anyway."
JIM: "We just went out last night and we

FIVE WELL-KNOWN LOVE OFFERINGS

This list of love offerings of the rich and famous was excerpted from *The Book of Lists* by David Wallechinsky, Irving Wallace, and Amy Wallace.

1. Pearls in Wine

When Mark Antony expressed surprise at the opulence of a banquet Cleopatra had prepared for him, she dropped two pearls of inestimable value in her wine and drank the concoction to his health, insisting that her tribute to him should far surpass the cost of the feast. After they became lovers, he presented her with Cyprus, Phoenicia, Coele-Syria, and parts of Arabia, Cilicia, and Judea.

2. Freedom

Suleiman the Magnificent, ruler of the Ottoman Empire, gave the enslaved Roxelana her freedom, as a love offering, and then married her. An observer wrote: "This week there has occurred in this city a most extraordinary event, one absolutely unprecedented in the history of the sultan's period. Suleiman has taken unto himself a slave woman from Russia as his empress."

3. Shakespearean Sonnets

Not Shakespeare, but the publisher who pirated the sonnets, wrote the dedication, "To Mr. W. H." The 154 poems are

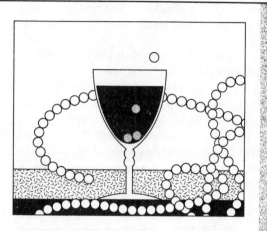

among the greatest love offerings of all time, but it is not known for whom they were written.

4. Sonnets From the Portuguese

Elizabeth Barrett began her famous sonnets when she first met Robert Browning, and they chronicle her reactions to their developing friendship and love. Browning learned of the sonnets early in 1847 after their son Robert Wiedemann Barrett was born. Elizabeth confessed to her husband, "I had written some poems about you."

5. A $10,000 Bicycle

"Diamond Jim" Brady presented actress Lillian Russell with a gold-plated bicycle complete with mother-of-pearl handlebars and spokes encrusted with chips of diamonds, emeralds, rubies, and sapphires. When Miss Russell went on tour, the bicycle —kept in a blue plush-lined morocco case —traveled with her.

352

never stay around and just rest anymore. I worked really hard today, you know."

Both of them think they are just defending their needs but, says Johnson, each feels that the other's defense is really an attack. Since both people feel attacked, they are likely to attack back any second now.

Let's backtrack a minute—surely this fight could have been avoided.

"Instead of each partner trying to prove that his or her need is more worthy than the other's," says Johnson, "the thrust should be toward accommodation. Both needs are fine—they just aren't compatible."

There are at least four ways to bridge the gap between Terry and Jim. The first way is for one of them to freely give up his or her idea and go with the other person's. Freely is the key word—the one who accommodates the other shouldn't feel pressured into it. He or she must know that a real choice exists. If Jim knows that if he doesn't go to the movie, Terry is going to pick a huge fight about something else, or make him pay in small, insidious ways (stony silences over that home-cooked meal?), then his choice can't be freely made.

Jim also has to feel that, over the long haul, Terry would do the same for him. If Jim believes he does all the giving in, then giving in is not a good choice at this point.

If Jim feels that he has a real choice to make, and that Terry would do the same for him at some other time, then a good way to avoid fighting would be for Jim to go to the movie. The best way, in fact, would have been for Jim to tell himself, "Sure, I'm tired, but Terry's a good egg— I'll just go to that movie." Then, he could have responded, "Sure, let's go," and Terry

never would have known that they had just been negotiating.

But, suppose neither partner was ready to accommodate the other so easily. Then, try choice two or three.

The second way to resolve a conflict without a fight is to compromise, says Johnson. They've been doing this all their lives, but sometimes Terry and Jim have trouble remembering how when they are in the middle of a fight. Compromise would go like this:

TERRY: "Let's go see a movie."

JIM: "I'm tired, and I wanted you to make us dinner so I could take a nap."

TERRY: "I could make us a quick dinner while you take a short nap, and then we could still catch a movie."

JIM: "Yeah, especially if we go to one nearby."

Choice three, *quid pro quo*, looks a lot like compromise. This, says Johnson, is when you each get all of what you want, but at different times. If they were to settle their conflict this way, Terry would cook dinner and Jim would promise that tomorrow night, they will go to a movie.

If none of these solutions works out, the final one is for Terry to go to the movies while Jim stays home and rests. "There is absolutely nothing wrong with this, as long as it doesn't happen so often that you never do things together any more," says Johnson.

"Doing things separately *sometimes* can actually strengthen a relationship," he adds. Why? Because doing things alone will give each of you the autonomy you need, and allow the intimacy you both want to flourish.

REGENERATE YOUR FAMILY BONDS

From TV talk shows to Sunday supplement sessions with sociologists, we've all been made aware of the impending demise of the American family. And while you may not have noticed the sound of epitaphs being chipped in marble, haven't you ever wondered what happened to the Waltons? If they were around now, would they be living in a condo, taking separate vacations, and seeing a family therapist?

Before giving the family photo album a decent burial, I called Dr. Donald Conroy, director of the National Institute for the Family, to find out what's gone wrong and what can be done. "To understand the gradual drifting apart of the family unit," he says, "we've got to go back to the eighteenth century. America was an agricultural society, where farm families really had to pull together to make ends meet. The family was where the young learned trades and other important information to help them get on in life.

"With little in the way of entertainment available, the family dinner table was where conversation and fun at day's end were to be had. At the occasional barn-raising party or harvest dance, families attended as a single unit, proudly making their entrance together and sharing the good times. For fun and for survival, the family was a necessity."

With the coming of the industrial revolution, factory work provided the farming man a chance to earn a less difficult living. So he packed up his family, sold the old farm, and made the jump to city life. There, families of similar ethnic background or religious beliefs formed close-knit neighborhoods, where tradition flourished. The menfolk worked together in a nearby factory, while the women were in and out of each other's kitchens borrowing a pinch of pepper, trading a favorite recipe, or enjoying a bit of juicy gossip. Meanwhile, when the children weren't learning their 'rithmetic in school, they were playing in the street right outside their front door.

While the family no longer needed to pull together just to survive, they were still bound together by their tradtions. But town life, with its taverns, theaters, dance halls, and diverse population, was beginning to provide other avenues of interest outside the home.

353

Bringing this history lesson up to date, Dr. Conroy continues. "From the 1960s on, the family has been put to the test of surviving through some rapidly changing social values and practices. Dual-career couples, changing sex roles, as well as greater mobility and the ever-increasing availability of entertaining and intellectual stimuli outside the home have made some former family interactions obsolete. Additionally, the high-tech, or information, age we live in has allowed us to lead lives that are bigger, faster, and more colorful without necessarily bringing us closer together."

Some of us probably can remember the whole family gathered around the radio or television, situated centrally in the living room, listening to "The Shadow" or watching Uncle Milty put on a dress. We laughed together, made jokes, and maybe even took votes on which program to watch next. "Now," says Dr. Conroy, "the typical American home is bristling with compact-disk players, televisions, telephones, video machines, computers, and personal cassette players. What we once watched, listened to, and discussed together, we now do apart in separate rooms."

I was beginning to get visions of Ray Bradbury's *Fahrenheit 451,* where the future consists of people sitting in unbroken silence before wall-high television screens. Before I got too carried away, Dr. Conroy shed a ray of hope on the situation. "Interestingly enough, we're beginning to find out that the very things that seem to be pulling us apart, isolating us, could also provide fuel for a better family relationship than was ever possible in the past."

How is that possible? Think about those farm families for a minute. Outside of an occasional roundtable discussion on tubers or whether they would have to shoot Eb's horse, what did they have to talk about? With little news to share and almost no time for leisurely studies, people back then spent time together, but did they grow together through shared knowledge and insight?

Now, with the world at our fingertips, each member of your household takes a daily plunge into a pool of new sights, sounds, and ideas, which they then bring home. It becomes your job to share your experiences with your family and get them to share with you.

The Skill of Listening

"Good communication," emphasizes Dr. Conroy, "is a primary attribute of a healthy family. And under this heading one of the most important skills family members can develop is how to listen to each other. We need to listen with our minds and our hearts, understanding what's being said and feeling the underlying emotions and concerns."

Leo Tolstoy once wrote, "Happy families are all alike; every unhappy family is unhappy in its own way." I asked Dr. Conroy what all these happy families have in common. "When they talk, they are direct and familiar. They're honest and constructive without being constantly critical. Family members appreciate each other and generally there is a real sense of purpose and commitment to preserving the family unit. Stress brings these types of families closer together rather than tearing them apart."

According to Dr. Conroy, we can either be crisis managers or fitness managers.

The former ride the crest of a wave, dealing with problems when they've reached a crisis point. Fitness managers, on the other hand, note family potentials, capabilities, and strengths, building on them and weeding out small disturbances ahead of time so that the crisis never arises.

Now, it's real nice to read about that rarefied air of the perfect family team, about meaningful communication and mutual appreciation. But somehow when we get right down to the everyday, we often treat our friends better than our family and relate more secrets to them than to our own flesh and blood. Why? "We get used to our family members," answers Dr. Conroy. "Taking our relatives for granted is one of the biggest things that can undermine good relationships in a marriage or a family."

To gain real breakthroughs in intimacy, what's needed is an experience that takes you and the rest of your family out of the everyday roles of father, mother, sister, and brother and makes you friends. You need to see each other in a new light.

I tend to favor creativity and humor as tools to take people out of context. A good laugh melts barriers faster than anything I know, while a work of creativity is always a window into the soul of the creator. Just walking around our offices I dug up some great suggestions for family activities sure to bring out the best in everyone.

"A giant family collage!" suggested one woman. "We took a Sunday afternoon, dug up all our old family photo albums and sprawled out on the floor of the den in a circle. Then we each took turns picking out favorite photos of each other and gluing them to a big poster board. When we were finished, we had it framed. Now it hangs on our living room wall. We had a

great time and I couldn't stop thinking that this was how a family should be."

The point is, when you're having fun together, you're learning about each other, appreciating each other in a new light that will make you closer in everyday life. Another family-fusing activity to try is making a video. Rent a camera for the night and let everyone take a turn shooting, directing, acting, and narrating. If you're stuck on how to start, try creating your own talk show ("He-e-e-e-e-errre's Uncle John!"). Set up a desk in the living room, start the camera rolling and welcome your first guest.

"A sense of playful celebration and humor are very important to the well-being of the family," agrees Dr. Conroy. "Another activity you might try is to start your own tradition." It could be a yearly celebration of the day you moved into your new house, or it could be something totally ridiculous, like an annual Groundhog Day Family Feast and Attic Cleaning Extravaganza. Stick to it each year and let no family member shy away.

In the end these silly and humorous antics are in fact carefully disguised acts of faith—faith in yourself that you possess a great deal of warmth, caring, and fun to share, and faith in your family that they'll take your lead, join in, and let their guard down. If you're wondering why you should bother, ask yourself, "Who do I turn to in times of trouble when there's no one to trust and the world's not with me?" Wouldn't it be nice to turn to those same people when things are fine and you just want someone around to share the good times?

The family is not dead, but a little intensive care wouldn't hurt.

M. G.

355

SEVEN SIGNS OF A HEALTHY RELATIONSHIP

Everyone can spot what is *wrong* with a relationship—"she's jealous," "he's selfish," "she monopolizes the bathroom when he's getting ready for work," "he leaves dirty dishes in the sink."

But what about healthy relationships, the kind where the bliss outranks the misery by a substantial margin? Because even the happiest of relationships aren't happy all the time (and conversely, even the most miserable couples haven't always got the blue meanies), some of us sometimes wonder just what really qualifies as a healthy relationship. Maybe we've got one and don't know it.

Part of this mystery stems from the fact that marriage and family therapists spend almost all of their time with troubled couples. Therefore, almost all of the current research on relationships focuses on the disturbed aspects. Amazingly few research projects have spotlighted healthy relationships. But the happily-ever-after partnership deserves equal time.

After talking with therapists and studying the latest research on the subject, we have discovered seven secret signs that may provide some enlightenment.

1. Independence

Ironically, healthy relationships begin with independence. In a study of happy marriages conducted by Dr. Paul Ammons, associate professor of social work at the University of Georgia, and Dr. Nick Stinnett, chairman of the Department of Human Development and the Family at the University of Nebraska, the two researchers isolated what they termed the vital marriage, defining it as one in which two people find their prime joy in life in each other, yet maintain separate identities.

When both partners have outside interests and don't depend on each other, the couple has a healthy relationship. That is not to say that each partner doesn't care about the other's interests. In fact, they maintain an enthusiasm about the other's work and hobbies. But they still function without the involvement of the other partner.

2. Giving People

In addition, partners in a healthy relationship are giving people. What Dr. Ammons and Dr. Stinnett found was that partners in a vital marriage are good nurturers who do not expect repayment for their good deeds. When a man rises early to make coffee for his partner, he does so because of the happiness it gives her. There's no tallying up for courtesies received. Taking care of a partner should result in the other partner's meeting a need in himself or herself to care and give.

No martyrs are allowed in healthy relationships.

3. Vigorous Sexual Activity

In a study comparing distressed and nondistressed couples conducted by two researchers at the University of Kentucky, statistics proved that the more sexual activity a woman has in her relationship, the more highly she thinks of herself. The same study showed that couples in happy marriages have about three times more sexual intercourse than unhappily married couples.

4. Constructive Fighting

Believe it or not, healthy relationships rely on this component. California therapist Lisa Frankel believes that couples should look at how they fight. "When you can't fight, " Lisa says, "something is wrong. Perhaps you're afraid to express personal feelings or sense a lack of permission to do so. Perhaps fighting led to chaos when you were growing up.

"After all, for many people, fighting means instability or even breaking up, so the message is that it's not okay to fight. Plus there are lots of negative role models around. In my family, you either blew up or cried.

"But in a healthy relationship," Frankel continues, "it's okay to be angry. It doesn't mean that the other person is bad. In an argument between people involved in a healthy relationship, there is no right or wrong person—you're just airing your feelings. This is the most important thing for people to learn: that fighting doesn't mean the other person is right or wrong."

For instance, Helen promised her husband, Peter, that she would cook dinner that night. After a nerve-racking day, Helen arrived home exhausted. "I'm too tired to cook, even though I know I said I would," she sighed, flopping down on the sofa.

His mouth had watered all day at the thought of Helen's walnut and ricotta manicotti, so Peter was both disappointed and hurt. It also seemed to him as though Helen had been too tired to cook for weeks. The result: an argument. But Helen didn't make Peter seem like a tyrant with obsessive demands, and Peter didn't imply that Helen was a lazy, thoughtless wife. After airing their feelings—Helen's frustration at her tough work schedule and Peter's culinary disappointment coupled with his yearning for time with his wife — the twosome ended their argument with Helen eager to cook for Peter as soon as she had time, and Peter's understanding that as long as Helen kept her job, it was unreasonable for them to plan elaborate meals at home during the week.

Which brings us to the fifth quality in a healthy relationship.

5. Open and Honest Communication

"And I mean honest in every sense of the word," reinforces Dr. Ruth Rice, a Dallas therapist who refers to herself as a "family life specialist."

"Contrary to what you read in Ann Landers and Dear Abby about how the other person is usually better off if you keep your mouth shut, I believe that you should be totally honest. If a woman comes home late because she was having a drink with a man, she should say so — not 'I was working late,' " Dr. Rice advises.

"Of course, honest communication may be extremely painful in some instances," she acknowledges. "Most people are really scared to tell the other one how they feel, because the end result could be separation or loss of intimacy. But in the long run, it's the best practice."

Dr. Rice is putting her belief system to the test in her personal life. "Rod and I buy each other lots of gifts," she relates, "and if I buy him a gift that he doesn't like, I want him to tell me. He bought me an ultrasuede suit for Christmas that I just didn't like. Because of our honesty, I was able to tell him that I didn't like it and return the suit and still feel okay, not guilty."

6. Trust

"When you have trust, you don't need to check up on someone. You have enough faith in the other person that you don't need to be a policeman," explains Frankel.

Dual-career couples often face strenuous tests of their relationship over the matter of business dinners with members of the opposite sex. Patricia, a journalist, was shocked to learn that her husband, an advertising account executive, has engaged in three one-night stands while on the road during their 12-year marriage.

When she began to travel while working on a book, however, Patricia experienced firsthand the loneliness that often sweeps over people who travel. She now accompanies her husband whenever feasible and encourages him to call her and express his loneliness. Although it took her some time to redevelop trust in his sexual fidelity to her, Patricia feels that her newly formed trust is more substantial than her earlier feelings.

Dr. Rice notices how the thriving singles scene in Dallas has affected her patients' trust in their relationships. One young married woman who works for an attractive unmarried boss had started going out for drinks on Friday evenings with her boss and other singles from the office.

The woman's husband came to Dr. Rice upset. His wife didn't want to end their marriage, and she did not want to give up going out for a drink on Fridays after work. What a couple must develop in a situation like that is trust.

7. Looking Forward to the Future

In a healthy relationship, there's talk of a future together. Talk of vacations, of housing options, of financial or family planning. Of doing things together because you *want* to.

Portland, Oregon, family therapist Peggy Sherr comments: "The word *commitment* gets overused sometimes. I prefer to say that you're making a choice to be together. In a healthy relationship, you realize that you are making a choice, and you make it every day. When you start feeling like a slave to the commitment, then it's not good anymore. The *choice* to be with someone must be renewed all the time."

AN EXCELLENT RELATIONSHIP WITH YOUR EX

How do you handle your child's high school graduation if you are divorced? In some families, the parents find each other's company so intolerable that if one goes to the ceremony, the other stays home. Others can manage to be at the graduation ceremony together, just as long as they sit at opposite sides of the crowd and celebrate separately.

Both of these groups fit the stereotypical image of the feuding ex-spouses; minimal and highly antagonistic contact. But there are many divorced couples who manage to get through events such as graduations very comfortably, even enjoyably, according to psychologist Constance Ahrons, and these couples may offer an alternative and healthier model for the roles of divorced men and women.

Ahrons, a professor at the University of Southern California, has been studying the relationship between divorced spouses for the past five years. She divides couples into four groups: fiery foes, angry associates (both described above), cooperative colleagues, and perfect pals.

Cooperative colleagues would probably sit together at the graduation ceremony and possibly go out to dinner together afterward, according to Ahrons. Perfect pals, who consider themselves good friends, would very likely plan a graduation party together.

Although perfect pals are the exception—only one out of eight couples in Ahrons's study fell into this category—they are not as unusual as you would think. And together with cooperative colleagues, they made up half of Ahrons's sample. Ahrons's study and a few others reveal a somewhat surprising finding: Not only do divorced couples frequently maintain a friendly relationship, but many of those who are not friends wish that they were.

Friends or Foes?

The common image most people have of divorced couples is warring partners fighting over finances and custody issues. This stereotype, perpetuated in jokes, movies, and television, has been accepted by society as the norm. The prevailing attitude is that "there's something a little crazy if you still have a good relationship with your ex-spouse," says Eleanor Macklin, a psychologist at Syracuse University. Even the words we use to describe divorced spouses, "ex" and "former," lack the capacity to indicate any kind of surviving relationship, Ahrons points out.

Many of the professionals who deal with divorce appear to share this stereotypical bias. In a 1978 study exploring the attitudes of clergy, therapists, and lawyers toward divorce, Rutgers University psychologist Kenneth Kressel found that they considered postdivorce friendship to be pathological—continuing attachment was perceived as an indication of distress over the separation, not realistic caring.

Why do people find it so hard to believe that a divorced couple can be friends? Ahrons says that society just isn't comfortable with the idea. "People believe that former spouses must, of necessity, be antagonists. Otherwise, why would they divorce?"

Anthropologist Margaret Mead had a theory about the source of this discomfort, which she summarized in an article in the book *Divorce and After.* "Any contact between divorced people somehow smacks of incest; once divorced . . . the aura of past sexual relationships makes any further relationship incriminating."

Some therapists tend to be skeptical about ex-spouses remaining friendly, according to Ahrons, simply because most of the couples who end up in counseling reinforce the feuding stereotype. As a result, the professional literature on divorce virtually ignores the positive value of a continuing friendship between former spouses.

Prevailing moral views have probably contributed to the stereotype as well. Until the past decade, Ahrons explains, divorce itself was viewed by large segments of the population as socially, psychologically, and morally aberrant. But now that divorce has become so common (even Ann Landers, the country's adviser on relationships and family matters, ended a long-term marriage), there is less of an emphasis on who was "at fault" or what was the problem with the marriage.

Many psychologists, such as Ahrons and Macklin, now view divorce as more of a transition than an ending and are focusing on how to help families adapt. It's estimated that at least one of every three children growing up today will have a stepparent before they reach the age of 18. With so many parents getting divorced and remarrying other parents, the traditional concept of family is no longer adequate, Ahrons says. She uses the term "binuclear family" to refer to the families created by divorce and remarriage.

Many people mistakenly hope to "reconstitute" the nuclear family when they remarry and end up excluding the nonresidential parents, says Margaret Crosbie-Burnett, a psychologist at the University of Wisconsin-Madison. "In this culture we tend to think that a child has to choose one real mom or dad. Of course it doesn't work, she says. "Kids can easily accept two sets of parents." Crosbie-Burnett found in her study of 87 "stepfather" families—families in which the mother had remarried and had custody of the children from the first marriage—that those who maintained a friendly, or at least businesslike relationship with their ex-spouses were much happier than those with hostile or unfriendly relationships.

Ahrons believes that it's perfectly healthy for divorced couples to have feelings of kinship and that they shouldn't be discouraged. She has been following 98 divorced couples for the past five years in her Binuclear Family Project, interviewing not only former wives and husbands but any new spouses or "spouse equivalents" as well at one year, three years, and five years after divorce. All of the divorced couples had had children together, and the average duration of their marriages had been 10 years. To be included in the study both spouses had to live in Dane County, Wisconsin, and the noncustodial parent must have seen the children at least once in the past two months. Of the 98 pairs, 54 had maternal custody, 28 had joint custody and 16 had paternal or split custody—in which each parent has custody of different children.

Based on the frequency and quality of their interactions, couples were divided into the four groups mentioned earlier. Perfect pals made up 12 percent of the sample. These couples enjoyed each other's company and tended to stay involved in each other's lives, phoning to share exciting news, for example. They were also very child-centered and tried to put their children's interests ahead of their own anger and frustration. Many had joint custody, and none were remarried or living with someone.

Ahrons interviewed one couple who actually shared a duplex apartment so that their children could come and go freely between their homes. The only drawback, they admitted, was lack of privacy, and they suspected that if one took on a new spouse or live-in lover, the arrangement might become awkward.

The largest group was cooperative colleagues, who made up 38 percent of the couples. They were not as involved in each other's lives as perfect pals, but they

managed to minimize potential conflicts, to have a moderate amount of interaction, and to be mutually supportive of each other. Ahrons sees them as the most realistic positive role model for divorcing couples.

Angry associates, who accounted for 25 percent, also had a moderate amount of interaction, but the interactions were fraught with conflict. This group was unable to untangle spousal and parental issues, thus setting the scene for fighting when they dealt with each other.

The archetypal feuding partners, fiery foes, made up 24 percent of the couples. They had as little interaction as possible, argued when they did interact, and did not cooperate at all in parenting. Ahrons suspects that this group many be underrepresented in her study since some of her criteria for inclusion would have ruled out many of the most antagonistic couples.

Lingering Anger

One of the major characteristics distinguishing the four groups was how they handled anger. Even perfect pals still harbored some anger over the divorce, but it was not a major part of the relationship and they were able to talk it out when it erupted. One said the relationship was "like having a good friend that you can still be angry with." Cooperative colleagues and angry associates had about the same amount of anger, but cooperative colleagues could separate the old spousal issues from parental ones, while angry associates could not. Fiery foes' anger was so overwhelming that it prevented any civil interaction.

Time, apparently, did not heal the wounds of divorce for the most antagonistic.

MAKING CONTACT

If a divorced couple who haven't been in touch wish to initiate contact or to improve their relationship, how should they proceed? According to Eleanor Macklin and Carolyn Weston, who have recently completed a study at Syracuse University of remarried women, it's extremely important to have the agreement of the current spouse.

"There must be a consensus within the marriage about what they can handle or tolerate," Macklin says. There can be no doubt that a person's primary allegiance is to the new spouse. The new spouse must be in on the decision and may even need to be involved in the inital contact. Some new spouses want to go along; others say, "Fine, have lunch or dinner together without me."

Macklin encourages divorcing couples to write their own "scripts" for the sort of relationship they'd like to have. "The traditional script has been the husband moves out, the couple no longer interact socially, and are hostile to each other, the father is usually considered 'at fault,' the kids spend most of their time with Mom and interact little with Dad."

Of course, it doesn't have to be that way, she says. It's up to each family to decide what is right for them. "You don't have to have weekly contact to feel like a family member," she adds.

One of Macklin's main goals is to help couples get past their anger. Psychologist Constance Ahrons also considers anger a crucial issue to be worked out. She teaches couples negotiation skills to overcome lingering animosity. "Therapy is helpful in the early part of the divorcing process," she says. "People can learn to build a new kind of relationship."

Although Weston encourages many ex-spouses to maintain contact, she realizes there are situations where it just will not work. If a spouse has abused a partner or the children or has serious alcohol or drug problems, Weston might be hesitant for them to initiate contact: "I think some sort of friendship is the ideal, but it's not always possible.

Ahrons found that angry associates and fiery foes were just as angry about the divorce three years later as they were one year later. And all couples became more distant over time; interaction and positive feelings decreased over five years.

Perhaps even more interesting than the actual relationships are the wishes of former spouses. Despite the fact that almost half of the couples in Ahrons's sample did not have a friendly relationship, in fact many wanted one. Almost everyone Ahrons interviewed wished that he or she at least were on better terms with his or her ex-spouse. They express sentiments such as these: "I really miss hearing about old friends and people he works with," "I would like her to share what's happening in her life," and "I wish there were less bitterness between us." And when asked

364

to describe an ideal parenting relationship, open and frequent communication between parents was often mentioned — even by the fieriest foes.

It's clear that a cooperative and friendly relationship between ex-spouses is beneficial to their children, but is it harmful to later marriages or romances? According to a study by Macklin and Carolyn Weston, a psychology doctoral candidate at Syracuse University, friendship between ex-spouses is not necessarily bad and can even be beneficial to a second marriage.

Macklin and Weston interviewed members of 60 stepfather families; none of the stepfathers had any of their own children living in the household. Based on an earlier study by psychologist W. Glenn Clingempeel at Temple University, Macklin and Weston suspected that those with moderate contact would have the happiest marriages. But they found that the more contact a woman had with her former husband, the happier the new marriage, as long as both she and her new husband agreed about the nature and frequency of contact.

They defined high contact as person-to-person contact more than once a month; moderate as contact at least once every six months; and low, less than once every six months. Thirteen percent of the wives had a least weekly contact with their ex-spouses and more than 60 percent had at least a moderate amount of contact. Interestingly, those who were most dissatisfied with their relationship with their ex-spouse wanted more contact, not less. And many new husbands, too, thought the wife should have more rather than less contact with her former husband. It

was very rare for a couple to be dissatisfied because there was too much contact or because a relationship was too friendly. Indeed, some new husbands were threatened by their wives' strong expressions of anger and frustration toward their ex-husbands. They believed that extreme anger represented a strong emotional attachment to the first husband — an interpretation with which the researchers tend to agree.

Why did frequent contact make for happier second marriages? First of all, Macklin says, "It works both ways. A happier new marriage may allow more contact with the ex-spouse." But the main reason, she explains, is parenting. Regular contact between former spouses usually ensures that the father will be more financially supportive and involved in routine coparenting. And new husbands are usually happier when they do not end up shouldering the entire burden of raising their stepchildren.

Marion, one of the women Macklin and Weston interviewed, is a case in point. She was devastated when her husband left her for another woman. But she decided that she had to put it all behind her and two years later began living with David, to whom she is now married. Eight years after the divorce, she and her ex-husband, Jack, are now on very good terms. Jack comes over sometimes to watch television with his two teenage sons and David, goes to baseball games with them, and even has keys to the house. Both Marion and David feel that it is very important for her sons to be actively involved with their father. They say that the boys get the best of both worlds, two fathers.

In Marion's case, continuing friendship with her former husband did not stop her from remarrying someone else. Are there situations in which lingering attachments prevent divorced men and women from replacing the former spouse? Ahrons found that perfect pals, those who interacted frequently, had never remarried. But she feels this was due to the couples' preoccupation with their children, not with each other. "These parents are so wrapped up in their children, they don't want to remarry for fear it will upset the balance." Another possibility, she says, is that outsiders see this tight-knit unit and are put off. For these couples, parenting issues are probably what draw them together.

But aside from the issues of coparenting, is there any reason for former spouses to maintain contact? More than one third of the couples Ahrons interviewed said that they would continue to communicate with each other even if they had no children. As one commented, "Fourteen years of friendship you just don't forget about."

In many ways divorce is more difficult for those without children, because they have no obvious reason to continue contact, says Eric McCollum, a social worker with the Menninger Foundation in Topeka, Kansas. He has counseled many people who dispute the conventional wisdom that a "successful" divorce is one in which feelings of attachment end or are converted to hostility. McCollum believes that "marital attachments do not end at divorce, rather they change in form and intensity." And any unresolved attachments can cause problems in later relationships. "The attachment can go underground," he says. "It may not be obvious, but it's still there."

He has encouraged some of his clients to contact their former spouses "in order to truly divorce." The goal is not to rekindle romance or hash out old issues but "to be together in a different way that allows them to go on." This may simply involve telling each other that they are not forgotten, forgiving the past, or reassuring each other that they have survived the divorce.

One of the women Macklin and Weston interviewed, Sally, left her husband, Allen, because he had a bad temper and physically abused her. She is now remarried to Martin but sees Allen about every two weeks when he picks up and drops off their son. Sally says she has no romantic feelings toward Allen but feels very awkward when they're together because they never really talked about the divorce. She is very timid about standing up to Allen and thought that her remarriage would help, but it hasn't and she is consequently disappointed with Martin. According to Weston, Sally needs to resolve some issues with Allen before she can have the relationship she wants with Martin.

Aside from resolving the past, some couples just want to keep up with each other. "A lot of these people are very good friends," Macklin says. "It doesn't necessarily stop just because the marriage stops." Although most divorced people don't want to resume a romantic relationship, it can be important to know that the person who shared part of their life is doing all right. "These people share history and family together," Ahrons says. "In many ways they have relationships similar to extended kin."

When asked about contact not involving their children, couples said it mostly consisted of phone conversations about extended family members, mutual friends, and new experiences. About half of Ahrons's couples talked about these topics once or twice a month. Fewer than one third talked about issues related to their former marriage, and many avoided discussing finances, a topic almost guaranteed to start a fight.

Almost none of the people in Ahrons's or Macklin and Weston's studies had "dated" or had physical contact or sex with their former spouses. "When we hear of this," Ahrons says, "it's usually right after the separation." The few who had lunch or dinner together said they arranged these meetings to talk about the children. But it was not unusual for these meetings to include discussions of mutual friends and family or personal issues. One of Ahrons's respondents said he would like to have dinner occasionally with his ex-wife but was afraid people in the community would get the wrong idea. In Ahrons's sample, nonparental interaction was most frequent among couples in which neither one had remarried. It was less frequent if both had remarried and rare if only the husband had remarried.

The Second Time Around

Not surprisingly, remarriage can cause a great deal of conflict between ex-spouses. According to Ahrons, the most conflict occurs when the husband has remarried and the wife hasn't—the most likely scenario after divorce. According to numerous studies, divorced men remarry more often and sooner than divorced women.

In the rarer situations when it is only the woman who remarries, the relation-

ship with the former husband is more likely to remain strong, according to Ahrons. One reason for this gender difference, she believes, is that new husbands are less threatened than new wives are by a former spouse and are therefore less likely to discourage contact. The issue, once again, revolved around parenting. Stepmothers are often very stressed and confused about their role as parent to their stepchildren, who rarely live with them, visiting only on occasional weekends and holidays.

Finances are another major reason, according to Crosbie-Burnett. When a man remarries it may be financially very threatening to his ex-wife. He may be more reluctant to support his former family if he is paying the bills for a new one. But when a woman remarries, it often unburdens her first husband financially and improves her standard of living.

Continued contact with the ex-husband was most important to women who had not made the decision to divorce, according to Weston and Macklin's study. On the one hand, this may mean that these women were still unresolved about the divorce and believed that any contact was better than none, says Weston, although there is another possible explanation.

A 1984 study done by psychologists Ellen Pettit and Bernard Bloom at the University of Colorado found that women are more likely to initiate a divorce when conditions have become really terrible. In cases in which just a few minor troubles lead to divorce, it's men who are more likely to initiate. Weston believes that if women wait to initiate a divorce until conditions have become intolerable, they have little desire to maintain a friendship once they're out of the marriage.

Certain factors can predict whether a divorced couple will be likely to maintain a friendly relationship, according to Macklin. The quality of the relationship before the divorce, not surprisingly, is one. If two people like and respect each other a great deal as individuals, not just as lovers, they are obviously more likely to remain friends. In addition, a couple's attitude toward divorce itself is important. "There are some people who believe that complete separation is the only answer," Macklin says. Emotional issues are another factor. Those who still harbor romantic fantasies, who are not happy in a current relationship, or who don't have one when the other spouse does are not good candidates for a friendly divorce.

The circumstances under which the marriage ended will usually affect whether a friendship develops, Macklin says. If it was not a mutual decision, or if there is still a great deal of lingering pain or resentment, friendship is unlikely. The quality of the new marriage and the self-confidence of the new spouse are also extremely important, as is the attitude of the family in general. Some parents will imply to their children, "You have to choose; you can't be loyal to two people," Macklin says. If spouses are especially close to their in-laws, it will encourage contact between former spouses. She points out that "many parents are extremely upset and hurt at the prospect of losing a son- or daughter-in-law." They believe that "we are family forever," regardless of blood ties.

Surprisingly, according to Macklin, neither the time that has elapsed since the divorce nor the presence of children predicts whether former spouses will remain friends.

Gary Ganahl, a psychologist at West Virginia University, has seen cases in which couples got along so well after their divorce that they moved back in together. In some instances, the reduced expectations following the divorce solve a couple's problems with control and independence. "They begin questioning their relationship and start to negotiate issues they haven't negotiated before," he says. Although it is very rare for divorced couples to move back in together, it is not unusual for some couples to find themselves getting along better after their divorce.

In Ahrons's study, 64 percent of the women and 52 percent of the men described their current relationship with their ex-spouse as superior to their relationship at the time of separation. The obvious question to many, then, is: "If a couple get along so well, why are they divorced?" Ahrons points out that just because a couple is getting along after a divorce doesn't guarantee that many of their original problems wouldn't resurface if they got back together. In some cases the end of a marriage reduces anxieties and expectations, so that on a more distant level a couple can get along fine. Crosbie-Burnett adds that working together "for the sake of the children" can often make a couple feel nostalgic. But despite these improved feelings, very few of these couples have any desire to reconcile. In Ahrons's study, more than 90 percent said they rarely or never talked about reconciliation.

There are couples who for whatever reason cannot be happily married to each other. As one of Ahrons's respondents said, "I still feel like I'm married to her sometimes, but I can't live with her." But even in such cases, Ahrons says, there may be aspects of the relationship worth preserving if there were a socially acceptable way of doing so. Macklin, who has maintained a very friendly relationship with her ex-husband, laments the fact that there is no term in our vocabulary to describe this type of surviving relationship. "You could call it 'brother-sister,' there is that kind of feeling, but obviously that's not quite right."

Although some people question the point of continuing a relationship if a couple has no desire to reconcile, Ganahl points out that "if a couple has children there is no question that they are going to have a continuing relationship." Keeping the relationship supportive and friendly benefits the children and in many cases can make life happier for the divorced couple.

On the other hand, Ahrons says, there are some situations where friendship between ex-spouses is impossible. The main point, according to all these researchers and specialists, is that it is not necessarily harmful for ex-spouses to be friendly. "Right now there are no positive norms or messages from society about divorce," Ahrons says. "Most people don't want to give up their total history, but there is very little sanction or support for their relationship to continue."

During the course of her interviews, Ahrons discovered that "no one had asked most of these couples positive questions about their divorce before. They had never thought of the concept of a binuclear family." She would like to provide a positive role model for couples who want to remain friendly. She thinks if people reacted to divorce with the expectation that relationships don't necessarily have to end, "maybe more spouses would be encouraged to have amicable relationships."

The main thing for everyone—therapists, friends, family, and couples—to keep in mind, Ganahl says, is that "relationships change, but rarely dissolve after divorce."

LEARN TO BE LIKED

"A sense of humor will hook me every time."

"Just having someone say hello to me goes a long way."

"I want to be looked in the eye."

"In my mind, someone who likes horses and dogs is automatically okay."

What makes you like certain people? Is it because they're sincere? Direct? Funny? Do they share a secret passion, or perhaps the same worries, as you? Do they care about you? Can you trust them?

Likable people seem to fit easily into just about any group. Their talent for winning friends allows them to take full advantage of the life-enhancing emotional support such social interaction offers. It's no wonder we may look at such people in awe, and perhaps even with a little envy, asking ourselves, "How do they do it?"

Luckily, researchers have asked that question, too, and come up with answers.

"The people who are successful in making contact with others have learned to give what they themselves would like to receive," says Dr. Arthur Wassmer, a psychologist from Kirkland, Washington, and author of *Making Contact.* "They give love to those by whom they would be loved. They respect those by whom they would be respected. They show their liking for people they want to like them."

Such people are likely to be more aware than usual of the impression they are making on others, with everything from clothes to body language to choice of words. Consciously or unconsciously, they have learned to behave in ways that give them an image of warmth and openness. They are giving off cues that say, "I like you and I want you to like me."

Those behaviors can be learned, Dr. Wassmer has found. He has taught them to professional counselors and psychologists, who use them to quickly establish good relationships with patients. He also teaches some of his patients these same skills, and has them practice in therapy groups and in real life, until the behavior sticks.

Learning social skills also can do a lot

to enhance self-esteem, which may be low in people who have a hard time making friends, Dr. Wassmer says.

"When the behavior changes, you start to have a different experience. You leave a party and say, 'Hey, those people really seemed to like me. Maybe I am likable.' So, the fear softens up, and at the next party you're a little more relaxed. You have an even better experience. And you say, "Well, what do you know? People seem to like me. I wonder what happened?' By the third or fourth experience, you're saying, 'Yeah, when I meet new people, generally they like me.' That's radically different from how you used to think."

Here's how to be liked by just about anyone.

Be an active listener. The shy person's frequent complaint is, "I never know what to say." But Dr. Wassmer says, "The way to making conversation is through the ears."

These five rules will help you become an active listener.

1. Listen carefully to what the other person is saying. Don't be worrying about what you are going to say next.

2. In your response, try to rephrase or restate the exact meaning of what has just been said.

3. Never ridicule or be sarcastic about someone else's comments.

4. Respond with questions beginning, "Do you mean . . . ," "Are you saying . . . ," or "Is this what I hear you saying . . . ?"

5. If a pause occurs in the conversation, ask a question of your own.

"Active listening gives other people the important gifts of respect, attention, and recognition, and leaves them with warm feelings toward the listener," Dr. Wassmer says. "It also alleviates the fear that you won't be able to think of something to say. The person you're talking to is telling you what to say every time he or she speaks."

Break the ice. Before you can listen to someone, you must get him talking to you. Most people do this by asking a ritual question, like "Where are you from?" or "How are you enjoying the party?" "Such questions seem like requests for information, but they are really conveying the message, 'I am interested in you' and 'I think I would like to know you,' " Dr. Wassmer says. It might scare you to do this the first few times, but remember: People are flattered and gratified by attention and interest.

Learn to ask questions. Don't panic during a pause in conversation because you feel it is your turn to think of some bright, clever, or profound thing to say, Dr. Wassmer advises. Instead, ask a question—the more obvious, the better. Give the other person a chance to be the expert.

Ask questions, too, when something said requires more technical information in order for you to understand it fully. Or when something said leads you to believe the other person could shed some light on a question in your own life, go ahead and ask. The other person will be pleased to help.

Tell others who you really are. Genuine contact is a two-way street. It requires that at some point you give something of yourself. You do this by learning to tell about your thoughts, your feelings, and your experiences. When you give of yourself, you make the ultimate statement of respect and acceptance of the other person. You are saying, "Here I am if you wish to come in my direction."

Tell about your job, a trip, or a project you're working on. The idea here is not to provide a travelogue or crafts lesson, but to share your experience, thoughts, and feelings through your description.

State a belief that is important to you. "Remember that the idea is to share yourself," Dr. Wassmer says. "This means your emphasis should be less on what you believe and more on what feelings and experiences led you to this belief." What you believe is a crucial key to who you are and can become an important way of sharing.

Talk about your hopes for the future. Let people know where you are by indicating where you're going. People are not interested in compiling performance statistics. They simply want to know you. When you share your hopes and dreams, you share a significant part of yourself.

Share a significant event from your childhood. This allows people to know you by sharing in the processes by which you became who you are. "It is not an experience itself, however, that forms your personality, but your thoughts and feeling in reaction to the episode," Dr. Wassmer says. "Try to convey not only what the experience was like, but also what it was like to be *you* having that experience."

Tell about a fear that you have. Revealing a point of vulnerability is an act of ultimate acceptance and trust. When you deliberately expose your fear to another person you are signaling that you trust that person not to hurt you.

Tell someone something you like or admire about him or her. "Socially withdrawn people usually do not provide posi-

tive responses to others because they feel uncomfortable having attention on them, even when that attention is positive and approving. So they assume other people feel the same way," Dr. Wassmer says.

The effect of this silence is often to raise the anxiety of others who have no way to tell if their behavior is pleasing or obnoxious to the withdrawn person.

"I really like you . . . It makes me feel . . ." Fill in the blanks as the situation warrants, but don't be afraid to be spontaneous! Such comments are far more effective when they're made at the moment you become aware of liking the other person. "Saved-up" responses, days or weeks later, may sound stale.

Tell someone that you like (care for, or love) him or her. A simple statement of affection is one of the most powerful combinations of attention and self-disclosure we can communicate, Dr. Wassmer says. You convey all the attending signals of respect, attention, warmth, and acceptance, and at the same time you disclose your own innermost feelings. Try, "John [or Sam or David or Maggie], I really like you very much. When I'm with you, I feel very free and full of life."

Don't worry about being "phony." You can't ever be anyone but yourself, Dr. Wassmer says. "If you want to make the mistake of thinking that your behavior *is* your personality, then you could claim that if you change your behavior you are not being true to your personality. But I think that's nonsense. The principle of cognitive behavior, which is the kind of psychology I practice, is that how people behave is pretty much the key to their experience. And if you want to change the way you experience things, you have to change the way you behave."

371

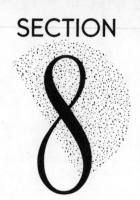
UNLEASH YOUR FULL POTENTIAL

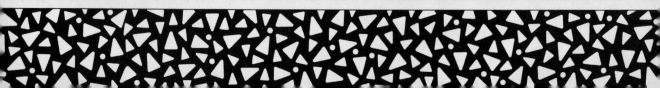

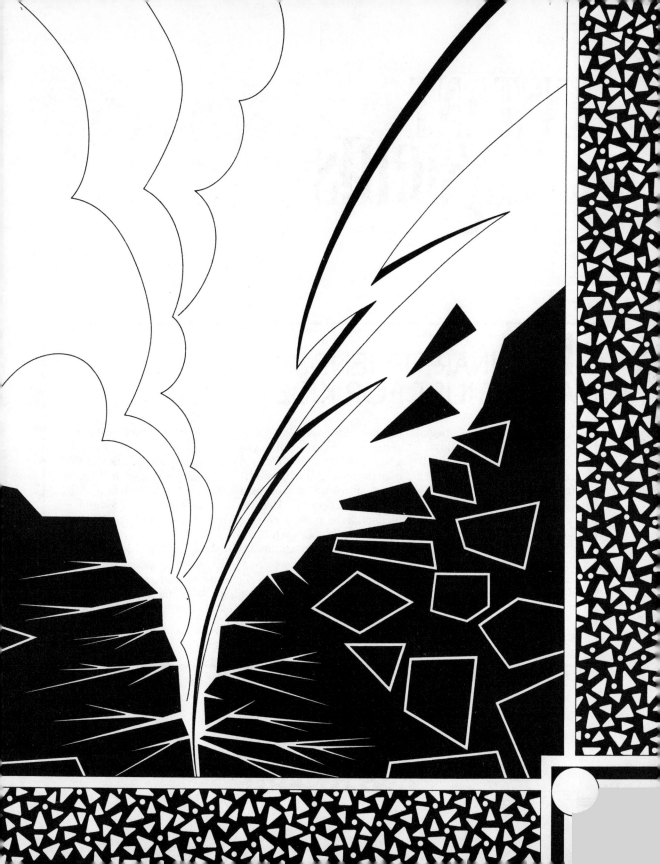

INSTANT INSIGHTS

IMAGINARY FRIENDS AREN'T JUST FOR KIDS

Remember that special friend you had as a child, the one only you could see? Well, recent research has shown there's an adult version of this phenomenon, and it can be used as a unique problem-solving device.

Social ghosts, as psychologist Mary Gergen calls them, are most often friends or family members that we're not in close contact with, but whom we talk to in our heads during the course of the day. While psychologists have traditionally viewed these conversations as a basically immature childhood hangover, Gergen suspected it was a universal as well as a beneficial experience. Her suspicions were proven correct when 75 of 76 college students answering her questionnaire admitted to imaginary conversations.

The real value of these tête-à-têtes comes in the form of practical problem solving. One woman who couldn't decide whether or not to accept a new job offer ran it by her boss in a fantasy conversation. In this way she was able to benefit from her boss's wisdom without actually having to tell her boss about the confidential offer. Besides their problem-solving abilities, social ghosts make great personal cheerleaders and can do wonders for boosting self-esteem and providing emotional support.

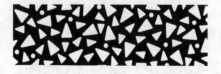

Two O'Clock Wow

A transcendental experience may be waiting just around the corner for you ... that is, if you're willing to stay up until 2:00 in the morning. Dubbed the "2:00 A.M. Wow" by psychologists Michael Persinger and Katherine Makarec of Laurentian University of Sudbury in Ontario, it's triggered when the brain's production of the chemical messenger serotonin drops, allowing for greater activity in the space perception and emotional centers of the brain.

The two psychologists were able to induce a sense of cosmic awareness in 200 people by placing them in a dim room with soft music and a gently flickering strobe light. As the subjects reported their experiences, electroencephalogram readings showed marked differences in their brain wave patterns. Increased theta wave production, a phenomenon that has been detected in Tibetan monks experiencing the deepest levels of meditation, was found to be a common feature of the "2:00 A.M. Wow."

That's The Purplest Music I Ever Saw

It could be that we are missing out on a very aesthetic aspect of the music we listen to: its color.

Synesthesia, the fusion of senses in which one evokes another, has been the focus of recent studies by Montreal composer Bruno Deschenes. But can it really be done?

After leading a group in guided imagery for six months, Deschenes not only thinks it can be done but hypothesizes that synesthesia occurs more often when listeners suspend the brain's more analytical functions.

Research done by neurologist Richard Cytowic seems to confirm Deschenes' theory. In his study, Cytowic found that blood flow decreases in the neocortex during synesthesia and increases in the limbic system. "The brain's higher information processing turns off during colored hearing and the evolutionarily older limbic system takes over," says Cytowic. "It's a less analytical, more fundamental way of listening to music."

Maybe in the future instead of singing the blues, we'll be seeing them.

TRAIN LIKE AN OLYMPIAN

A swimmer speed races in his living room. A tennis hopeful perfects his serve on the bus ride across town. A dancer adds spin to her pirouette in the tub.

What's going here? Mental rehearsal. It can perfect your game.

Consider Olympic gold medalist Greg Louganis. His mental rehearsal was downright rigorous. Before he stepped on the platform to dive, he imagined the dive just as he wanted it to be, step by step, 40 times.

What did it get him? The distinction of being the only Olympic diver to score a perfect 10 in international competition.

THIRTY MINUTES A DAY TO OPTIMAL FUNCTIONING

Give yourself the gift that makes you better each day: a 30- to 45-minute time-out.

That's the advice of Dr. John Clarke, a Harvard-trained cardiologist and current chairman of the Himalayan Institute of Yoga in Honesdale, Pennsylvania.

Spend some of the time conditioning the body and some of it quieting the mind, using either relaxation or meditation techniques, he says. Together, the body conditioning and the mental discipline will help free you from the internal chatter that separates you from your potential for greatness.

"The more successful you are at reaching deeper and deeper levels of quiet, the greater your opportunity to reach that innate creativity, to uncover your decision-making skills, as well as improve your physical and psychological health."

To keep you on track, ask your family to support and reinforce your efforts, Dr. Clarke says.

KUNG FU IN THE SURGICAL SUITE

Checking out your fellow physicians for their use of good martial arts technique is not something the average doc spends a lot of time doing.

But it comes naturally to Dr. Yu Lap Yip, chief of surgery at a Hong Kong hospital.

And when he toured ten hospitals in New York, he discovered that these ancient Asian arts could be a big help to American surgeons. Not by using the forceful methods of kung fu to make incisions without the need for scalpels, but rather an "internal," serene, and graceful variant known as T'ai Chi.

By extension, his advice could be well used by everyone who must stand on their feet or sit in a chair, for hours on end, using great concentration.

The problem he saw among surgeons was terrible posture. *Unnatural* posture. "They hunched their backs, twisted their necks, shrugged their shoulders, and stuck their elbows out. They were so absorbed in what their hands were doing and their eyes were seeing that they seemed to have forgotten the feeling of their own bodies."

The result of this awkward posture, (including lots of leaning instead of replacement of the feet) is enormous muscular tension, stiffness of the neck and shoulders, and low back pain.

The solution? A small dose of T'ai Chi principles. Always keep the spine erect, says Dr. Yip, the neck and head in alignment with the spine. The shoulders relaxed. Elbows close to the sides. Feet planted firmly and securely on the ground. Don't bend your neck, hunch your shoulders, slouch, or work on something that is not easily reached using good posture.

He admits it isn't easy to do that without practice, suggesting in the *British Medical Journal* that "perhaps T'ai Chi training should be incorporated into the training of every surgeon."

A little dose might also do wonders for many office workers, technicians, artisans—just about everyone.

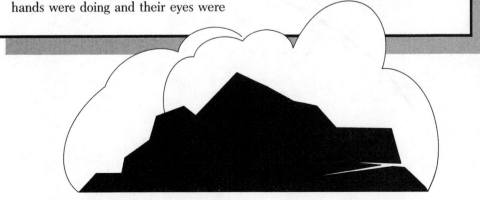

SUBTRACT YOUR CHILLS WITH ARITHMETIC

Solve this: What do you normally do when you get chilled? Probably you reach for a sweater, turn off the air conditioner, or turn up the heater.

Now figure this: next time you're cold, reach for your child's math book.

When subjects in an ice-cold lab were chilled through and through and nothing could stop their chattering, the best chill-queller was not a cup of hot coffee, but a card brimming with rows of numbers to be added, say physiologists at the University of Minnesota Medical School.

Researcher Robert Pozos paid university students $25 to dress in shorts and a light top in his hypothermia lab. When the students were sufficiently chilled and quivering, Pozos gave them a card with double digit numbers to add. "When they did mathematics, shivering shut off," Pozos says. Students given a blank card continued to chatter away.

The researcher speculates that this effect can be produced by a change in breathing: When you do mental calculations, your breathing slows down.

ABOUT THAT RAISE

When's the best time to ask for a raise?

That depends upon the strength of your argument and your boss's mood, says Herbert Bless, a research associate at the University of Mannheim in West Germany.

In studies exploring the effect of mood on information processing, Bless found that people tend to evaluate information more thoroughly when they're mildly depressed than when they're euphoric.

So if you think you've got a good case, approach your boss when she's feeling a little down. If your argument is weak, wait until she's in a great mood. She just may be distracted enough to miss any holes in your argument.

THE SWAN SONG PHENOMENON

Many of the world's greatest composers apparently were never told that we hit our creative peak before thirty, according to psychologist Dean Keith Simonton of the University of California at Davis. What he has christened the Swan Song Phenomenon is the fact that many of these composers produced their best music in old age and even at death's doorstep.

Using a computer, Simonton analyzed 1,919 pieces by 172 different composers using a set of seven criteria and comparing the results with age. While these "swan songs" scored lower in melodic originality, they scored much higher in repertoire popularity as well as aesthetic significance.

LET THERE BE CREATIVITY

Congratulations, you were creative today. Oh, you don't remember being creative? But didn't you stick a ruler under the window with the broken sash to hold it up? And weren't you the one who crumbled up bran muffins to use in the meatloaf when you ran out of bread crumbs? Surely you remember repairing your eyeglasses with that paper clip.

So, what did you think you were doing? Making do, you say? Well, that's creative. "Any time you force things together that don't usually go together, you're being creative," says Dr. Linda Organ, creativity researcher and associate professor at the University of Southern California.

She says that all of us are naturally creative, but lots of times, we don't give ourselves enough credit. How about you? Have you ever come up with a theme for a party, or an unusual costume to wear to it? Thought up a game to play with a child or a pet? Propped up one leg of a table with a book? Found shapes or pictures in a cloud? Told a story about something that happened to you in such an entertaining way that your friends laughed and begged to hear more? If you answered yes

to even one of those questions, according to Dr. Organ, you've been creative—and you have the potential to answer yes to all the questions as well as thousands of others.

Bet you feel pretty good now. That's one of the benefits of being creative. There are lots more, too, and we'll get to them in a second. But first, close your eyes and imagine how it would be if you were much, much, more creative than you already are. What would you be like?

First off, you'd probably trust your own intuition and be full of opinions and ideas, says Dr. Organ. You'd have a good sense of humor, an active imagination, and you would see many possibilities where now you often see only one or two. What's good about that? Well, the person who can put together a set of Tinkertoys a thousand ways will be entertained by them for a lot longer than the person who only sees one way of putting the toys together. Life is like a jumbo set of Tinkertoys.

Creativity could make your problems easier to solve, your relationships more open and fun, and your long, empty Sunday afternoons full to overflowing. "You'll achieve your full potential," says Dr. Mary

Murdock, assistant professor at the Center for Studies in Creativity at State University of New York at Buffalo, "especially in terms of your self-image and mental health." Basically, if you let yourself be creative, you'll be the kind of person you'd like to know.

Here's the good news: You can be more creative than you are now. All it takes is a little practice.

Creativity's Four Aspects

"Think of creativity as having four components," says Dr. Organ. "If you go after one of them, you'll automatically get better at all of them."

Fluency. This is the ability to come up with many ideas in relation to one situation. You might want to come up with uses for a seashell, for instance. Some obvious answers could be to use it as a paperweight or a decoration, but the idea is to go further. Maybe it could just as easily be a planter, a funnel, or a vase.

Flexibility. The capacity to look at the situation from a whole new angle is flexibility. You could break the shell, for example, and use it to cut something. Or you could grind it up and use the calcium in it.

Elaboration. You elaborate by adding details to the situation, perhaps by getting lots of shells and making a lamp or a serving dish out of them.

Originality. This is what we usually think of when we think of creativity — the ability to come up with a completely new, never-before-tried, super idea. Totally unique examples aren't easy to come up with. You could make the shell into jewelry,

THE LAUREL AND HARDY SCHOOL OF CREATIVITY

Given a candle, a box of tacks, a book of matches, and a cork board, how would you attach the candle to the board so that the candle could burn without dripping wax on the floor?

If you're having trouble, watch a comedy or tell some jokes with friends and then try again. People who had just watched a funny movie found that question easier to answer than those who had watched a film about math, says Dr. Alice M. Isen, psychologist and professor at the University of Maryland, who conducted the study. In fact, anything that puts you in a good mood, from finding change in the coin return of a public phone to winning a video game, will increase your creativity, she says.

One possible explanation for this phenomenon, says Dr. Howard Lieberman, a New Jersey neurosurgeon, is that good moods are a result of an increase in the frequency and rapidity of electric connections in the brain. "Mood elevating drugs cause people's thoughts to flow more rapidly," he says. "They may not be coherent, but there will be more of them and they will be connected in ways they weren't before. A good mood works the same way but better, allowing coherent, fluent thoughts, the hallmarks of creativity."

Still stumped for the answer? Empty the box of tacks, pin it to the board, and use it as a candle holder. Now that's flexibility.

but that's been done. Maybe you could use the shell as a shovel . . . but that's been done. How about wearing it on your face as a funny nose?

381

(continued on page 384)

How Creative Are You?

Here's a quick test to give you some idea of how well you're fulfilling your creative potential. Most of it is excerpted from the book *How Creative Are You?* by Eugene Raudesepp.

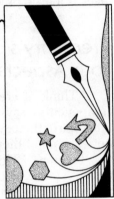

1. Draw 30 small circles on a piece of paper. Now, in 2 minutes, turn as many as possible into small doodles of different objects. One, for instance, might turn into the top of a wine glass. Drawing ability doesn't count, but originality does. That means you shouldn't end up with 30 faces, each with a slightly different expression. (This exercise was suggested by Doug Stewart in his May 1986 *New Age Journal* article "Thinking Sideways.")

2. For 1 minute, make a list of all the possible uses that you can think of for a brick.

3. How do you feel about the following statements? Circle the number in the column that best describes your feelings.

	Agree	Don't Know	Dis-agree
1. I'm attracted to the mystery of life.	+2	0	−1
2. For most questions, there is one right answer.	−2	0	+2
3. I prefer specific instructions to those that leave many details optional.	−1	0	+1
4. I can become so absorbed in my interests or work that I lose track of time.	+1	0	−1
5. I find I'm often turned to for advice and reassurance.	+1	+2	0
6. I prefer tackling problems for which there are precise answers.	−1	0	+1

7. I often get my best ideas when doing nothing in particular.	+1	0	−1
8. I feel that I am considerably different from other people.	+1	+2	0
9. In evaluating information, the prestige or trustworthiness of its source is more important than its content.	−2	0	+2
10. People who use strange or unusual words do it to show off.	−1	0	+1
11. I have many hobbies.	+1	0	−1
12. Sometimes I'm sure that other people can read my thoughts.	−1	0	+1
13. People who seem unsure and uncertain about things lose my respect.	−1	0	+1
14. In groups, I occasionally voice opinions that seem to turn other people off.	+2	0	−2
15. It doesn't bother me if people do not like me.	+1	+2	0
16. I'm a very reality-oriented person.	0	+2	+1
17. There's nothing wrong with showing off a little now and then.	+1	0	−1

Scoring:

1. Give yourself 1 point for every picture you drew. If you finished early, give yourself 5 points extra.

2. Give yourself 1 point for each use you thought of.

3. Add up the values for each of your answers.

37 and over — Exceptional. You're obviously a very creative person. You know the benefits of being creative, and you know that you can always improve on your abilities.

36-24 — Good. You have a strong grasp of how to think creatively. Practice this skill and soon you'll amaze yourself.

23-13 — Average. You've shown you have the potential to build on and proven that you could be a lot more creative.

12-0 — Not up to snuff at all. Read the chapter and then try again.

Obviously, learning to be original is tough. But the great thing about looking at creativity this way is that you can become more original by practicing being more fluent and flexible.

So, suppose you have a free evening and no idea what to do with it. You're bored. Well, that's great. Boredom, say psychologists, often leads to creativity. Now, instead of banging your head against the wall and saying over and over, "I have to be creative, I have to be creative," try practicing fluency. Come up with as many entertaining plans as you can. Don't jump at the first solution you come up with— being solution-oriented blocks creativity— and don't worry about whether your ideas are practical or even possible until you've got at least twenty. You might get your friends to help you come up with ideas. You're sure to find something fun to do, and you'll have done a creativity exercise without even trying. The exercise is called brainstorming, and the most creative people do it all the time.

"Creativity is a skill," says the president of Princeton Creative Research, Eugene Raudsepp. "And like any skill, if you don't practice, it atrophies."

The first step in practicing your creative skills is to make the process as easy as possible. Don't put unnecessary blocks in your way. That means keeping a pad and pencil handy to write down your ideas (if you come up with lots of good ones in the shower, you could even install a piece of lucite and a grease pencil over the soap dish, suggests Roger von Oech, author of *A Kick in the Seat of the Pants*. It means waiting until the 11 o'clock news to first turn on the TV for the day; and it means letting go of your fears of sounding stupid, looking weird, or being the first to do something new.

Step two is simple: Think a lot. Here are some ideas to get you going.

● When you run into a problem, describe it to yourself in different words to find out what it really entails.

● Ask yourself "What if . . ." at least once a day. For example, "What if people could fly?"

● Keep a shoe box full of interesting and funny articles, plans for projects, and spur of the moment ideas.

● Be ready to find something you weren't looking for, says von Oech. Remember when you went to the library to get a book your neighbor recommended and found a great one on the shelf underneath? That kind of thing will happen all the time if you're open to it.

● In a conversation, pretend you're the person you're talking to.

● Change your focus, von Oech suggests. If you're usually visually oriented, pay attention to smells. If your typical style of action is logical, try being emotional or intuitive for a change.

Games People Play

Getting more creative isn't something you have to do alone, either. Here are some ideas for parties and get-togethers.

The Dictionary Game

One of you find a word in the dictionary that no one else knows. The rest of

GREAT MINDS THINK IN STRANGE WAYS

Creative genius can strike at any moment and in any form. Samuel Taylor Coleridge found one of his greatest poems, "Kubla Khan," in a dream. This is what he wrote about the event, which began after he took some heavily opiated medicine and fell asleep in his chair:

> The Author continued for about three hours in a profound sleep, at least of the external senses, during which time he has the most vivid confidence that he could not have composed less than two to three hundred lines; if that indeed can be called composition in which all the images rose up before him as things. . . without any sensation or consciousness of effort. On awakening, he . . . instantly and eagerly wrote down the lines that are here preserved.

The sad part of the story came after that, when a man from a nearby town, Porlock, rang his doorbell and insisted on talking to him for nearly an hour. Coleridge had only written down part of the poem before he was interrupted; by the time the man from Porlock was gone, he had forgotten the rest.

Sometimes great ideas come to writers while they are awake, arriving almost mystically in their complete and perfected form. Sir Charles Tennyson wrote in his 1949 biography of how poet Lord Alfred Tennyson came up with his most famous lines on a ferry:

> During the twenty-minute crossing over to Yarmouth from Lymington, on his way from Aldworth to Farringford, there came to him, almost in a flash, the most famous of all his lyrics, "Crossing the Bar." He unfolded a used envelope and jotted the 16 short lines roughly down on the inside of it. . . . After dinner that night he showed the lines to Hallam, who said: "That is the crown of your life's work." He replied: "It came in a moment."

Then again, as often as not, genius is achieved purely by accident. This story about James Joyce comes from Richard Ellman's 1959 book about one of the greatest authors of the twentieth century:

> Once or twice he [Joyce] dictated a bit of *Finnegans Wake* to [the much younger Samuel] Beckett, though dictation did not work very well for him; at the middle of one such session there was a knock at the door which Beckett didn't hear. Joyce said, "Come in," and Beckett wrote it down. Afterwards he read back what he had written and Joyce said, "What's that 'Come in'?" "Yes, you said that," said Beckett. Joyce thought for a moment, then said, "Let it stand." He was quite willing to accept coincidence as his collaborator.

SOURCE: *The Oxford Book of Literary Anecdotes*, edited by James Sutherland (New York: Simon and Schuster, 1975).

you make up definitions and write them down so they sound like one that could be real. The person with the dictionary reads all the definitions including the real one, and the rest of the group votes for the most likely entry. You get a point if anyone votes for your made up definition, and if you vote for the real one.

Story Round-Robin

One person begins to tell a story. After a sentence or two, the next person continues the story from where the last person left off, using the same characters and setting, but with no other restrictions. Keep going around the circle and listen with delight and dismay as your idea for a romantic boy-meets-girl tale gets twisted into an adventure with the sewer monster.

Proverb Frenzy

Get together with friends and try to come up with original "proverbs" to express your views on life. Better yet, spend the evening speaking in original proverbs. Is it dinner time? Try this one: "Food for the body brings forth nutritious thoughts." Do you want someone to close the window? Try saying, "Cold winds blow over the soul," or "An open window invites disaster."

BLUEPRINT
FOR FULFILLMENT

You're reading this section because you'd like to do something more with what you've got. Psychologist Abraham Maslow in the 1940s called this quest self-actualization, the drive to do what you feel best fitted for, to become the most you can be given your particular talents and limitations.

Self-actualized people are happy people. Look at Bruce Springsteen and Mother Teresa, and as different as they are, see the parallels. They've developed what they do best, they're doing what they want to do, and are admired for it.

That sense of being able to choose how you spend your time is a key to your happiness. Self-fulfilled individuals arrange their time so they're using more of it to do what they want to do, for the joy of it—rather than doing what they feel they *have* to do or *should* do says Dr. John Neulinger, a nationally recognized expert in leisure studies. "It's not the activity that matters, but the reason why you're doing it.

"A lot of people are caught up in the confusion between what they want to do, and what they actually do," adds Maryland psychiatrist Barry Sultanoff. "The son may not be like the father, for example, yet he's expected to follow in his footsteps. It takes a leap of courage to go with what he really wants to do. A lot of people are living life mostly on 'shoulds.'"

Go with What You're Good At

You've heard it a zillion times. "You'll do best at what you love best." But somewhere along the way, some of us have trouble putting this into practice. So we mold ourselves to fit into the structures we see out there: the jobs listed in the want ads, the hobbies our friends have. We stop short of figuring out ways to shape what's out there to fit *us*.

That was Bonnie's problem, at first. Teaching was a profession she knew existed, and she thought she'd like working with kids, so she became a teacher. She wasn't in the field all that long before she realized it was the wrong career for her.

388

With the help of a counselor at Coil, Ballback & Slater, a California career guidance firm, Bonnie discovered that "everything she really enjoyed doing was outside of her work: planning parties and socializing," says partner Ann Coil. So Bonnie chose to explore media events planning.

That led to a job planning entertainment for the local Visitors and Convention Bureau. Then Bonnie landed a job in supplier relations, organizing parties and TLC-type programs to help large companies keep on friendly terms with their suppliers and vendors. These days, Bonnie is head of community relations for a very successful shopping mall.

"She really evolved a whole career path for herself," says Coil. "And got a salary increase with each new job." All because Bonnie realized she loved bringing people together.

What's Stopping You?

Some of us have a hard time going after what we want for the simple reason that we don't have a clue as to what that is.

That can happen for any number of reasons. Sometimes, the confusion is temporary, brought on by crisis: death of a loved one, divorce, loss of a job.

"People who are self-actualizing at one time can come up against one untoward event, and then they withdraw, they get stuck," says Dr. Robert Conroy, director of the William Menninger Center for Applied Behavioral Sciences in Kansas. "They're relatively self-satisfied, relatively productive. What they have to do is to work through that mourning process of loss. We see that often in our clinical work."

Sometimes the problem goes deeper. It has to do with what we're taught—or not taught. Maybe in grammar school we learn that conformity brings success. Maybe we grow up watching our folks spend their free time going to the movies or out to dinner, and it doesn't occur to us that camping, hiking, or rappelling are within the realm of possibility.

"Our range of experience and exposure is more limited than people believe," says Geoffrey Godbey, a professor in Pennsylvania State University's Department of Parks and Recreation. "We like what we know. We don't always know what we'd like. To a remarkable extent, people are limited to what they've been exposed to."

Another problem is that we may be sabotaging ourselves.

Dr. Baila Zeitz, a cognitive behavorial psychologist with practices in New York and New Jersey, says she's often amazed at the "incredibly creative ways people find to hold themselves back. These are people with incredible talents and abilities who have virtually tied themselves up in their own underwear for years."

"There's a two-word sentence called 'I can't,'" adds Dr. Zeitz, whose career path led her from wife and mother, to technical writer, to psychologist before she found her niche. " 'I can't.' A statement like that comes from not caring enough about yourself. Talk back to those excuses. What's the evidence? Other people have managed to do it under all kinds of circumstances."

But more often than not, we don't have a clue as to what we'd like because we never stop to ask ourselves. So we

(continued on page 396)

WHAT AM I DOING?

You know what you'd find fun. The problem is squeezing it in. Those everyday obligations seem to gobble up your waking hours.

Sounds like you could use some analysis — time analysis that is. Dr. John Neulinger, an expert in the field of leisure studies, has just the thing for you. He calls it the What Am I Doing? or WAID log for short. He designed it to help individuals measure how much time they're spending on activities they choose freely, and how to increase it.

The log on page 390 shows how to record a day's activities. If the information is to be of use, you'll have to keep a log for a decent duration. A month's worth probably will begin to show you a pattern.

Be sure to record the day's activities by the next day, while your memory is clear.

To use the log, begin with column 1. Select the hour you woke up and fill in your primary activity for that hour. Then hour by hour, fill in your primary activity. If the activity lasts more than an hour, go to the hour indicating when it ended.

Column 2 asks you to indicate where, using a number code. If it is in your home, write 0; if done while commuting or traveling, write 1, and so on. The codes are listed below the log.

Column 3 asks you to indicate how many people you spent the hour with. Again, look below the log for the codes.

Column 4 asks you to rate the degree to which you freely choose the activity. Writing 100 here means the activity was solely your choice while 0 means you had no choice at all. Use either number, or any number in between that reflects your degree of choice.

Column 5 asks you to indicate why you chose the activity. Did you do it for the sheer joy of it, or just to avoid a negative consequence? If you did it for the first reason, write 100, if for the latter, write 0. Again, choose a number that reflects the degree to which self-satisfaction movitated your decision.

Column 6 asks you to indicate how you felt doing the activity. If you enjoyed it, write 100. If you found it a real drag, write 0. Choose whatever number is appropriate.

When you've filled in the log, move to the "Summary Data" section. Under "Where," total up the number of 0's, 1's, 2's, and so on. Do the same for the "With How Many" column. Now move to columns 4, 5, and 6. Add up your numbers in each column, then divide by 24, to arrive at the mean.

The mean score will show you how much choice you've allowed yourself and how much satisfaction you derive from your activities. If the ratio of satisfaction to drudgery is too low, it's time to make some changes. For some possibilities, see the table "Name Your Game" on page 392. The time you spend doing the log will allow you to see where the real time eaters are and what activities you can eliminate so you can begin adding more satisfying ones.

For more information on the WAID log, write to Dr. John Neulinger, The Leisure Institute, R.D. #1, Box 416, Dolgeville, NY 13329, or call (315) 429-9563. For $12.50, he'll send you a booklet explaining the WAID log in detail.

(continued)

WHAT AM I DOING? — *Continued*
WAID LOG

Time	STEP I				STEP II		
	Activity	Where°	With How Many†	Choice You - 100 Other - 0	Reason Own Sake- 100 Other - 0	Feeling +100 − 0
Mid-night						
1 A.M.						
2 A.M.						
3 A.M.						
4 A.M.						
5 A.M.						
6 A.M.						
7 A.M.						
8 A.M.						
9 A.M.						
10 A.M.						
11 A.M.						

Day logged: □ Mon. □Tues. □Wed. □Thurs. □Fri. □Sat. □Sun.

Date of day logged (TARGET DAY): _____ / _____ / _____
(month)   (day)   (year)

°0- in your home
 1- commuting or traveling
 2- at place of employment or self-employment
 3- at school (formal or informal educational institution)
 4- other

†0- alone
 1- with one other
 2- with two others
 3- with three others
 4- with four others
 5- with five others

| Time | STEP I | | | | STEP II | | |
	Activity	Where°	With How Many†	Choice You - 100 Other - 0	Reason Own Sake- 100 Other - 0	Feeling +100 − 0
Noon						
1 P.M.						
2 P.M.						
3 P.M.						
4 P.M.						
5 P.M.						
6 P.M.						
7 P.M.						
8 P.M.						
9 P.M.						
10 P.M.						
11 P.M.						

SUMMARY DATA

0 ____ 1 ____ 2 ____ 3 ____ 4 ____	0 ____ 1 ____ 2 ____ 3 ____ 4 ____ 5 ____	
		Mean Choice	Mean Reason	Mean Feeling
24	24	

NAME YOUR GAME

Custom-tailor your interests and skills so they help you meet other personal objectives. Here are some possibilities. The lower part of the table is blank so you can try your hand at it.

Interest or Skill	Alone	To Socialize	To Serve
Giving Advice	Be a freelance columnist	V. at a tourism information bureau	Be a board member at a nonprofit agency
Baseball	Collect cards	Join a league	Coach Little League
Sculpting	Work in a studio	Devise performance art projects in which you collaborate with other artists	Teach inner-city kids
Cooking	Experiment at home	Organize a gourmet dinner circle that meets regularly to share food and talk	V. for Meals-on-Wheels or a local soup kitchen
Horses/Riding	Ride solo in woods or on beach	Take part in horse shows, take group riding lessons	V. expertise to A.S.P.C.A., organize night neighborhood patrol
Foreign Cultures	Travel solo, be a freelance travel writer	Give lectures, organize group travel	Help organize ethnic pride festival for your town
Swimming	Swim early morning laps at the pool	Join a swim team, take swimming or scuba classes	Coach handicapped kids, join water rescue team
Deductive Reasoning Skills	Solve mental challenge puzzles, plot out a mystery novel	Join debate society or chess league	Serve on a community ad hoc board
High-Risk Adventure	Sail or fly solo	Ride the rapids or skydive	Join rescue squad
Acting	Create a one-person show, do mime or impressions	Audition for a play, be a movie extra	Do a public service spot, perform in nursing homes

NOTE: V. stands for volunteer.

To Rub Elbows with the Rich and Glamorous	To Make Money	When Your Budget Is Tight
Become a leisure counselor or financial planner	Start a consulting business	Endless possibilities, talk is cheap
Organize celebrity games for charity fund-raisers	Buy and sell cards, join the pros	Organize company team, play stickball
Join art museum board, frequent gallery receptions, get gallery to show your work	Seek commissions or grants, teach	Sculpt with soap or found objects
Become a restaurant critic, teach cooking on your own cable show	Open specialty foods store, Start a catering business	Join a food co-op, discover the joys of picking your own, grow an herb garden
Play polo	Be a jockey, breed and sell horses, teach horseback riding, be a groomer or trainer	Exchange stable duties for riding privileges
Become a diplomat, represent your company at international conferences	Get a foreign service job, start specialty tour business	Find a foreign pen pal
Join exclusive swim clubs, lifeguard at swanky resorts	Be a lifeguard, teach, coach at college level	Buy a season pass to your municipal pool, find a safe lake or free beach
Join a public policy think tank	Become a research scientist, private investigator, or any kind of analyst	Endless possibilities
Go on safari or other expeditions in exotic locales	Become a stunt person or an ambulance driver, perfect a trapeze act	Go cliff-diving
Be a theatre critic, snag a leading role, entertain at corporate conferences	Go pro, do commercials, act in corporate training films	Outside of classes, most activities don't require money

(continued)

NAME YOUR GAME — *Continued*

Interest or Skill	Alone	To Socialize	To Serve
Photography	Endless possibilities	Join a class or club, organize a photo exhibit	Do photo essay of social problems, help nonprofits with publicity
History/Preservation	Research your family tree, develop expertise by reading, write essays for journals	Join a society, give lectures, take classes, go on archaeological digs, collect oral history from the elderly	V. for a local preservation group, compile community history
Bodybuilding	Set up a home fitness center	Compete, join a gym	Teach kids with low self-esteem
Marine Life	Create an aquarium, explore tidepools	Learn to scuba dive, join oceanic society, go whale watching	Become a marine biologist, V. for Earthwatch

To Rub Elbows with the Rich and Glamorous	To Make Money	When Your Budget Is Tight
Freelance for celebrity magazines, do fashion or portrait photography	Be a photojournalist or commercial photographer	Join a club, see if someone will lend you equipment or darkroom privileges
Head up a centennial celebration commission, join executive board of history museum	Teach, work for a history museum, become an archaeologist	Few of these activities cost money
Model, hire yourself out as a trainer for starlets	Model, endorse product lines, sell exercise equipment	Work in a gym in exchange for free use of equipment
Lead scuba tours at Club Med-type resorts or in exotic locales	Be a marine biologist	Snorkel

drift, caught up in the day-to-day, week-to-week routine, never really focusing on where we'd like to go. And the years pass.

Cycle Breakers

One way to make a new start is by breaking free of the patterns that keep you stuck. If you're the type who keeps saying "I can't," how about trying an Outward Bound outing or some other test-your-mettle-against-the-outdoors program for a quick boost of confidence?

Mike G., a manager in a computer products company, found himself skiing in hip-high snow, and blazing a trail in blizzard conditions after he signed on for his first guided cross-country skiing and winter camping tour of Yellowstone National Park. He was cold, uncomfortable, and exhilarated. "I felt as good about myself as I ever have in my life, when that week was over," he says. "Something like that definitely tells you you can do whatever you put your mind to. You can rise to the occasion."

"The way humans work, there is a tremendous interconnection between emotions, behaviors, and thoughts," says Dr. Zeitz. "If you engage in behaviors that give you evidence 'yes, I can,' it tends to generalize into other areas. Motivation follows action. It does not precede it. Action by its nature is an incremental process. The key is to do something."

Exercise can help break that cycle, too, because it's a natural at dissolving depression. Acquiring some upbeat friends can also help. Who do you know who has a real passion for life, a can-do attitude? Who's got a hobby you've been meaning

to check out? Ask. Bribe. Wheedle. But get them to teach you what they know.

Ready, Set, Action!

Buy a multisection notebook and a folder. Or spring for a large diary.

The other tool you'll need right now is a local newspaper. If you don't subscribe to one, get a neighbor to pass along the old, preferably unclipped copies, for at least two weeks.

The purpose of the exercises below is to help you focus inward, where fulfillment starts. Later, you'll direct your focus outward with an eye toward finding the options best for the you you're in the process of discovering.

Exercise 1. This one's easy. Clip from your newspaper every item on community activities: notices of speakers and seminars, club listings, announcements of adult education programs, activity directories, entertainment offerings, the recycling guide, all of it. Two weeks ought to give you a decent sampling. File the clips away for now. You'll get back to them later.

These next exercises involve thought and some writing. Before you groan, realize that these are at the heart of those costly life-planning seminars and institutes and you'd have to do them there, too. Don't panic about the writing; it doesn't have to be anything fancy. Just be honest with yourself. No one has to see what you write unless you invite them to. You can tackle these in any order.

Exercise 2. "Before I die, I want to. . . ." What do you have to accomplish so you could die, satisfied you've fulfilled your dreams? Be as wildly imaginative as you want. After you finish, make a list of what you've already done, what you have yet to do, and steps you need to take to lead you in that direction.

Exercise 3A. "If I had $100 million to spend...." For the first part of this exercise, forget philanthropy. Concentrate on yourself. It's okay. Really. Now, reread what you've written. What's important to you? How are your "purchases" connected? If, for instance, you've listed a cabin in the mountains of Vermont and a hideaway home in Kauai, you probably love natural beauty, the outdoors, and travel.

John Crystal, career-counseling pioneer and head of the John C. Crystal Center in New York, remembers what happened when Richard B., a 45-year-old electrical engineer, did this exercise during one of his seminars. "I'm going to be a doctor! In an office overlooking the Long Island sound," Richard had said. And that, Crystal reports, is exactly what the man did.

Exercise 3B. "If I had $100 million to spend..." This time, you can't spend a cent on yourself. Will you give it to the local environmental group to clean up the groundwater? Underwrite a new movie or play? Donate it to AIDS research? Send your kids to China until they're all grown up? Reread what you've written and scan for clues. What's important to you? What do you value?

Exercise 4. Write a life diary. This can be powerful. The drives that indicate your future potential have not been dormant until now. They've shown themselves in what you've done best, and enjoyed doing the most.

Write a minimum of 25 pages, but go as long as you'd like. You can bounce back and forth in time, if that's easier. Be sure to mention any schooling, where you've lived, what you've done in your free time, jobs you've held, accomplishments that make you proud, and how you felt about all of it.

After you finish, set it aside for a few days. Then play detective as you reread it. Notice any skills that keep surfacing. Underline them. On a separate sheet of paper, make two columns: "Things I've Done Well and Enjoy," and "Things I Choose Not to Do (or Have) Again." Then fill in both lists.

When Maria, age 30, was first assigned this exercise at a John Crystal workshop, she doubted that her "boring little life" could fill a page, even if she triple-spaced the type. But by the time she got to page 110, she "discovered this woman I never met before. She's absolutely lovely! And she's me."

Tailoring for a Good Fit

Good going. You've got a clearer idea of what you like, what you're good at, and what you consider important. Let's sharpen the focus even more so you can really zero in on the most compatible activities. It's not enough to say you think running is cool. Do you do it to socialize or to spend time alone with your thoughts? Are you a sprinter or a marathoner? Do you crave competition or hate it?

Three key concepts for determining the right form of an activity are: values, balance, and substitutability.

Keep your *values* and any personal objectives in tune with your actions, or

Testing ... 1, 2, 3, 4

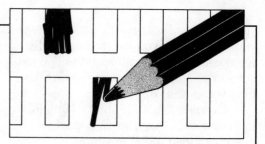

Remember those aptitude tests they gave you in school? The ones you needed to fill in with a no. 2 lead pencil?

Now you can take them at home, return the completed exercises and receive an analysis and recommendations. How useful are they? Career counselors differ in their assessment. John Crystal, career counselor pioneer, thinks you'll do better asking yourself what you want to do. Others find them useful.

Among those available by mail are:

• Guide-Pak, which includes the California Psychological Inventory and the Strong-Campbell Interest Inventory. $25 postpaid. Write to Behavoirdyne, 994 San Antonio Road, Palo Alto, CA 94303, or call (415) 857-0111.

• Career Interest and Ability Inventory. $27.50 postpaid. Write to Chronical Guidance Publications, P.O. Box 1190, Moravia, NY 13118; or call (315) 497-0330.

• Self-Directed Search. You score and analyze it yourself. $5.50 postpaid. Psychological Assessment Resources, P.O. Box 998, Odessa, FL 33556; or call (813) 968-3003.

Dr. Baila Zeitz, New York and New Jersey psychologist, likes the Johnson O'Connor tests best. These you can't take at home. But the Johnson O'Connor Research Foundation has testing centers in 15 different cities. The cost is $450 for three half-day sessions. The foundation can be reached at (212) 838-0550. The tests, which take two sessions, explore everything from idea production to tonal memory. A test administrator interprets the results at the final session.

you'll literally end up at war with yourself. Maybe you love to socialize, but you while away the hours at home doing needlepoint. Why not join a quilting bee, or start one? Or maybe you're a writer who's overdosing on the cynicism and narcissism of the literary crowd you move in. Why not volunteer to teach someone to read, and share their excitement as they learn to recognize words on the printed page?

On to *balance.* A well-balanced work/leisure plan will supply you with the essential ingredients your psyche needs to be well nourished. Your job, for instance, ought to offer you sufficient challenge, some degree of control, opportunities for creativity, and the ability to demonstrate competence and be recognized for doing a good job.

If your job is lacking in any of these areas, and you're not about to change it, find a leisure activity that compensates. Maybe you feel anonymous in your job, so seldom does anyone acknowledge your contribution. Acquire an activity you can master that will put you in the limelight. How about a magic act or a comedy routine? Maybe you want to become the local expert on salt-water fishing.

Or maybe your work is so theoretical, you find yourself needing to produce something solid in your off hours. How about landscaping a garden, building dollhouses, or amassing a stamp collection?

Substitution is a concept that gains importance as your circumstances change. You can fit activities to alterations in budget, family demands, physical capabilities, or geographic location.

Nora Britch, a leisure counselor based in New York, had a client who used to love to horseback ride, something she felt less free to do as a single parent with a 2-year-old child. So Britch suggested she substitute hiking, which allowed her to enjoy the outdoors while spending time with her daughter.

Amy loved to ski and ice-skate until her knee gave out. Now that she's gotten her ski buddies to take up canoeing with her, she feels less like she's missing out.

Time to Explore

Take out your notebook. Write "Shopping List" on a clean page. List skills you want to use or exercise. Note any personal objectives or goals you want to fulfill. Examine whether you need to compensate for goodies you're not getting from work. And write down any activities you need to replace with appropriate substitutes. Mark these with an "S."

Now it's time to go idea shopping. Start with the newspaper clippings you've been saving. Does anything appeal to you,

or prompt some ideas? Write them down.

The library is your next stop. Go on a day when you've got several free hours and feel relaxed enough to browse. Bring your notebook so you can jot down the ideas, addresses, and phone numbers you'll want to keep.

If you're after some new ideas about recreation, see if your library has *The Leisure Alternatives Catalog*—a fun compilation. Skim adventure travel books. Leaf through the associations directory and write down the addresses of national organizations that interest you, because they may be able to put you in touch with a local chapter. Pick up hobby magazines and regional publications. Ask if there's a subject file on any subjects of particular interest. The library probably will have catalogs of local adult education programs.

Career-improvement ideas can be gleaned from catalogs listing short-term college seminars, or those identifying scholarship, fellowship, and internship opportunities. Browse through the special interest magazines, trade journals, even the yellow pages of your phone book. Look through business directories and pay particularly close attention to business journals for your region. The vertical files will help once you've narrowed your interests.

Getting Going

Ideas are colliding in your head. But before you let your enthusiasm sweep you and your charge card into the local sporting goods shop or piano store, think rental.

"See if you like it," advises Britch. "I always tell my clients to hook up with an association. Anybody who has ever done anything has made a club out of it. If you

399

400

can, hook up with people who live in your area. They're usually really nice people. They might be able to lend you equipment." Or give you tips on what to acquire and how.

As you begin to add new activities to your life, take notice of how the changes feel. One secret of many achievers is they take time each day, or every few days, to review how they're spending their time and whether or not it's leading them in the direction they've set for themselves.

"The people who are most satisfied with their lives are the ones who have a few things to do that they love to do, and are willing to sacrifice the alternatives," says Godbey. "They often do less instead of more."

Once you get underway, remember to be patient with yourself.

Creating a fuller life takes practice. "If I gave you a tennis racket, you wouldn't be a pro that same day," says Dr. Conroy. "Recognize that you don't have to make absolutely drastic changes. People change in millimeters."

WHEN ADDITIONAL HELP IS USEFUL

There are times when it's just plain better to bounce your ideas off a professional. Sometimes, a little reinforcement makes the difference between a life-changing move and no change at all.

Career counseling firms that stay on top of the jobs available, particularly the newer and more offbeat openings, may help cut your research time. They can also teach résumé-writing and interviewing skills.

Ann Coil, a partner in Coil, Ballback & Slater, suggests that you grill the guidance agency you're thinking about hiring. "Make sure they spell out very clearly what you are getting in the program—what the content is, how many hours it lasts, what program materials you'll get."

Prices for career counseling services vary widely. Your local college may be able to schedule you in free, or may charge you a nominal amount. Business-oriented programs, on the other hand, can run into the thousands.

Check to see if your local college career guidance office or professional guidance firm offers SIGI PLUS, a powerful little computer program that has you explore your interests, aptitudes, and values by asking you a series of questions. Your answer determines the next question. SIGI PLUS, developed by the Educational Testing Service, of Princeton, New Jersey, is so complete, it can show you 1,600 possible occupations and even lists salary averages.

Leisure consulting is a bonafide business these days, too. If the idea intrigues you, but your yellow pages don't list the service, ask your local Parks and Recreation department or university for a referral.

MAKIN' MUSIC

An interesting tale I picked up at a conference on spirituality had to do with music and an order of monks living high in the French Alps. A large part of their daily regimen consisted of singing Gregorian chants, simple but resonant liturgical music that originated in the seventh-century church. When the abbot of the order decided to eradicate the chanting, the monks fell under a strange malady, leaving them weak and listless. At the suggestion of a perceptive doctor, the chanting was reinstituted a few months later and with it the monks were cured. They literally sang their way back to health.

I'm a musician myself. A violinist. While I won't quite say an aria (or a concerto) a day keeps the doctor away, there are a few special points to be made about music.

In every culture, no matter how complex or simple, there is music. Compare Americans with the bushmen of the Kalahari desert. We watch cable TV, they hunt wild antelope. But, we both compose, play, and enjoy music. While the unusual clicking noises the bushmen make orally might not hit it big on American Bandstand, it answers their need for rhythmic/melodic stimuli. On the other hand, I suspect that American Bandstand would have the bushmen running for cover.

There is anthropological and historical evidence that music has been around for at least 30,000 years. Music is a building block of civilization right up there with agriculture and the development of language.

Many great musicians and composers have performed remarkable achievements in this field at an advanced age. Giuseppe Verdi composed his famous opera *Falstaff* when he was 81. Pablo Casals was giving cello concerts in his nineties. Vladimir Horowitz made a world tour in his eighties. And when the critics raved over his Moscow concert, they weren't judging him in the "virtuoso pianists over 80" category. They were saying that Horowitz is the best there is. Let the youngsters weep with envy.

Everyone either wants to play a musical instrument or regrets having given one up. Okay, that isn't quite a proven fact, but I've yet to meet anyone who wouldn't like to belt out a tune or two, even if it's a tour de force in the shower. Seriously, I play in public a great deal and every person I've spoken to after a performance has mentioned a desire to play. The only thing stopping them is self-doubt.

Starting on the Right Note

Why take up an instrument at this stage in life? (*a*) to spite your neighbors, (*b*) because hang gliding is too dangerous, (*c*) in case they ask you to play the national anthem at a Mets game, (*d*) Guy Lombardo would have wanted it that way, or (*e*) because playing an instrument stimulates both the creative and logical parts of the brain and requires them to interact. Additionally, it exercises coordination between eye and hand. The creative satisfaction that playing music provides can be enjoyed throughout life and will help you to retain mental lucidity in later years. It also gives you a reason to stick around and unnerve your grandchildren with all that lucidity.

If you picked (*d*), you're sentimental, but wrong. If you picked (*a*), you're still wrong and kind of nasty to boot. Surprise! It was (*e*). And it's all true. But as usual, it's not always easy to start something that's going to do you some good.

First things first. What do you want to play? If a particular instrument's sound has already made off with your heart, far be it from me to talk you out of it. If you're unsure, level of difficulty might be something to consider. Any instrument takes dedication to play well, but some are easier to learn than others.

At the top of the torture list is the violin as well as viola, cello, and string bass. Because I was 8 years old when I started, the fact that my parents temporarily lost their sanity when I practiced afforded me limitless delight. But if you're not keen on recreating World War II fought entirely by alley cats, pass on the strings initially.

French horn, bassoon, and oboe are also not the easiest instruments to jam on at first. If you're proud of your lungs, however, a saxophone or flute is not a bad idea.

Piano and guitar are two of the most popular instruments for a number of reasons. They are friendly to the beginner, sound great without accompaniment, and are at home in either a classical or pop vein.

Whatever you choose, don't go nuts right away. Rent, don't buy. You may have second thoughts about your choice and don't want to find yourself stuck with a snap decision. None of these instruments make useful household appliances. When you do go shopping, ask your local music store salesman about his rental policy. He's used to dealing with junior high school marching bands. Believe me, he will love renting an instrument to someone who won't stick chewing gum on it.

While you're at the music store, find out about lessons. Many stores give lessons right on the premises. If they don't, they should be able to direct you to a teacher in the area. Remember, they want you to like your instrument . . . so that you will eventually buy it. They'll be very helpful.

Concerning music teachers: Just about any instructor worth his weight in metronomes will be able to show you the fundamentals, teach you how to read those little black dots, and fortify you with some music theory. The important thing to do is find a teacher you like and respect.

Practice That's Practically Easy

Okay. You've got an ax (that's hip talk for your instrument) and a teacher. Now it's time to practice. Again, don't go nuts. It's a little like physical exercise. You've got to work your way up to a long session or you'll burn out. Start with ½ hour a day and see how it goes. If at all possible, make it the same time each day. You'll find that a regulated schedule will help you practice better.

Before you sit down to practice, clear your mind of the day's problems. Then, when you pick up your instrument, concentrate on every note you play. Not only will you improve faster, but your daily workout will become something akin to meditation, providing you with a kind of musical stress control and peaceful sense of purpose.

A word of warning. You'll occasionally reach points in your advancement where things seem to level off and you're just not progressing as quickly as you'd like. It's all right. Achievement plateaus are to be expected. Keep plugging away. With perseverance you will eventually regain your forward momentum.

Now, I can't promise that Carnegie Hall will be pestering you for a recital, but so what? You'll be having fun, you'll be exercising your mind and spirit, and you'll be doing something most folks only dream about. When you've become confident of your playing skills, find some other people to play with. There are thousands of late starters out there with more zeal than many a recital-worn pro. Put up a sign in your apartment building or on the community bulletin board. Get together and form an impromptu Wednesday evening chamber group. As you pick up your instruments, remember: One of the finest things human beings can do on this earth is make harmonious sounds together.

M. G.

403

WEEKENDS WERE MADE FOR REGENERATION

Several months ago, I was in the midst of my Monday morning slump when I ran into my boss in the hall looking as energized as I did pooped. He'd just returned from a week at the Golden Door Spa in California, where daylong schedules of planned exercise in conjunction with well-balanced meals had worked a very regenerative effect on him. While he admitted that such an intensive schedule might get tiring over a long period of time, an occasional "tune-up" could do wonders.

As he was describing his visit, an idea began to form in my somewhat foggy mind. While most of us might not have the time (or in my case the cash) to do a week at a spa, there's no reason why we can't do a mini-spa for body and mind at home on the weekend. I decided to give it a try.

First, I made no plans for the weekend: no visiting and no shopping, and the broken garbage disposal could wait until next week. If you decide to do this, don't deliberately cancel an important or pleasantly anticipated engagement, it will only weigh on your mind all weekend. Wait for a time when you have nothing important to do and try and keep it that way.

Second, Thursday night, on the way home from work, I stopped off at the library and picked up a couple books I'd always meant to read but never got around to. At home, using *Rodale's Basic Natural Foods Cookbook,* I mapped out a schedule of healthy, well-balanced meals for the whole weekend. If you're like me, you sometimes don't have the time that you'd like to plan and cook yourself a really nutritious menu. Now's your chance to be your own dietitian for the weekend. Do a little reading and try to arrange the best possible combination of foods from Friday night straight through to Sunday evening.

Friday evening: Head out to the supermarket, health food store, and anywhere else you might need to go for supplies. Try to plan your food and sundry needs carefully so that you can grab everything you need for the whole weekend at once. An important part of this mini-spa is to achieve a continuous flow of regenerative activities free from everyday hassles.

Later, at home, it was time to transform my house into a personal regeneration zone. The first stop was the refrigerator. I've found that when I make a promise to do myself some good, it helps to seal the deal with physical action. In this case, I took all the food that had collected over the week and relegated it to the bottom shelf in the vegetable drawer, where it would be out of sight for a couple of days. In its place, I put all my weekend food in easy reach.

Unplug the Television

The next step was the television. I made room for it in the closet. While there are some worthwhile programs on TV, a good book still gives your mind more of a workout. You don't have to banish the tube to the closet, but again make a physical gesture, such as unplugging and turning it toward the wall. You'll think twice before reactivating it for a fix.

Dinner. Time for the first of your carefully planned, health-conscious meals. If you have a stereo, cook to some fine music and let your mind wander. I always suspected that there was a philosopher hiding in every chef, and I have to admit I did a bit of speculating while the soup simmered. Light some candles, get out the good dinnerware, and enjoy a leisurely dinner.

Afterward, I took a brisk 30-minute walk to burn off a few calories and just plain see what the moon and stars were doing. When you get back from your walk, settle down with a good book. When I say a good book, I mean one that pleasantly challenges your imagination without making you feel like you're fighting for the meaning of each sentence. For my choices, I picked a rather fancy-looking volume of Wordsworth's collected poems and a beat-up copy of Albert Camus's *The Stranger.* Part of the regenerative principle is enriching your capacity by utilizing your internal resources. The complex layers of meaning provided by the written word spur your mind's cognitive processes far more than the one-dimensional snap plots often found on TV. Also, a book forces your mind to create a mental image, while TV provides one for you.

Go to bed early. 10:00 P.M. should find you tucked squarely in bed with the alarm set for 6:00 in the morning. While I hate to use a cliché that's been needle-pointed into thousands of pillows, Ben Franklin had something when he said "Early to bed, early to rise . . ." Maybe this kind of sleep schedule rings true with an evolutionary need to rise with the sun. Or maybe it's just that morning is a time of new beginnings so the more of it you have, the better you feel. Take a shower and then hit the road for a 30-minute walk. It's a different world out there: clean, fresh, and quiet. Since most people are still asleep, it's your world to do with as you please. Make plans, dream a little bit. It's almost impossible to have any worries while drinking in that cool, sharp air.

Now that you've worked up an appetite, head on home and make breakfast. Eat it near a window that lets the sunlight in and make plans for the rest of the day. Got a hobby that you never seem to have time for? Absorb yourself in it today. I spent the rest of my regenerative morning playing my violin.

Monet for a Day

After lunch, I suggest another walk. It's great exercise and one of the most contemplative sports I know. When you get back, try your hand at a new form of expression. It could be painting, music, wood carving, or flower arranging—just as long as it's a way of saying something. Part of the success of our society hinges on mankind's need and talent for communication. Trying a new form of communication will direct your mind into unexplored patterns of thought. I tried painting. While the Louvre hasn't been phoning me day and night, I enjoyed myself and experienced a period of heightened concentration that left me thoroughly relaxed.

After a creative afternoon, I filled in the time before dinner with an aerobic workout. If you've got a regular exercise program, by all means stick to it over the weekend. If you don't exercise regularly, don't worry. A pair of ½-hour walks a day will get the heart working in a sensible way that won't have you aching the day after. If you're not in the habit of walking frequently, a quick call to your family physician for an official okay might not be a bad idea.

Dinner. Stick to your menu. Afterward, relax with the book you started last night. Or you may just want to lounge around doing nothing in particular. It's all right. Call it your freestyle meditation period. Doing nothing is a carefully cultivated art that we seldom allow ourselves the time to practice. Make sure to hit the sack early and do a solid 8 hours of sleep.

Sunday, start the morning with another sunrise walk. I won't go through the whole day, since you're probably get-

ting the hang of it. Just a few simple rules. No television, no newspapers (unless it's the comics or crossword puzzles), and if you don't have to go anywhere, no cars. The idea is to create a miniature retreat where you can shut off the normal concerns of the outside world and focus completely on yourself: a shot of concentrated regeneration to put you in good standing for the days ahead. The only thing I would add is a period after dinner to plan for the week. What needs to be done? Where are the trouble spots? No need to go into depth, but a quick review can give you a feeling of confidence and control.

When Monday finally rolls around, you might discover several things. First of all, you'll feel great. Not only were you good to your body and mind, but you'll feel a sense of accomplishment from planning and carrying out your weekend project. You may also enter the new week knowing a little more about yourself.

Of course each person's regeneration weekend is going to be a little different, but try to include these basic ingredients somewhere along the line: good nutrition, exercise, "early to bed, early to rise," introspection, quiet surroundings, and some creative activities. Although I did my weekend alone, it'll work just as well for a couple and can actually do wonders for bringing two people closer together. But whether you're a solo act or a duet, give it a try. If you like it, do it bimonthly. If you're really ambitious, then by all means do it once a month. One warning. Don't be too cheerful on Monday morning: Most people aren't going to understand it.

M. G.

LATE BLOOMERS

No matter what you're doing with your life now, if you don't like it, you could be doing something else.

That idea may seem revolutionary, preposterous, or just plain unrealistic. But it's not. If you're retired and not doing anything, you could find an absorbing, meaningful hobby, start a business, or get a job. If you're doing work you no longer like, you could go to night school and learn to do different work, or transfer the skills you already have into a more satisfying job. If you've been working without pay, you could get paid, and if you've been working for pay, maybe it's time to try working for free.

Consider these examples of older achievers profiled in "Late Bloomer," a radio series produced by Connie Goldman, an independent radio producer who creates programs and educational cassettes on issues and images of aging in America.

Aged 73, Jacob Landers recently became a lawyer. He spent most of his life as a high school superintendent, but he retired after a series of heart attacks that eventually led to open-heart surgery. After his recovery, he heard his lawyer's daughter talking about law school, which she had just begun to attend, and realized that that was what he wanted to do, too. Today, he works for a foundation in New York City that is concerned with the legal rights of the elderly.

Thelma Tulane had always wanted to dance, but at age 80, living in an old-age home, she figured that dream was best left behind. Then she attended a workshop led by Liz Lehrman, a younger woman who believes that anyone, at any age, can and should dance. Thelma joined Lehrman's company, Dancers of a Third Age, and now, at 88, is on tour with the group.

Ralph and Bernie Kleinschmidt are athletes, though they are 71 and 65, respectively. After Ralph retired from his government job and then had a heart attack a number of years ago, he and his wife decided the time had come to get in shape. Now they travel around the country, competing in the Senior Olympics. Ralph's game is horseshoes while Bernie competes in the high jump, discus, shot put, and the 1-mile walk.

Alert, Active, and Involved

"Through my study of changes throughout life, I know a gentleman who at age 57 took up ice dancing," says Dr. Warner Schaie, professor of human development and psychology at Pennsylvania State University. "He's 66 now, retired, and spending a great deal of time participating in ice-dance competitions. Several other older people have managed to write books that they successfully published and a number of people, after retirement, opened up consulting firms.

"These people have something that gives new meaning to the last part of their lives," says Dr. Schaie. "They are typically more alert than those who sit around watching television. Their minds stay sharper and they usually are in better health because they have reason to take care of themselves."

Not only do achievers have alert minds and interesting dinner conversations, but they actually live substantially longer than those without interests, says Dr. Donald Super, professor emeritus of psychology and education at the teacher's college of Columbia University. "People who retire without any special interests are likely to die sooner than those who retire with continuing interests," he says. "And of those who do survive, the ones with interests are happier than those without."

Of course, he adds, someone could retire without an interest, get one after retirement, and still have the same benefits in happiness and longevity as someone who's been active all his or her life. So it's never too late.

Then what holds people back in unsatisfying jobs or boring retirements? Myths. Ever since we were kids, we've been taught that the older you are, the more you need to be taken care of, and the less you can learn. So when we get to "old age" (whatever that may mean for us) we automatically think it's time to hang up our boots and settle in under the electric blanket, without even checking how we feel about it first. The good news: Scientists have proven again and again that what we were taught was wrong.

First of all, most older people are reasonably healthy and perfectly able to take care of themselves. Only about 20 percent of Americans over age 65 have even a minor physical impairment (like arthritis) that limits their activities, according to a spokesperson for the National Council on Aging. And over 65 percent of older Americans have no physical limitations at all.

Older but Wiser

What about the idea that, as an older person, your work won't measure up to that of your younger colleagues? "A lot of people think that if you're older, you're untrainable, but research shows that isn't true at all. If you've been using your mind throughout your life, the chances are that your mental ability is not going to get any worse with age," says Dr. David A. Waldman, an assistant professor of management at the State University of New

York at Binghamton. He and his partner, Dr. Bruce Avolio, found that job performance goes up with experience—and experience tends to be linked with age.

"Athletes can play pro sports longer than most people think they can," says Dr. Waldman by way of illustration. "A 40-year-old player can, in reality, be as good as a 24-year-old player. An older pitcher may not be as strong, but he has more finesse. He understands the players better and the game better."

Prepare Now, Bloom Later

If you're in your forties or fifties, late blooming may seem like the last thing you need to read about—your life is so full of raising your family and working that you don't have time for—or even want—one more thing. That's understandable, but when your current commitments lessen up, there's a good chance you'll have trouble making the transition into a different kind of lifestyle. That is, unless you plant the seeds now.

How do you prime the soil for blooming later? "People who do not develop interests throughout their lives find it difficult to develop them late in life," says Dr. Warner Schaie of Pennsylvania State University. But developing interests doesn't have to be a tremendously time-consuming process. Besides, it's fun. Here's what three people in your age group are doing now to prepare for later.

Dr. Howard Lieberman, 53, of New Jersey, writes the rough draft of a poem or two every night, and has collected a prodigious stack of them already. "It takes about a week to finish each poem," he says. "So I'll have a lot of writing to do once I stop working so much."

His wife, Denis, 49, is learning to read Russian in her spare time from a grammar book she got out of the local public library. "I don't plan to have much free time until I'm 70," she says. "I should have the hang of it by then. Then, when I'm an old woman, I can sit at home reading Pushkin and doing translations for publishing houses."

Louise Avalon, a 46-year-old bookkeeper and office manager of Staten Island, New York, is planning, too. She's planning to keep working forever. Already, she's on her second profession—she started as a full-time homemaker. Now she's preparing to become either a computer programmer or a lawyer when her youngest child goes to college in two years. "My mother is 82 years old and she's still working, so I feel as if I still have another 30 or 40 years of active life," says Avalon. "I'm taking an introductory computer course now. When I started, I felt as though I was being admitted to the inner sanctum of learned people. Before that, computers were incomprehensible to me.

"Going to school, I found out that I'm smart and I didn't know that before. That's what's really going to help me make the next 40 years interesting and productive."

410

What does change with age is our way of solving problems and thinking about situations. "People's abilities to solve practical problems increase with age," says Dr. Steven Cornelius, associate professor of human development at Cornell University, "while other abilities, particularly abstract reasoning, tend to show a decline." Answer this one quick: Which come up more often in real life, practical problems or abstract ones? You got it—practical ones.

Nonetheless, some people do feel they can't learn as quickly as they used to, or that their intelligence really has taken a nosedive in the past few years. Well, maybe it's true. "For many individuals, the major reason for declining mental competence is that they don't use their minds," says Dr. Schaie. But it's not too late even for the worst slugabeds. He continues: "We have ample evidence to show that people who have declined can be brought back up to where they were previously if they develop a more stimulating lifestyle."

More stimulating means finding an absorbing interest (or three) and diving in. But if you want a slower start, Dr. Schaie says, "There is a positive correlation between playing skilled games and your level of mental competence. So bridge players are better off than bingo players, and bingo players are better off than the person who stays home and doesn't do anything at all."

The bottom line: Scientists have shown that any age is a good age to start a new job, business, hobby, or project. And the fact of the matter is, lots of people are already doing it. "Today, it's very well-documented that people have serial careers," says Dr. Marsha Sinetar, an organi-zational psychologist and author of *Do What You Love, the Money Will Follow*. "That means that over a lifetime people might do two or three things," she adds. "It's possible because we are living longer with better health than ever before, we have better educations today, and personal computers have increased our individual capacities."

In many ways, an older person is even at an advantage in a new endeavor. Older people are often financially settled, with grown children who may be out of school. They are often settled emotionally as well, with secure relationships and social circles.

"There was this myth that older people going back to school couldn't keep up with younger people," says Barbara Bring. She went to school at the age of 46 to become a psychiatric nurse after running an antiques business for 15 years and raising a family for most of her adult life. "But the minute I got into school, I realized I would do very well. I had much better concentration than the younger people. The young girls had a social life they wanted to keep up with, and a lot of them were holding down small jobs at the same time. The older women were not as old as myself; they still had children at home and were often single mothers. I didn't have those handicaps. As a result, I became the top student in the class."

Bring didn't just jump into her new career. "I realized that I had outgrown my store," she says. "I wanted it to be a bigger, more prestigious business, but I didn't have the capital to invest to make it that. I gave my situation a lot of thought. I went away on a long vacation and read a very good book about people changing their lives.

When I came back from that vacation, I had made up my mind that I was going to change careers. I was 45 at the time."

Three Stages of Renewal

Obviously, wise choices and realistic plans can help you achieve your goals. Dr. Michael Perelman, coauthor of *Late Bloomers: How to Achieve Your Potential at Any Age*, divides the process of "blooming" into three parts: realization, quest, and fulfillment.

1. Realize You Want More

The first challenge is to identify the major components of your life that are unsatisfactory. "Some people look to a career or hobby to provide excitement that really is missing in their marriages. So you have to find out what the main area is that really needs change," says Dr. Michael Nichols, author of *Turning Forty in the Eighties.*

"If it's your career, the thing to do is try to improve it in place. Maybe you can change the nature of what you're doing, work harder, or work smarter. You should give this process about three to six months. If it works, then you've solved your problems and you haven't taken any risks. If it doesn't work, then you have a clearer idea that your dissatisfaction is definitely where you work," says Dr. Nichols.

If you are retired, maybe you haven't given retirement a chance. Learn how to have fun, enjoy your financial independence, and perhaps try volunteer work before you rush out to get a new, paying job.

2. Begin Your Quest for Information

Once you've found that whatever you are currently doing is not what you want to be doing, the next step is to find out enough about yourself to know what you'd really like to do, and what activities are suited to your personality.

"Ask yourself what would really be satisfying. Some people get seduced into occupations they don't love by high pay or prestige. But when you get into midlife, it's too late to put up with that crap any more," says Dr. Nichols. "Ask yourself what activities you enjoy. Talk to your friends and talk to yourself. Think about the activities you like, not the job you're looking for.

"If you are considering starting a business or large community project on your own," adds Dr. Nichols, "look for hard, concrete evidence in your past that you are an autonomous person. I think most of us, though, need to be part of a team or an institution. If you are this kind of person, don't make the mistake of going out on your own. There are plenty of things you can do with some kind of institutional support."

Here's a quick checklist by Dr. Super of some of the characteristics of people who have succeeded in starting a new career or project later in life than usual. How many do you have?

The successful late bloomer has:

● The ability to see that failure is only temporary.

412

- The courage to try something new.

- Encouragement or support from a friend, associate, or mentor.

- Patience. This person plugs away in a modest way and builds up confidence with modest successes until a real success comes along.

- Persistence. This person works at problems until they are solved.

- Previous success in other domains, such as homemaking or some paid work.

- Substantive interest in the new activity.

- Willingness to believe that he or she can do well.

3. Fulfill Your Goals

Once you know what you want, and feel fairly certain that it's suited to your personality, the final step is to go out and get it. But go for it the right way. "If there's one thing you should do when looking at a major change in your life," says Dr. Perelman, "it is to break up your end goal into discrete parts and take pleasure in the process of reaching the goal. If you focus too much on the end goal, you will get discouraged and give up without ever reaching it."

If your goal is a new job in a different field, Dr. Nichols suggests that most people will be better off if they look discreetly. "Don't alert the people where you are that you are unhappy and want to leave until you are absolutely ready to walk out the door," he says.

Your best bet is to explore a new situation without losing the one you've got. A part-time job or a temporary leave of absence from your current job are luxuries that can make a world of difference.

Obstacles to Overcome

Beware of the I've-found-my-niche trap: This one can trip you up before you even get started, making you think if you've got *one* of the basic requirements for a full life, you've got them *all*. Or, you can get caught in this trap after you find a new interest; if you make it your whole life, before you know it, you'll be back in the old rut again.

"It's an error to look to one area of your life to provide all your satisfaction and meaning," says Dr. Nichols. "You don't need just a hobby. You need a hobby, friends, and relationships. You need to have fun and you need to do something for people.

"What happens to the person whose only satifaction in life is a job, when she retires? Or the person whose only pleasure in life is family when the children grow up and the spouse dies of a heart attack? By the same token, if your only happiness in life comes from running long distances, you're going to be in big trouble if you get an injury," says Dr. Nichols.

Another pitfall is the I-want-another-honeymoon trap. Whenever you start something new, there's an initial burst of enthusiam. You love what you're doing because it's fresh and interesting and the people you're doing it with love you because you're fresh and interesting. Soon enough, though, they'll start to take you for granted. Hopefully, you'll still like what you're doing, but the brand-new shine will have worn off a bit.

At that point, says Dr. Nichols, lots of people start to miss what they left behind. The trick is not to get tied up in regrets. It no longer matters whether the choice you made was 100 percent correct. "Get involved in your present situation," says Dr. Nichols. "The secret for enjoying any situation at all is to be as fully involved as possible." That's the secret for late blooming, too.

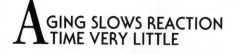

AGING SLOWS REACTION TIME VERY LITTLE

Most of us accept without question that our reactions get slower and slower as the years go by. But scientists who question that axiom are finding a surprising answer. Their research is showing that age actually slows your reactions very little.

Harold P. Greeley, Dr. Alexander G. Reeves, and co-workers at Dartmouth Medical School, found that people lose only about 1.4 *thousandths* of a second in reaction time each year after age 20. At that rate, your reactions would slow by only 1/10 second in 60 years.

The researchers measured reaction time using an innovative system developed by Greeley, a biomedical engineer. The subjects sit before a screen displaying red lights. They're asked to step on a pedal when the lights turn green. Electrodes measure the time it takes for the light to be perceived by the brain, and the time it takes for that message to be sent to the motor center of the brain (the part that controls movement).

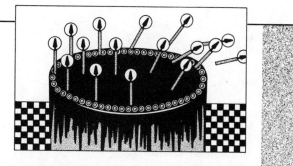

That's called the central reaction time.

Dr. Reeves did find significant slowing of reaction time in people with diseases of the nervous system, such as Alzheimer's disease. But healthy individuals maintain their quick reaction times throughout life.

"We are finding that in normal people, aging is more of a psychological perception than a physiologic change," says Dr. Reeves, who is chairman of the neurology department at Dartmouth. "The use of reaction time is a paradigm—we were really testing cognition, or thinking. Generally, 80-year-olds solve problems just as well as 20-year-olds, given just a little more time. People who eat good diets and continue to exercise and be involved in their environments may even improve their brains' power of cognition.

Resources for Renewal

Unless otherwise indicated, the following organizations are the national chapters of large networks or groups. They can send you information and direct you to local chapters that you can join.

Organizations for Older Adults

ACTION
806 Connecticut Avenue NW
Washington, DC 20525
(202) 634-9135

(Become a foster grandparent, a retired senior volunteer, or a senior companion through this group.)

American Association of Retired Persons (AARP)
1909 K Street NW
Washington, DC 20049
(202) 872-4700

(This national program puts out *Working Age* newsletter and produces a whole stack of pamphlets to help older people stay informed and do just about anything. Write for a list of publications, including a list of universities that offer free tuition to senior citizens.)

Displaced Homemakers Network
1010 Vermont Avenue NW
Suite 817
Washington, DC 20005
(202) 628-6767

(Join various local programs for support and/or retraining.)

Elderhostel
80 Boylston Street
Suite 400
Boston, MA 02116
(617) 426-7788

(Offers week-long college experiences to senior citizens. Take courses all over the country and abroad. Domestic programs cost approximately $230 for a week, and financial assistance is available.)

Gray Panthers
311 South Juniper Street
Suite 601
Philadelphia, PA 19107
(215) 545-6555

(Become an activist and fight social and economic injustice, especially as it deals with the elderly.)

National Center on Arts and Aging
National Council on the Aging, Inc.
600 Maryland Avenue SW
West Wing 100
Washington, DC 20024

(This national program puts out a newsletter, *Collage*, which documents art-related activities of older adults and can provide information and support for starting activities of your own. Not a membership organization.)

National Hispanic Council on Aging
2713 Ontario Road NW
Washington, DC 20009
(202) 745-2521

(Learn to do, or take advantage of, job training and advocacy for the Hispanic elderly.)

National Indian Council on Aging
P.O. Box 2088
Albuquerque, NM 87103

(Offers job training and advocacy for Native American elderly. Not a membership organization.)

Older Women's League
1325 G Street NW
Lower Level B
Washington, DC 20005
(202) 783-6686

(Join older women engaged in political and social work aimed at giving older women control over their lives.)

Peace Corps
806 Connecticut Avenue NW
Washington, DC 20525
(202) 254-6886

(Older people with needed expertise are encouraged
to apply for two year-long overseas appointments.)

SAGE
208 West 13th Street
New York, NY 10011
(212) 741-2247

(Join gay and lesbian senior citizens in support
groups and social programs. A New York-based
membership group that will refer people to other
local organizations where they exist.)

Service Corps of Retired Executives
1129 20th Street NW
Washington, DC 20416
(202) 653-7561 or 1-800-368-5855

(Join other retired business people in advising small
businesses for free.)

Volunteer — The National Center
1111 North 19th Street
Suite 500
Arlington, VA 22209
(703) 276-0542

(Become a volunteer — myriad opportunities, but
start by checking out the Retired Senior Volunteer
Program.)

Your state office on aging.

(Every state has an office set up by the governor or
the state legislature to help older people in a variety
of ways. Contact them to find out what services they
offer. The office is located in your state capital and
may be called the Commission/Council on Aging,
Aging and Adult Administration, Aging and/or
Adult Services, Department/Office of/on Aging,
Aging and Community Services, Division for Aging
Services, or the Department of Elderly Affairs.)

Directories of Educational Funding Sources

These directories of places to get
funding for school are available through
your local public library. Be sure to get
the most recent edition. (List compiled
by the American Association of Retired
Persons.)

An Independent Sector Resource Directory of Education and Training Opportunities and Other Services. Washington, D.C.:
Independent Sector.

*Better Late Than Never: Financial Aid for
Older Women Seeking Education and
Training.* Washington, D.C.: Women's Equity
Action League (WEAL).

*Directory of Financial Aids For Women:
Scholarships, Fellowships, Loans, Grants,
Awards, Internships.* Santa Barbara,
California: Reference Service Press.

*Directory of Special Programs for Minority
Group Members: Career Information
Services, Employment Skills Banks, Financial Aid Sources.* Garrett Park, Maryland:
Garrett Park Press.

Foundation Grants to Individuals. New York:
The Foundation Center.

*Money Business: Grants and Awards for
Creative Artists.* Boston, Massachusetts: Artists Foundation.

*Paying for Your Education: A Guide for
Adult Learners.* New York: College Entrance
Examination Board.

HOW TO BE A LEADER

No one has to ask Elaine Petuch Zettick to lead. She just can't help herself.

"When I see a need, I usually think I know how it can be done better," says Zettick, a surburban Philadelphia business, civic, and political leader. "I set my goal and I go all out to achieve it. When I hit a golf ball, I want to drive it as far and as straight as I can. I'm that kind of person.

When we read comments like this, we often get the impression there's something almost superhuman about the people who choose to lead.

Truth is, there is often very little difference between the people who sit in folding metal chairs and the people who run the meetings.

Traits You'll Need

Experts who have studied leaders have identified their most successful traits. Some are obvious; some less so. We can't promise you that by learning every skill that you'll be a leader, too.

But if you have the desire to take a leadership role in helping your community, your business, or your family, much of what the experts have learned may help you along. Here is some of their best and most practical advice.

Have a Dream

This sounds obvious, but it isn't to a lot of would-be leaders whose clubs, businesses, or service organizations drift about with no particular goal or aim.

"Effective leaders all have a good sense of their group or organization," says Burt Nanus, professor of management in the school of business at the University of Southern California. "They know what's going on in their organization, where it's been and where it's going."

One way to develop a vision is to visualize your group five years from now. What do you see? What will the group have accomplished in five years with you at the helm? Whatever your goal, lock onto that dream and don't let go.

When Candy Lightner, founder of Mothers against Drunk Driving (MADD), focused on her dream, it was an outgrowth of tragedy. Her 13-year-old daughter, Cari, was killed by a drunken driver. She wanted to get drunken drivers off the road, and she has never given up on that goal.

Thanks in large part to Candy Lightner's vision, MADD has become a powerful grass-roots lobby group. The dream is still very much alive.

"I am actual, living proof that you can make a difference," she says. "And there are hundreds of people out there, housewives who were never before involved in the political process. Now they're writing public-service announcements, lobbying legislators, testifying in the courtroom for MADD."

Set Your Style

"The underlying thing that makes an effective leader is the ability to ask oneself, 'How do I want to be led?'" says Jerald Vaughn, executive director of the International Association of Chiefs of Police and sought-after lecturer on the subject of leadership. "Think about the kinds of qualities you like to see in a leader, then tailor your approach to that. Very few people want to be led by a bad leader."

The absence of effective leadership locally and nationally drew Zettick into public life. She worked in three presidential campaigns.

Later, her concern over local leadership led her involvement in community issues. Zettick's persistence and commitment led local politicians to ask her to run for supervisor in her town. She ran and won.

A few years later, she became so concerned about what she considered divisive leadership in county government that she set about trying to recruit people to run against the incumbents. In the end, the party asked *her* to run. "For some reason, things got turned around, and I became the candidate," she laughs. "I went on to win and become the first woman commissioner of my county, and the first woman chairman of the board of commissioners."

Be Enthusiastic

You can tell others about your great vision for the future, but without passion your vision is just another passing fancy.

"Really good leaders are like little boys in the sandbox, having so much fun it doesn't seem like work to them," says Nanus, coauthor with Dr. Warren Bennis, fellow University of Southern California management professor, of *Leaders: The Strategies of Taking Charge*, a programmed audio course (SyberVision). "Leaders are effective at communicating that enthusiasm to others. If a leader feels good about what he's doing and he's having fun, that has to be communicated, too, along with the message."

Assume You Can Do It

Think about how you have been raised, the values that have been handed down to you by your parents and teachers, the things that are important to you. And consider, too, an experience that far too many people fail to appreciate—running a household.

"You can be a leader within your own home," says Lightner, "by virtue of the example you set for your children, your patience, and your tact. The quality of being all things to all people really begins in the home—chauffeur, home-maker, cook, confidant, friend, discipli-narian." Most of these skills—"all except cooking," Lightner says with a laugh—provide the basis for leadership in many other areas, from civic activities, to home-and-school associations, to local politics.

Consider Yourself Fail-Safe

Effective leaders don't accept failure, and they don't allow setbacks to knock them off course. According to Nanus, lead-ers learn from their mistakes and move on. "They really don't believe in failure," he says. "The word isn't in their vocabulary."

If you play it safe, you won't fail, but you won't get to where you're going either. And that's the difference between a good leader and a bad one.

"There are some people who watch things happen," says Vaughn. "There are others who wonder what happened. Lead-ers *make* things happen."

Don't Be A Tyrant

If you want power, call the electric company. "Leadership is not what peo-ple think it is—poking, prodding, and manipulating people," says Nanus. "It's really energizing people, pulling people in the right direction. Good leaders don't issue commands or send out a stream of memos. It makes the people under them feel dependent and saps their energies. A leader finds ways to help other people realize their potential."

Look for Opportunities

Recognize that all the leaders are not at the top. "One of the things I tell my students," says Nanus, "is that there are more opportunities to lead in an organiza-tion than they think. In most organizations, the person willing to take the initiative can be a leader."

Being a leader also doesn't necessar-ily mean you must be a leader all the time, in every facet of your life. During the day, for example, you might be a schoolteacher, one of thousands in a large city district, taking your marching orders from the principal and superintendent. At night, you could be chairman of the teachers' union, sitting across the bargain-ing table from the school superintendent in contract talks.

Recognize Others' Accomplishments

A good leader appreciates the peo-ple who follow.

"There's a role to play for those who follow," says Vaughn, "as well as for those who lead. The important thing a leader has to remember is that it's the followers who are doing the work and making the leader look good. A good leader recog-nizes accomplishments of others."

If, in the end, you decide to try your hand at leadership, there may be intangi-ble but nonetheless worthwhile benefits.

"The rewards of leadership are purely personal," says Vaughn.

Zettick and Lightner concur.

"I've always gotten a sense of satisfaction knowing I've been able to effect a change, to make a name for myself," says Zettick. "That's the ego part of it. But that's not what you're thinking about when you go out to do things. You think, maybe I can help, maybe I can do it better."

For Lightner, the rewards of leadership are intensely personal, deeply felt.

"I can think of no greater honor to Cari," she says. "Nobody will ever be able to take away the thousands of lives that MADD has saved. I'm very proud of that. I'm proud of me."

THE REGENERATIVE ENVIRONMENT

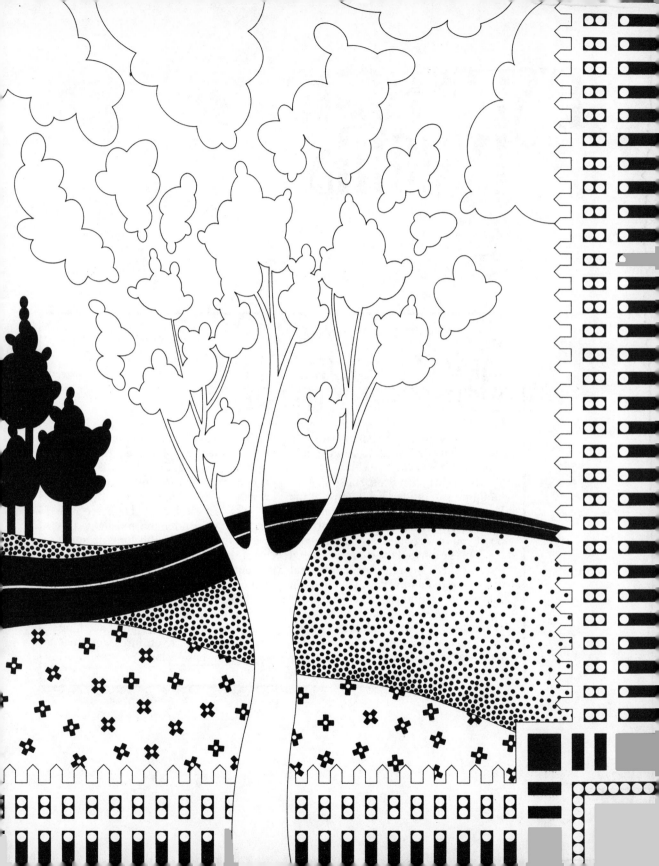

INSTANT INSIGHTS

Rev up your WORKOUT WITH RED

If you want to put more power into your workout, try installing a red light in your exercise room.

A study by Dr. Scott Hasson, assistant professor of physical therapy at the University of Texas Medical Branch at Galveston, suggests that red light may boost your energy and muscle strength.

Dr. Hasson said the study was based on previous research that shows that colors like red and yellow, which are in the upper frequency range, increase arousal, while low-frequency blues and violets tend to have an inhibitory effect.

The handgrip strength of 14 volunteers was tested in darkness and under red light, white light, and blue light. A load cell attached to the handgrip device measured force. Electrodes attached to each volunteer's arm measured electrical activity in the muscle.

The test was repeated on three successive days. Under the red light, the electrical activity in the forearm muscles of the volunteers was an average 14 percent higher than it was under other light conditions.

Why does red light have this property? Dr. Hasson thinks it may be instinctual. "Red and yellow have long meant 'warning.' Even birds don't eat anything in those colors."

WARNING: GOOD ART MAY BE DANGEROUS TO YOUR HEALTH

Planning a European vacation? Just to be safe, pack the smelling salts—you may just find yourself to be one of a handful of foreign visitors who faints at the sight of ancient art and architecture.

These few are more than emotionally moved by the beauty of art; they experience dizziness, confusion, depression, persecution, and loss of identity when gazing at a Botticelli, Giotto, or Michelangelo.

Called Stendhal's syndrome, this disease is being researched by a Florentine team led by psychiatrist Gabriella Magherini at Ospedale Santa Maria Nuova.

Most affected are men and women aged 20 to 40, research shows. The disease has been labeled as cultural gluttony by Magherini's associate, Stefano Crivelli. "It's as if they (visitors with Stendhal's syndrome) want to consume the art and take it home with them," he says.

Local people are more cynical of the disease and blame visitors' emotional overreactions on the heat.

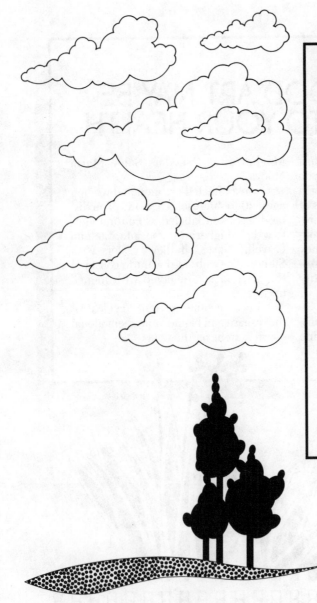

A NOSE FOR HAPPY MEMORIES

The next time you want to entertain some fond memories, you may want to make sure you're surrounded by pleasant odors. A study performed by researchers Howard Ehrlichman and Jack Halpern at City University of New York, seems to show that memory retrieval is affected by what your nose is retrieving from your present environment.

College women were asked to recall memories cued by neutral words while being exposed to a pleasant odor, an unpleasant odor, or no odor at all. Upon completion, the women who were exposed to the pleasant odor produced a significantly greater percentage of happy memories than did those in the other two groups.

Home, Sweet Home

Over a long period of time, a laboratory rat can be conditioned to withstand ever-larger injections of heroin. Eventually, the rat can nicely survive a dose of the drug large enough to kill an unconditioned animal in a matter of seconds.

But if that same rat is removed from the familiar cage where the injections have been administered, and given the same dosage in a strange environment, it will quickly die.

The crucial role of environment in withstanding stress has barely been investigated in humans.

In one study, Japanese immigrants to California who maintained strong ties with traditional Japanese culture were found to be much more resistant to heart disease than those who didn't—even when both groups were eating the same rich American diet. The survivors, evidently, had "detoxified" the strangeness of their new homeland by enjoying some of the familiar comforts of their old homeland.

Black Brings Out the Villain In Us All

Do clothes make the man? According to research done at Cornell University it can in some circumstances. That is, if the clothes are black and the man happens to be in the National Football or National Hockey Leagues.

Apart from being the color of formal dinner wear, black is associated with evil and death in virtually all cultures.

Wondering whether black clothes might change a person's behavior, researchers Mark Frank and Thomas Gilovich studied football and hockey teams that wear black uniforms to see if they were any more agressive than their nonblack uniformed competition.

A review of penalty records showed that teams wearing black ranked near the top of the list in both sports. Not only that, but teams that switched from nonblack to black uniforms experienced an immediate increase in penalties.

Why? Perhaps black-garbed players regard themselves as more aggressive. Then again, it could be that referees unconsciously believe that guys in black are the bad guys.

RETUNE YOUR MOOD WITH A SOUND PRESCRIPTION

Blindfold a friend. Then pull out your key chain and give it a few shakes. Ask your friend to identify that sound. There's a good chance the answer will be "keys." But the right answer would be "jingle" since that was the *sound* that the keys made.

This isn't a plot to fool your friends, but rather a simple illustration of what sense we tend to rely on the most: sight. Even when we hear a sound without seeing its cause, the first thing we do is try to visualize an object. This cultural bias toward sight even shows up in our language. Which do you say more often, "I see what you mean" or "I hear what you're saying"? Is there an auditory equivalent to the word in*sight*?

While we are constantly aware of the appearance of our surroundings, there is a second environment—an invisible one composed of sound—that we seem to notice only when it's incredibly beautiful or extremely annoying. But whether we're listening to a Bach sonata, a rabid jackhammer, or any of the millions of sounds in between, certain transformations are occurring in our bodies on both a mental and physical level. Understanding these changes allows us to rearrange the aural environment. We can protect ourselves from "junk food" noises and boost our mental well-being with a "sound" prescription.

Have you ever found yourself getting a little annoyed at your spouse or children for no reason at all? A pair of experiments performed in 1981 might provide a clue to the mystery of the souring personality. In the first experiment, a researcher with his arm in a cast dropped a pile of books on the sidewalk in the path of passing pedestrians. Another researcher operated a power lawn mower on the grass several feet away. The first researcher, looking very much in need of assistance, then tried to pick up his things. When the lawn mower was silent, 80 percent of the passers-by stopped to help. When the mower was on, only 15 percent stopped.

In another experiment, students were asked to evaluate job applicant résumés.

The average starting salary recommended by students in a quiet office was $1000 a month. In a noisy office (70 to 80 decibels), that average dropped to $900.

Sure, obnoxious sound can spill the milk of human kindness, but who has a lawn mower tearing up the living room carpet 24 hours a day? According to Dr. Steven Halpern, California composer and music therapy researcher, it doesn't take a lawn mower to get on your nerves. It can be a sound as subtle as the humming of the refrigerator. "You can be sitting there reading a book or watching TV, not really paying attention to the refrigerator. Then when it suddenly shuts off you breathe a little easier and your shoulders relax. It's only then that you realize you had been steadily getting tense because of a sound you weren't really listening to."

Noise has been blamed for high blood pressure, ulcers, increased risk of heart disease, and as shown by the previous experiments, a sour personality. "Some studies suggest it may even make a dent in the human sex drive," says Arline L. Bronzaft, chairperson of the Noise Committee of the Council on the Environment of New York City.

Your home probably doesn't produce the kind of noise that's going to do you serious harm. But noise that seems tolerable on the surface may be causing subconscious irritability. Remember, 70 to 80 decibels was enough to make those students stingy with the cash. Could it be that the sounds of the television, the blender, and the refrigerator are all subtly conspiring to make you less than the sweet, understanding person you know yourself to be?

The Downside of Decibels

427

Let's start with the decibel (dB), the unit of measurement for the pressure sound creates. (For trivia buffs, the decibel was named in honor of Alexander Graham Bell.) One decibel is the softest sound the average person can hear. A dripping faucet measures about 45 dB while a rocket taking off can go as high as 180 dB. The following is a list of familiar sounds and where they rank on the dB hit list.

- Refrigerator: 50 dB
- Ordinary human speech: 60 dB
- TV or stereo at normal volume: 65 dB
- Window air conditioner: 60 to 75 dB
- Blender: 65 to 80 dB
- Noisy restaurant: 70 to 75 dB
- Vacuum cleaner: 70 to 80 dB
- Electric shaver: 75 dB
- Busy traffic: 75 to 85 dB
- Alarm clock: 80 dB
- Subway train: 85 to 105 dB
- Screaming child: 90 to 115 dB
- Live rock concert: 90 to 130 dB
- Jackhammer: 100 dB
- Chain saw: 100 dB
- Motorcycle: 100 dB
- Automobile horn: 110 dB
- Loud thunder: 120 dB
- Jet engine at takeoff: 120 to 140 dB
- Fire siren: 140 dB

This is where it gets a bit tricky. It might seem that if your refrigerator puts out 50 dB, then a siren is only a little less than three times as loud at 140 dB. But if you've ever been scared right out of your shoes by a siren, you know this is not the case. Actually, the increase is logarithmic, as Maurice H. Miller, professor of audiology at New York University, explains: "While 90 dB is equal to the sound of a train roaring into a subway station, 100 dB equals the sound of 10 trains pulling into the station simultaneously, and 110 dB represents 100 trains."

While a television plus a refrigerator plus a screaming child don't add up to 215 dB, together they become louder than the separate parts. Think about how many noise makers you have around your house sounding off at the same time. Is it any wonder that you find yourself getting a little snappy at family members?

If you suspect yourself of being a sound victim, here are a few tips from Dr. Halpern's book, *Sound Health*, to help you help yourself to a little peace and quiet.

● To reduce noise, you can put foam pads under blenders, mixers, food processors, typewriters, and the like.

● You can use sound insulation and vibration mounts when installing major appliances like dishwashers, clothes washers, and refrigerators.

● Before buying new appliances, compare the noisiness of different models and select those that are quieter.

● Be especially careful when purchasing children's toys that make loud and sharp sounds. Some explosive-type sounds can cause permanent damage to young ears.

● When you are looking for your next home or apartment, take into account sound factors such as airport noise, traffic noise, and noise leakage from neighbors' homes or apartments, especially at common walls.

● Additional carpeting, rugs, draperies, and wall hangings will absorb sound and pay an added bonus in heat conservation.

The Soothing Sound of Music

Now that we've safeguarded ourselves from junk noise, let's turn our attention to a sweeter sound of life—music. Whether it's a snatch of Beethoven's Fifth on an aspirin commercial or five bars of "Dixie" honked out by the horn of a Ford pickup with Texas plates, we hear music every day of our lives. And the best part is, it comes in as many "flavors" as the ice cream from Baskin-Robbins.

Jazz, classical, bluegrass, pop, Irish reels, gospel—the list could go all the way down this page and up the next. As a matter of fact, there's probably a wider selection of music in your record collection than there are prescriptions in your medicine cabinet. And like medicine, we often take a dose of one kind of music or another when we're feeling a little out of sorts.

But while we've all managed to gain some comfort from a sweet bit of Bach or a quick pick-me-up from a favorite song, it is only in recent years that music has been created to consciously benefit the mind and body.

New Age is the phrase currently used to describe this music. Almost always instrumental in nature, subtle and peaceful in form, it covers everything from bamboo flutes recorded near a waterfall to spacey synthesizers as expansive as a clear and starry night. At the forefront of this new movement is Dr. Halpern, creator of anti-frantic music.

"There are times when you just want to put on some music, kick back, and really listen to it," says Dr. Halpern. "That's fine. But many times we have music playing in the background while we're writing, reading, or working at home. Or we put it on specifically to relax. The problem is that most music was just not designed for these situations and can actually get in the way of our original intentions."

The first problem with the compositional nature of most music, especially classical, is what Dr. Halpern calls a sense of expectation. "The foundation of Western music is one of tension and release. As a passage begins and steadily builds in intensity, your anticipation level builds with it. You're waiting for the big payoff, the release. And when the climax finally comes, it starts all over again except that you automatically start the next cycle at a higher tension level."

Since you're always waiting for the big beat to kick in or the chord pattern to resolve itself, you end up in a state of "future tense" rather than "present relaxed." Where New Age music in general and Dr. Halpern's compositions in particular differ is they provide a constant level of fulfillment. The notes are arranged so that each one answers a need rather than creating one.

Of course this makes for a kind of music that we're just not used to hearing. "When my best-selling tape *Spectrum Suite* was first released, there were a few people who actually became tense and uncomfortable while listening to it," recalls Dr. Halpern. "I was a little puzzled until I realized that they were listening to the music in the same way they listen to all music, anticipating the big payoff. When it didn't come, they were left unsatisfied."

If this is going to be your first tango with New Age music, you'll need to acclimate yourself. It's actually a great experience. Pick up one of the tapes mentioned at the end of this story. If you've got a Walkman, use your bed as a launch pad. If not, pop it into the stereo in the den, dim the lights, and lie comfortably on the floor. Don't think about anything in particular, just let the music float you along. Feel it with your body and mind. Do this for about 15 minutes the first couple of times you listen. After that, put it on whenever you like, for relaxation or even as background music.

Missing the Beat

One thing you will notice is a lack of beat. "Any external beat sets up a rhythm entrainment phenomenon in the body that literally takes hold and manipulates the heartbeat," explains Dr. Halpern. "I was working with a group of nurses once and needed to graphically show them how external rhythms can force unnatural rhythms on the body. I had them all lie down on the floor and monitor their pulses while I pounded out a beat on the lecture stand. As I changed the beat, their heartbeats speeded up and slowed down right along with me." With pieces such as *Spectrum Suite,* the lack of imposed rhythm allows the body to choose the internal rhythm it finds most natural.

Considering the effects of rhythm and the anticipation response, it's easy to see how music, when not carefully chosen, can actually be an annoyance. It can even assure you a one-way ticket to the wrong side of the bed in the morning. "Personally, I find that waking up to the wrong music makes me feel like I only got 2 hours of sleep. My reactions are slower and I'm irritated all day," admits Dr. Halpern.

If you use a clock radio to sound the alarm, it really becomes a matter of potluck as to what song starts your day. "And what the D.J. has in mind is seldom what you have in mind," adds Dr. Halpern. Fortunately technology has given us a cure for the morning show blues—cassette alarm clocks. You can find them at the same stores that sell alarm clock radios. The difference is that you get to *choose* your wake-up sounds. Pop in a tapeful of soothing music and suddenly there's only one side of bed—the right side. "Basically, it's the difference between jumping into a cold lake and easing into a warm bath. They both wake you up, but one does it with a lot less stress," notes Dr. Halpern.

Whether you're looking for relaxing sounds, unobtrusive background music, or a way of masking some of the trying noises of daily life, New Age music has a lot to offer. A few years ago, you might have had a hard time finding it, but with consumer interest running high, just about every record store has a bin or two devoted to New Age. If you can't find it at the record shop, try your local metaphysical bookstore. A quick look through the pages of *New Age* magazine will also offer you a wide mail-order selection. Here are a few of Dr. Halpern's picks to get you on the road to healthy listening experiences.

- Kitaro: *Silk Road* (Canyon Records)
- Steven Halpern: *Dawn* (Halpern Sounds)
- Paul Horn: *Inside* (Golden Flute)
- Iasos: *Interdimensional Music* (Interdimensional Music)
- Emerald Web: *Valley of the Birds* (Bobkat Productions)
- Deuter: *Haleakala* (Kuckuck Records)
- Georgia Kelly: *Seapeace* (Heru Records)
- Paul Winter: *Common Ground* (Living Music Records)
- William Aura: *Auramusic* (William Auramusic)
- Mark Allen and Friends: *Summer Suite* (Rising Sun)
- Dallas Smith: *Stellar Voyage* (Rising Sun)
- Schawkie Roth: *You Are the Ocean* (Heaven on Earth)
- Daniel Kobialka: *Timeless Motion* (Li-Sem)
- Michael Stearns: *Morning Jewel* (Continuum Montage)
- Paul Warner: *Waterfall Music* (Waterfall Music Records)
- Environments: *Ultimate Seashore* (Atlantic)
- Solitudes: *Spring Morning on the Prairies* (Solitudes)
- George Winston: *Autumn* (Windham Hill)

LIVING IT UP DOWNTOWN

Listening to people talk about cities, you get the feeling that no one really knows what the word means. "Cities are wonderful, exciting places." "Cities are dirty and dangerous." "City people are the friendliest in the world." "They're all wierdos. I wouldn't walk on 42nd Street if you paid me."

Of course, part of the reason there are so many conflicting ideas about cities is that there are so many different types of cities. But they all have one thing in common: they're a mix of delightful and disgusting. What if you could somehow zoom in on the good stuff and compensate for the seamy side? You'd be living in a Superburg.

Here's a two-step project that can make your city-living experience a super one. Step one is to start to really like the city—a bad attitude will only get you into the big-city blues. So, let's figure out which of your ideas about urban life are products of positive thinking and which are moldy myths you should toss out.

Myth: Urban dwellers have no friends and feel anonymous.

Fact: This is bushwah. Of course city folk have friends. But the way they have them is a little different from the friendships of people who live in smaller areas. "On the average, the larger the community, the less likely it is for people to be on a first name basis with other people in the immediate vicinity—like the mailperson and the neighbors," says Dr. Claude Fischer, professor of sociology at the University of California at Berkeley.

But, he adds, city dwellers have plenty of friends who don't live right next door. Those friends are often people who resemble them in terms of interests, background, and occupation, says Dr. Fischer. People who live in cities tend to have specialized friends—one friend to see movies with, another to talk to about problems, and a third to shop with.

A resident of New York city, Betsy Andrews, finds Dr. Fischer's description valid: "I have some friends who know each other," she says, "but we don't usually end up in a big group and we don't live near each other. I tend to do things with one person at a time and then I won't

431

see them again for a month. Living in the city isn't like "Cheers," with everyone hanging out together in a bar all the time."

Not knowing the people who live near you can make you feel anonymous, but counting up the friends you have all over the city should counteract the problem. Charlotte Wang, a biologist and a longtime resident of San Francisco who recently moved to Boston, offers this perspective on anonymity: "Walking outside at lunchtime, I don't know anyone I see, so of course, I feel anonymous. But by the same token, in my work environment, I don't feel anonymous. Since my workplace could not exist anywhere but in the city, it is just as much a part of the city as the street. And I belong there."

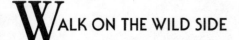ALK ON THE WILD SIDE

Picture yourself creeping silently through the underbrush, clad in khaki and boots, flashlight in hand, stalking a wild animal. Once you find it, walk around the block and down a cool glass of O.J. at your favorite city deli.

Sound like a fantasy? City naturalists know that the urban safari is a reality. In New York City alone, you can see muskrats and foxes by day, and owls and flying squirrels by night. And that's just the beginning: A pair of red-tailed hawks nested in a small park surrounded entirely by tall buildings near the apartment of Norman Stotz, a member of the board of directors of New York's Audubon Society.

"And this past spring," he says, "there was a pair of peregrine falcons—the fastest bird in the world—living in mid-Manhattan on the roof of the Waldorf-Astoria." They feed on pigeons, Stotz adds, "which is fine; we've got plenty of food for them."

In other cities, there are raccoons, opossums, and even coyotes. "And you do occasionally read a story about the moose that wanders into a New England town," says Stotz. "A critter gets a bit confused, and it's liable to show up anywhere."

To start your own expeditions, bring friends, flashlights, and binoculars, and explore parks, wooded areas, around evergreens, and in open areas near woods. Or, get on the trail with guidance and possibly expert-led tours from your city's urban park ranger program. Find out if your city has one by calling the parks and recreation department of your city government. (In New York City, call (212) 397-3091.)

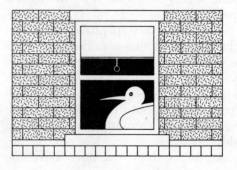

Wang also knows more of her neighbors than most city folk because she made an effort to meet them. "I know the people in my building," she says, "because a couple of weeks ago I needed a telephone book, so I knocked on everyone's door to find one. I said, 'I just moved in upstairs and I need a telephone book.' That's a good way to meet people because it's perfectly socially acceptable."

The fact remains, though, that some people are lonely in the city. Some researchers suggest that the loneliest people are those who don't do things outside of their homes that bring them into contact with other people. Almost no one knows their names or who they are, and that can lead to a frightening sense of isolation. Fortunately, the cure is simple: Go out and get involved in a club, a job, or a community organization. Find out what's available from a local paper.

Myth: City residents have a high rate of depression and mental illness.

Fact: Depression and mental illnesses are not particularly prevalent in cities. In fact, they are slightly more common in rural areas.

Dr. Jonathan Freedman, a professor of psychology at the University of Toronto, surveyed thousands of urban and rural Americans about how happy they are. "The major thing I found," he says, "is that people in the city are just as happy, if not happier, than people who are not in the city."

And in 1974, Dr. Leo Srole, professor emeritus of sociology at Columbia University, finished a 20-year-long study in which he followed the mental health of a group of people living in New York City during the entire study. He found that 72

AMERICA'S TOP TEN METRO AREAS

What's the difference between an okay city and one that's really a great place to live? Well, a mild climate's one. And low crime and unemployment rates are pretty important, as well as low living costs. A great city just wouldn't be great if it didn't have super health care, education, transportation, and recreation. And a stimulating array of concerts, museums, and movies tops off a city that's really tops. Well, the folks at Rand McNally and Company rated 329 metro areas on all these counts, averaged the scores together, and came up with the 50 best places to live. Here's the top ten.

1. Pittsburgh, Pennsylvania
2. Boston, Massachusetts
3. Raleigh-Durham, North Carolina
4. San Francisco, California
5. Philadelphia, Pennsylvania
6. Nassau-Suffolk, New York
7. St. Louis, Missouri
8. Louisville, Kentucky
9. Norwalk, Connecticut
10. Seattle, Washington

percent of them either stayed the same mentally or actually improved, despite the many mental disabilities the city has been rumored to cause.

One payoff of living in the city: There are many hospitals, clinics, and therapists, so mental, emotional, and physical illnesses can be quickly and easily treated.

434

Myth: It's dangerous to live in a city—if a mugger doesn't get you, high pollution levels will.

Fact: Let's settle the crime question first. Yes, in some very large cities, the crime rate is higher than in the suburbs and rural areas. But the country is where murder and violent crime rates are surprisingly high, says Kenneth Wilkinson, professor of rural sociology at Pennsylvania State University. "The long-term pattern in this country is that the rate of murder in rural police jurisdictions is greater than in most cities," he says. "The smaller the city, the safer. The reason: In rural areas, people tend not to have many acquaintances; too many intimate relationships with not enough casual contacts actually *adds* stress."

So, if you're in a small city, count your blessings. For those of you who live in large cities, simple safe-city practices can help you avoid most problems.

"My approach is that I don't walk alone at night," says Wang. "I also read the pamphlets that say to walk briskly, look straight ahead, and act confident, and I do all those things. They make me feel better.

"If I'm going out at night, I either try to go with someone or I drive somewhere and stay in a lighted neighborhood," she adds. "Another way I get around without the walking at night problem is riding a bicycle. I feel much safer on bicycle because I'm going much faster—I can get away from the bad guys quicker."

When you're on that bicycle, though, try to avoid riding right behind buses and trucks. Same goes for running. Dr. Benjamin Honigman, the emergency room direc-

WHAT WOULD YOU MISS MOST?

"Tell them to appreciate what they have now, before it's too late," exclaimed one woman we surveyed. No, she wasn't talking about your health or wealth—she meant the wonderful amenities of the city. We surveyed 27 ex-city dwellers about what they miss most now that they're living in the suburbs and the country. Here's what headed the list of longed-for urban comforts.

1. A variety of restaurants.
2. Ethnic diversity.
3. Easy access to theatres showing a wide variety of movies.
4. Lots of different kinds of food stores.
5. Many types of musical events and offerings.

What they don't miss at all: crowds.

tor at the University Hospital of the University of Colorado Health Sciences Center, says, "If you run or exercise in areas where you come in direct contact with exhaust, you are obviously getting much more exposure than is good for you." The early symptoms of overexposure to carbon-monoxide are nausea, blurred vision, and headaches.

But don't worry—they'll go away after a short time. The best bet, says Dr. Honigman, is to exercise in parks, on roads without a lot of traffic, and in well-ventilated indoor gyms, especially on high-pollution

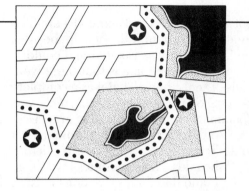

Takin' the 10¢ Tour

Can you imagine being backstage at the Metropolitan Opera House, sitting in Louise Nevelson's living room, or being among the very first ever to enter the World Trade Center? Folks who tour New York City with Adventures on a Shoestring can — because they've done those things and more, all for just a $3 fee and yearly membership dues.

Howard Goldberg founded the tour group in 1963 when he wanted to visit the *Herald-Tribune* but was told he needed at least 15 people to get past the receptionist. He put a one-line ad in the paper and found 65 people waiting at the appointed meeting place. The organization was born.

If you live in or visit New York a lot, you can stop reading for a minute and call Goldberg for his brochure. But if you don't, close your eyes and try to think of all the places in your city you'd like to visit. The storage rooms of the city's historical museum?

The hospital viewing room during open heart surgery? The airport's control tower?

Well, why not? Follow Goldberg's example and give some of your city's more interesting people and places a call. Explain that you've organized a group of individuals who would like to have a tour and, if possible, meet with whoever runs the place. Once you've set up the tour date, advertise through word of mouth, flyers, and an ad in the paper. Have people meet you at the site of the tour. Who knows? Twenty-five years from now, you may find yourself, as Goldberg did recently, in a helicopter high over your own beautiful city, pointing out the sights to members of your own tour organization.

days. Don't stop exercising outdoors altogether, though — it's a great way to meet people safely.

Myth: The crowds and noise in cities are unhealthy for human beings.

Fact: Crowds aren't bad for you — they're stimulating. They make all emotions — good and bad — seem more intense, according to Dr. Freedman, and they add excitement to everyday life, says Dr. Srole.

"The high volume of human contacts in the city is a stimulus — a stimulus for the good," says Dr. Srole. "In India, monkeys run around free. A psychologist did a study on these monkeys and found that those in the city behaved in a much more animated fashion than the ones out in the country. There's really no question that the urban environment is much more stimulating in many, many respects."

If the crowds do get to you, one way to cope is to find a retreat. "In San Francisco, I found lots of retreats," says Wang. "There was a beach a 2-hour drive away at the

436

foot of a cliff on the Pacific Ocean. The great thing about this beach, besides the fact that it was isolated and couldn't be seen from the road, is that there were loads of seals there. That was a complete escape. For a temporary escape, there was a botanical garden right in San Francisco.

"And sometimes the problem isn't being in a city, but being in a particular city," she adds. "So sometimes I would go to city B and find things that don't exist in city A, like a better nightclub or a unique restaurant."

If noise is a problem, the solution is even simpler. Give yourself some time without any. Bill Greenburg, a CPA who lives in New York, installed double-thick windows in his apartment. And New Yorker Andrews just leaves the radio off when she gets home.

The trick to winning in the city-living game, says Dr. Freedman, is to accept that the city *is* a city. "Every community has something to offer, and you should take the community for what it has to provide."

Thirteen City-Loving Strategies

Now that we've got your anti-urban attitude straightened out, the second part of the two-step super-city project is to dance outside and do something that will make you really love your city. Think up your own ideas, or give some of ours a try.

1. Plan a block party.

2. Have dinner on the roof of your building.

3. Be a tourist in your own town. Call up the visitor's bureau and ask them what's hot in the city.

4. Turn Japanese and plant sunflowers outside your building. The Japanese have them along highways because they know sunflowers soak up scads of nitrogen dioxide from cars and trucks.

5. Plant hardy wildflowers between your house and street. You can buy seed mixtures in cans at garden stores.

6. Shop in a farmers' market instead of the supermarket. Studies show that ten times as many social contacts happen in outdoor markets as in supermarkets.

7. Visit the major corporations in town, check out the displays in their lobbies, and pick up some free samples of their products.

8. Write a letter to the editor of the local paper about an unusual hot spot you've found in town.

9. Conduct your own contest for most beautiful garden or window boxes in town. You be the judge and award a letter of commendation to the winner.

10. Make like the gamesters in New York and set up a card table with a checker, chess, or backgammon board on a busy street at lunchtime. A small sign—"Free Game"—will reel in playing partners in no time.

11. Plant a tree. Or get together with your neighbors and turn your uninviting local park into a lush arbor. Check with City Hall to see if funds are already earmarked for this kind of thing.

12. Meet your next-door neighbors.

13. Start a community garden—grow an urban utopia along with your cucumbers.

TRAVEL FOR THE SOUL

No one appreciates home like the footloose traveler. Every ramble and excursion that fills the eyes with novel sights gives fresh insight into the uniqueness of the familiar. It's a polishing act, kind of. With every trip, another layer of mental dust is blown away. Things you have known for years seem to mysteriously change. You realize that nothing is static, but can be reinterpreted over and over. Even that potted plant on the kitchen table. Or that potted opinion.

Travel regenerates each of us in different ways. Every so often, I need something to astonish me. Baffle me. I need to have the hands of habit tied so that I can reach out for something new. I need to have the mental chorus of do-this-and-do-that drowned out so that I hear the uncontrolled gush of the here-and-now.

I need the memories, too. Memories that are not antiques but living parts of you like your vocabulary. You can call them up, relive them, share them. How good it is to sit in your chair and think, I remember the Japanese baby in its mother's arms whose eyes suddenly opened as wide as mine because she had never seen a Caucasian in her life. I remember walking through the dusty streets of an Indian city with two million people and two traffic lights and never being stared at, never hustled or begged at, never feeling afraid, not even in a slum where 10,000 people live on 3 acres, because the people are so proud, and then rethinking my notion of what poverty and crime are all about in American cities. I remember trying to walk across a log 10 feet over a rushing mountain stream in Switzerland and freezing up, paralyzed with fear, watching a pair of 65-year-old women cross nimbly in front of me, and the leader of the ramble coming back for me, saying: "Rest your fingertips on my back and follow me across," and I did, and suddenly the fear evaporated like mist. I remember hiking along a trail out to the Na Pali coast in Hawaii, and standing there on the very last spot of land, looking at the emerald green valley 2,000 feet down and the clear sea just beyond and thinking this was the most beautiful place I'd ever seen and saying to my fiancée, "Let's get married right here," so we did, at that very moment.

And all you travelers, you have your memories, too.

Travel for the soul, I call it. Travel

that takes you to as many wonderful places inside you as it does outside you.

But travel—even for the soul—has its practical side, too. Here, I'll go through some pointers that have worked for me.

Let your mind wander before your feet. To find out about unusual travel opportunities, you can't depend on the big vacation bargain ads, the charter trips, or the average travel agent. First, go to a bookstore and browse through some thick travel books, the kind that describe hundreds of hotels, inns, campgrounds, villages, national forests, hikes, and obscure restaurants. (About 80 percent of what they say is true, or close to it.) Then, look for the little ads for unusual travel in the back of magazines for gourmets, hikers, and generally sophisticated people. Write for every brochure even if what they offer doesn't sound too appetizing. (To get you started, we have some suggestions at the end of this section).

Best of all, talk to your friends. People who have been on fabulous trips love to share their experiences. They will give you the best tips of all.

Don't be afraid to travel with a small group. Sure, you're the independent type. But going with a group has so many advantages you may be better off. First, having an experienced guide will get you over your fear of traveling in a strange place where they may not speak your language. Then, your guide will know the best places to go, and may well have friends and contacts in the area who can make your visit much more meaningful.

Every trip I've been on with groups provided plenty of time for individual poking around, shopping, and the inevitable foray for ice cream. The other people in

the group are fun to be with, anyway.

Talk to the organizers of the trip by telephone. Find out not just the itinerary, but the texture of the trip. Are many hours going to be spent touring historical landmarks? If there's hiking, just how challenging is it? What's the vertical gain of mountains to be hiked? How warm is the water at the beach? How much time is spent on buses? Let the organizers know what you like to do, and see if your vision of the trip matches up with theirs.

Go easy on history and museums. At least that's my personal preference. Nothing is so exhausting as a couple of hours shuffling through a museum. It's harder on your legs than a walk up and down hills. Ditto, cathedrals, forts, and palaces. Will they really recharge your spiritual batteries . . . or just grind your engine? I'd rather spend my time prowling through a good local flea market.

Expect the unplanned. If you leave home thinking that everything ought to be perfect from the get-go, you are bound to wind up frustrated. Experienced travelers know that goof-ups and delays are inevitable. I've conditioned myself to just kind of float through those moments. Usually, I speak up—sometimes loudly—but inside I'm saying "What's the difference?" Airlines and customs officials may be able to disjoint your schedule, but you, and only you, are in control of your mood. Relax. Go with the flow, even when you can't see where it's going—or if it's going at all! Things will work out.

Enjoy a full-course vacation. The experience of a vacation doesn't begin with the boarding call. The "appetizer" of the full-course vacation is the books you read before you ever leave home. Not so much the see-this/see-that books, but those that tell you about the culture of your destination. Mind-stretching in itself, that kind of reading will deepen and intensify your on-the-scene experiences.

Keep a diary. I always carry a spiral-bound notepad that I can easily slip in and out of my back pocket. At every opportunity, I yank it out and write down detailed descriptions of what I've seen and done. Sometimes I stop along a sidewalk to jot down what I've just encountered in a shop. Goods, prices, dialogue, the works. In restaurants, I make note of every dish. On mountain tops, the distant views and the whip of the wind. At night, I fill in more details and record my impressions of the day, the place, the people met. That kind of diary-keeping quickly sharpens your senses and leads you to a fuller interplay with your environment. Later, your notes will bring back memories of your trip with a startling immediacy.

Be security conscious. Some cities and even whole countries are known for purse snatching and wallet picking. The most frequent story I hear is leaving a purse wrapped around a restaurant chair and not remembering it until 5 minutes later, at which point it has vanished. Here are some tips to make thievery less likely.

● Carry your valuables in a little zippered pouch, the kind that attaches to a belt. You may want a two-pouch deal; one for money, the other for an instamatic. Always wear the pouches in front of you. Keep small bills in your front pocket, so you don't flash a big wad when you buy a newspaper.

● Never leave money in your hotel room. If you can't carry it, put it in the hotel safe.

● Never leave anything that even *looks* valuable in a locked automobile.

● Don't wear gold chains.

● Ask your innkeeper where it's safe and not safe to go by day and by night. But remember that most robberies occur in places frequented by tourists. That's why I recommend carrying money—and everything else—securely fastened to your body. That way, you won't get cramps from clutching your pocketbook all during lunch.

Personally, I have lost far more things around the house than I have traveling around the world. In fact, my only experiences along these lines have been the opposite of thievery. In Toyko, a waitress came running down the street after me because I'd left too many yen on the table. In Hyderabad, India, a hotel keeper ran out of the hotel as I was getting into a motorcycle-cab to go to the airport. Had I forgotten to pay for the last glass of juice? No, it was the sneakers I'd given to the 10-year-old boy who cleaned my rooom. The man wanted to be absolutely sure they were really a gift.

So although there are verminous types who will take advantage of a foolish or distracted traveler, there are far more people who will go out of their way to help and protect you.

Now, we want to tell you about some trips that are good examples of "travel for the soul."

M. B.

WALKING THROUGH JAPAN

I'd already walked some 75 miles or better through the streets, lanes, mountain paths, and boulevards of Japan, but now I hesitated to set foot outside. We all stood there, eight Americans poised in the foyer of the hotel, milling around nervously, fussing with our clothing. That was the problem—we didn't have any. Only robes covered our bodies—thin, cotton *yukata* with blue-gray striping held together with a simple linen sash. On our bare feet, slippers.

Already feeling slightly conspicuous in a town almost never visited by foreigners, the idea of parading down the busy main thoroughfare in these getups seemed outrageous. True, the Pacific Ocean was just across the street, over the seawall. And true, they'd told us that here in the mineral-water resort town of Shirahama in southern Japan, it was perfectly acceptable to promenade in your "jammies." But as I peered outside, all I could see were men wearing crisp blue suits and black shoes, a kind of national uniform in Japan. Not so much as a pair of walking shorts.

Well, *"Bonzai!"* I mutter and we all start off. We haven't taken but a single step when the hotel staff begins screaming and grabbing their hair. What's wrong? Is this robe business all a big joke? No, just the opposite. And one of our party, it seems, has made a terrible mistake. The trouble is with Barbara, now surrounded by Japanese making frantic gestures. Is something showing? No, we learn from our guide and translator. Barbara, being left-handed, has made the terrible mistake of fastening her robe with the right side over the left. And what's so terrible about that? In Japan, robes are fastened that way only on the dead, it's explained. Barbara, not wishing to do an imitation of the walking dead, retires to make a quick adjustment. Then we're on our way, shuffling along in our slippers, trying to keep our robes in place as the ocean breeze whips around our bare legs.

Sun, Surf, and Steam

Ten minutes later, our bravery is rewarded with the discovery of outdoor hot mineral baths set smack on the ocean. Hot water tumbles down over stones coated with a rainbow of mineral deposits and splashes into rock pools. I toss off my robe, slip through the steam and ease my walk-weary body into the favorite Japanese tranquilizer: the hot bath. There we soak and paddle, surrounded on three sides by rock walls, the fourth open to the Pacific Ocean and its waves that lap against the rocky ledge. Behind us rises a steep cliff in which are carved three images of Buddha, and statues of gods with vessels of flowers at their feet. Above, big brown sea hawks circle and circle. When the heat finally becomes too much to bear, I step out of the pool, walk to the ege of the Pacific and let the ocean spray cool me off as my eyes search the horizon. Somewhere out there lies home, seven time zones and many mind zones away.

A Different Kind of Town

I had come to Japan with eight other Americans, including Anne, our Japanese-American guide and translator. I know nothing about Japan and couldn't speak a word of Japanese except "Benihana of Tokyo" (which, I discovered, in Tokyo is called "Benihana of New York"). But I had a great desire to see this nation, where a population over half as large as the United States' population lives — and thrives — on a land mass about the size of Montana. Then I learned of a small San Diego travel firm, called Intimate Glimpses, founded by walking enthusiasts. They had organized trips to Japan, designed to let you see the country as the Japanese do, staying only at Japanese inns, called *ryokans,* where essentially no English is spoken, and no Westerners ordinarily visit. Using six inns in as many cities and villages as home base, we'd go out on foot every day to walk for miles through the fall foliage of mountain paths, the thronged and gaudy Ginza, the sacred shrines, fish markets, noodle parlors, and backyard rice fields of Japan.

To me, a fitness vacation is always best. Not just for walking or cycling or whatever your form of exercise, but because such trips have an air of discovery, of warmth and intimacy — and always the unexpected — that makes a vacation so memorable.

An Unexpected Picnic

We're hiking through the Japan alps, a short hop over a mountain, to the next village. Under our feet, what is called "The Stone Tatami," a woven mat, in effect, of stones carefully fitted into place by local people. Hundreds of years ago, they knew, great Japanese samurai had traveled over this very path, and volunteer labor has now rebuilt it. Around us, a grove of bamboo, each tree a different shade of silvery green or pale yellow.

"In case there's an earthquake," says Anne, "duck into the bamboo grove. According to the Japanese, their roots are so strongly intertwined that the ground cannot be torn apart. And the trees are so flexible that they can't be knocked over." Only later do I realize how much the Japanese people are like the bamboo grove.

We wind out of the deep forest and are passing a village when we spot a small shrine, mostly hidden by trees. There are shrines everywhere in Japan, but there's some special charm to this one. We all pause from our hike to enjoy the serenity of what turns out to be a small cemetery, deep in green shade, the stones overgrown with lichens. Then we notice that there are happy voices coming from behind the adjoining shrubs. Peeking through branches, we see a picnic going on. Anne concludes it's a festival held by members of a Buddhist temple. Then they become aware of our presence, and we feel awkward having intruded on their holy grounds. But several of the women immediately approach us, take us by the hand, and insist we join their picnic. Another blanket is put on the grass, and in moments we are surrounded by smiling faces pouring us hot cups of tea, serving us platters heaped with thick triangles of savory rice studded with vegetables, mushrooms, and tiny pieces of pork. Then plate after plate of a lightly pickled medley of cabbage and vegetables. It's delicious: delicate and crunchy, and I can't get enough—although finally I do. Anne explains this kind of dish is made only in private homes, never restaurants, and is fermented using by-products of the rice harvest. Filled with good food and good vibes, we offer a prayer at their flower-wreathed Buddha, leave a donation for the temple, and with a flurry of deep bows, handshakes, smiles, and waves, take our leave to head on down the mountain to the next village.

Mt. Fuji and the Health Engineer

Up at 4:00 A.M., thanks to jet lag and a couple of roosters clocking in for the day. It is perfectly black so there is nothing to do but lie there snuggled between *futons* on the tatami floor, head surprisingly comfortable on a pillow of rice hulls. By 6:00 A.M., we are outside, where an early-morning fog is slowly lifting itself from the cabbage patches and rice fields like a levitating blanket of gauze. And then, as if from nowhere, Mt. Fuji suddenly appears massive, majestic, and solitary, its perfect volcano shape crested with streamers of snow that dazzle in the light of high dawn.

By seven, we are back at our little inn—not much bigger than a boarding house—in time to meet another guest, a Japanese construction engineer who is leaving for work. Anne, our guide, discovers that he lives an hour away, but is staying here for a while to supervise a local job. And that's not just to avoid the annoyance of the long commute. It's important, he says, to be perfectly rested, fit, and healthy when you are responsible for 150 people. Must be a really big construction job, Anne

suggests. No, I only have 40 people working at the site, he says. *No comprendo,* says Anne in Japanese. "The 150 people are the families of the workers," the engineer explains. "I am responsible for their welfare, too," he says, and goes off to put in another 10- to 12-hour day.

Easy Walking in a Strange Country

Japan is a lark for the rambler. There are remarkably few places where you don't feel perfectly safe. Walk down a side street in Kyoto after dark and the worst you have to fear is bumping your head on a low bridge not designed for tall Americans. Violent crime and robbery are, by our standards, almost nonexistent. Stores do not bother with security guards, mirrors, or package checking. Indeed, owners of small shops often leave their stores wide open while they go in the back room to eat or rest. You may have to walk into their living quarters to rouse them if you want to make a purchase. The herds of bicycles parked on the sidewalks have wheel locks, but none are fastened to a post. One inn we stayed at in the major city of Kyoto, had no room keys. All this with virtually no policemen walking beats.

Nor does the walker in Japan encounter any panhandlers or hustlers, abandoned buildings, broken windows, spray-can graffiti, or jalopies rusting in alleyways.

What the rambler does see is workers picking up every last scrap of street litter with their hands. Great packs of uniformed students on class trips—behaving like Boy Scouts. Old people who may smile and bow at the sight of a foreigner. Small children who chirp *hello!* and wave. Ramblers even have their own gods — tiny roadside shrines with ancient, weathered statues whose spirits are said to protect the traveler. Often someone has put fresh flowers at the god's feet. And over his head, a red woolen cap, as if it were a child that needed to be protected from the cold.

A good place to go for a walk.

The Sea of Trees

Put Japan on a drawing board and it won't work. There are simply too many people and too many mountains in too little space. A planning committee would reject it out of hand.

But somehow Japan does work. And it works in ways that give the Western visitor new thoughts about his own homeland. The Japanese, you see, are a team. A family. Everything is *us*, not him or me. Sure, the subways and streets can get crowded, but it's crowded with *us* — so what is there to get uptight about? Sure I could steal something — easily — but how could I steal from *us?*

Rather than retreating from a crowded society to survive as an individual, as we might imagine doing under such circumstances — perhaps as we already do — the Japanese survive by holding on to those around them.

This haiku was written on a hill near Mt. Fuji.

> Where a tree cannot grow
> the green forest sings.
> Root holds root,
> leaves dancing.

The hill overlooks a dense wood — called the Sea of Trees — that has managed to grow out of an old lava bed nearly devoid of topsoil.

— ■

M. B.

(*Editor's Note:* For more information on walking tours in Japan and Europe, write to Intimate Glimpses, Box 6091, San Diego, CA 92106, or call 619-222-2224.)

ADVENTURE UNDER THE TALL SAILS

Last summer I lived for a week with 34 strangers in an area smaller than a tennis court. We each plunked down $360 for the opportunity. There were no bathrooms to speak of. And every day, someone screamed in agony.

We also laughed and sang late into the night. We ate and drank like fools. We read good books, taught each other crafts, and thought about our lives. At the end of it all, we felt relaxed, rejuvenated, and ready to recommend it to friends.

Our "tennis court" was the *Mattie*, a century-old schooner that once shuttled lumber, coal, and granite up and down the Atlantic seacoast. In 1939 she was still going strong, but the practice of trading by sail had weakened considerably. So in that year she became a "dude schooner," taking on city-legged vacationers at

Camden, Maine, and traipsing them out around the off-shore islands. Today there are 15 such boats—best known as wind-jammers—operating off the coast of Maine, and three others elsewhere in New England. Every summer, they make a lot of people very happy.

Almost everything about my schooner, the *Mattie*, was still back in the nineteenth century—including the plumbing. There were no showers. There were three communal "heads," each consisting of a lone toilet with a long steel pipe of a handle that, when pumped several times, would more or less flush it. Fresh water for washing was located in two oak barrels on the ship's deck. Every morning, my fellow passengers and I would ladle some of the water into our plastic basins and wash up—right out there in the open. That was our first radical adjustment in matters of personal hygiene.

The Price of Hygiene

But that was nothing compared with the ordeal of getting an honest shower and shampoo. There was no choice but to jump overboard. Now, in Maine, the Atlantic is unswimmably cold. The passengers who jumped in would roar with pain as they hit the water. Then they climbed out, lathered up, jumped in again, and screamed again.

Sleeping conditions were similarly rustic: Bunks tucked in cabins below deck. The cabins were cheek by jowl with the heads. By midvoyage (trips last Monday morning to Saturday noon), our cabins got understandably stuffy. Each night, more people began sleeping up on the wooden deck of the ship, rather than in the cabins

below. Blessed were they who had brought sleeping bags. The brochures tell you a sleeping bag is optional, but I'd say it's mandatory. The night air in Maine is as cold as the sea.

Doesn't sound like a formula for happiness, does it? Even the hard-core campers among us groused a little. But most of us refused to let it bother us, maybe because we knew it was a necessary part of the total experience. We were roughing it for a purpose. We didn't want a luxury cruise. We didn't want to be pampered, or fed pâté five times a day, or go bowling aboard a floating city. Those things isolate us from where we are.

On the *Mattie* all those isolating things are stripped away. On a ship smaller than a tennis court, there's simply no room. For five and a half days I sat on the wooden deck of a dot in the ocean, subject to fog, sun, wind, and storm. At times I had the feeling I wasn't even on the ship. I was living at the top of the sea, at the bottom of the sky, sharing an existence with buoys, channel markers, rocks, and gulls.

Feeling that way at some places on this earth would be no great thrill. But because the Maine coastline is incomparably beautiful, such intimacy with the environment is a joy eternal. On a normal vacation in Maine, you point at things through the windshield, or through the picture window in a motel room, and say, "Isn't that picturesque?" Maybe you buy a painting of a lighthouse with waves crashing on the rocks, to hold onto what you saw. But on the *Mattie,* you spend a week *living inside the painting.* The mountains sloping down to the sea. The cozy harbors. The white sails furling. The constantly changing weather. The spangle of sunlight or glow of full moon on the water.

The islands. Woods. Pastures. Farmhouses. Wildlife.

The pure unstinting beauty was what I liked most about my trip on the *Mattie* last summer, and most of my fellow passengers felt the same way. Annette, an emergency room nurse in Boston, told me she liked "the sun, being outside and on the water all the time; the fresh air, rain, cold, hot — the different weather." Ann, a mental health counselor in Erie, Pennsylvania, said she liked "the peace, the beauty, and how incredibly free from the usual worries it was." Judy, a Congressional lobbyist, had a droll way of putting it: "I enjoyed not being around shopping centers."

Annette, Ann, Judy, the other passengers, and the crew of five were the other wonderful part of the trip. We came from as far away as California; we ranged in age from 17 to 60. There were six couples; the rest were singles...a majority of ones. About two thirds were women. Most of us hit it off well together. Every night before dinner we had a spontaneous happy hour: We'd drag out the bottles we had brought on board, and treat new friends to our Old Grand-Dad.

To say a little more about the number of singles on board: It's no wonder. A windjamming cruise is a perfect solo vacation. You meet new people under the best of circumstances; you eat, talk, and play as a group. It's impossible to feel awkward about being alone. In fact, it's almost impossible to be alone.

Night and Day

Where does a windjammer sail in five and half days? It all depends on the winds, the weather, how sleek your ship is, and whether it is equipped with radar (imperative for sailing through the all-too-common Maine fog). Windjammers drop anchor at a different harbor each night — places with names like Dark Harbor, Pulpit Harbor, and Swan's Island.

A crew of four does the sailing, but nobody would go anywhere if the passengers didn't help out with jobs like raising the anchor or lowering the sails. In the process, you get an inkling of what sailing is all about, and you can get to literally "know the ropes": the profusion of hempen rigging on a traditional sailing vessel.

The fifth crew member is the cook. All the cooking is done on a small wood cookstove below deck. Charming and awe-inspiring. Luckily, we had a cook who triumphed over the adversity, and we ate massive quantities of delicious food. Simple food. No pâté.

Given all the adventures of a windjamming cruise, you might get the impression that it's not a good vacation if you need to relax. Not true. All I can say is, one of my fellow passengers was a high-powered man of 45 who owns a New York fabric supply company. On the fourth day of the cruise I caught him bouncing around the ship playing pirate like a small boy and growling "Arrgh, maties!" Now that's what I call unwinding.

We all unwound; we all hated to see the trip end. We swapped home addresses and phone numbers. One of us said to our captain, "I'll bet you don't get many groups as nice as this one." And he smiled as he looked out over the wheel and said, "On the Friday of just about every trip, someone comes up to me and says, 'Isn't this the best crew of people you've ever had?'"

Laurence Stains

446

THE OTHER HAWAII

We're not far from the end of the world.

I can see it from here, in fact—a stone rim that vanishes into mist down at the other end of this high, wildflower-spattered valley, where the clouds are forever massing and dispersing, and great rock shapes appear and then disappear, as if passing from matter into mist and then back again.

What a strange, savage, beautiful place this is!

We seem to have pitched our tents on Mars. Around us, in the day-bright moonlight, we're surrounded by black, glassy slabs of old lava flows, yet the air is so heavy with moisture there's a ring around the moon. Above us the unfamiliar stars wheel in and out of clouds, eerily brilliant as if imagined by Van Gogh.

For the umpteenth time on this trip, I have to remind myself where I am. This *isn't* Mars, or the moon or someplace in Idaho. This is Hawaii!

An Undiscovered Star

We're on the island of Maui, camped at 6,800 feet, down inside the volcanic crater of Haleakala, a 4,000-foot-deep hole almost big enough to swallow Manhattan. Earlier that day, the five of us had descended from the crater's 10,000-foot rim—which soars above cloud level, like a rocky island floating in a sea of clouds— and walked 8 miles to this spot. We passed through terrain as majestic and desolate as an undiscovered star. At certain eleva-

tions, almost nothing grows except the amazing silversword, a plant that looks like an extravagant, silvery chrysanthemum and grows nowhere else on earth except Hawaii. Later, a dense fog started rolling in—and suddenly we were on the Maine seacoast, walking through what looked for all the world like bayberry, blueberries, and pearly everlasting.

It was all so strange—and so little of it seemed to fit my classic mental postcard of Hawaii, land of the hula, the luau, and the sunset coconut palm.

But what's more, this Hawaii I was discovering kept changing from one thing into another with such frequency and speed that it dizzied the brain. These islands, I was beginning to find out, have dozens of microclimates and microecosystems all crowded into a very small space, the way New York City has microcultures that change every few blocks.

In the red sandstone gorges of Waimea Canyon, on Kauai, I thought I was in the mesa country of Arizona; in the fawn-colored grasslands of Lanai, where a herd of grazing giraffe or zebras would have looked perfectly at home, I might have been in Africa; up among the towering pines around the base of Mauna Kea volcano, on the Big Island, I could have been in Colorado. Only the bamboo forests and jungle waterfalls of Maui really fit the Hawaii of legend (and old Elvis movies).

But it was the "real" Hawaii—or Hawaiis—that I'd come a quarter of the way around the world to see.

And what better way to do that than

by two weeks of close-up contact with the place—camping, hiking, skin diving, sailing, and generally getting Hawaii in my hair, in my shoes, and all over my hands and face?

Easygoing, Outdoorsy

The five of us who'd signed on for this "13-Day Hawaiian Adventure" first met beneath a giant wall map of Kauai, "the garden island," in that island's little airport in Lihue. There was Jim, a pixie-ish 42-year-old accountant for a Boston scrap-exporting firm; Elaine and Debbie, two meat-cutters from a supermarket in Boulder, aged 40 and 28; Nancy, 33, who managed a medical lab in a Houston hospital; and me, a 33-year-old writer from Pennsylvania.

For me, a veteran nonjoiner, the notion of flying all the way to Hawaii to join a group of strangers on an organized, two-week vacation put me a little on edge. But we weren't strangers to one another for more than a few minutes, and once our hosts Karen and M. J. appeared, I suddenly realized how nice it was to turn the worry and the details over to somebody else.

Karen Fong, a Chinese-American emigre from Pittsburgh, was our cheerful and competent guide, accompanied for the first few days by M. J. Bilgrav, who with her husband Zane operates Pacific Quest, the small outfitting business that organized our trip. Ours was a fairly typical group, Karen told us—easygoing, outdoorsy—though smaller than most. (During the busy seasons, winter and summer, groups range in size up to 16.) Also, though most trekkers range in age from 38 to 45, about a quarter are over 50.

The trip was set up to be a sort of get-acquainted tour of four of the six islands you can visit—Kauai, Hawaii, Maui, and Lanai, with brief stopovers on Oahu for air connections.

About half our nights we spent in unheated cabins with real beds, in state or national parks (one night we stayed at a creaky old hotel), the other half in comfortable, roomy tents. We had access to regular restrooms and showers (not always heated) every night except the one we spent in Haleakala. So all in all, we weren't exactly roughing it—but we were still a long way from room service.

Except for one night at a glitzy seafood restaurant in Lahaina, and a delightful backyard luau at the home of Earl and Audrey, two Hawaiian schoolteachers, we ate Fong's finest camp cooking. Breakfasts were hearty, with eggs, coffee, sweet Portuguese bread, or local fruit, like fresh papaya sprinkled with lime; a slight trail lunch of sandwiches and "gorp" (dried fruit, nuts, and M&Ms); and our well-earned evening meals, including vegetables, fish, meat, sweet potatoes, or local fruit. One night Karen whipped up a delectable dish of *sashimi*, raw yellowfin tuna (what the locals call *ahi*) in garlic, soy, onions, and brown sugar.

The Exhilaration of Exploration

But the real focus of the trip was the exhilaration of exploring those amazing islands on foot, tramping along the sea cliffs, or up a jungle trail with only a day pack slung over your back. The longest we walked in a day was 10 miles (the pace was always easy and conversational); other days we walked the beach or snorkeled among the reef fish for as long or as little as we liked. But wherever we went, the sheer astonishment of the place, and the drama of its contrasts, made for endlessly interesting walks.

Our first day on Kauai we left our camp in Kokee State Park in heavy rain and mist. Three miles later having hiked over steep, densely forested hills riotous with *lantana* and the pink passion-fruit flower, we emerged on a grassy bluff overlooking the black towers of Kauai's Na Pali coast—on a brilliantly sunny day. We had lunch there in the sunshine, watching white-tailed tropical birds wheeling deliriously over the cliffs, and then headed homeward—into heavy mist and rain. Overhead, we could see a division clear as some aerial DMZ: on one side, blue sky, on the other, rain.

Hawaii, it turns out, has two natures—one wet, one dry. On the wet side of the islands you'll find the lush paradise of Tarzan movies, so fertile that leaves grow to fabulous size and even sheer rock faces are green. Dramatic, rain-laden cumulus clouds sweep across the Pacific on the trade winds, collide with Hawaii's volcanoes and dump their cargo into these valleys, making some spots (like Mount Waialeale, on Kauai) among the wettest places on earth. But so little rain gets over the mountains that the other side looks like a very different movie—definitely a Western, set in a sun-blasted landscape of prickly pear cactus, mesquite trees, and black, naked rock.

On the big island of Hawaii, the desolation is of a different sort, caused more by volcanic activity than lack of water.

Hawaii, in fact, is an island still in the midst of creation by fire. One of Kilauea's vents has been spewing magma hot enough to melt steel about once a month since 1963, and evidence of this fearsome geological turmoil is all around. Hiking into Kalauea Iki crater one day, there was a burnt smell in the air, and acrid, sulfurous steam poured out of cracks in the lava bed.

Another day, on Maui, we hiked back up a steep valley to Waimoku Falls, up a narrow footpath that got darker, denser, and more humid as we gained elevation. Dawn-of-time tree ferns 10 or 15 feet high hung over the trail like dinosaur fodder. Old lava stones impassive as the great heads of Easter Island and half buried in moss tilted out of the mountainside. We passed through a towering bamboo forest, under giant old mango trees, past things I've seen growing only in shopping malls, all blown up to tremendous size. Then we reached the falls—a thin, silvery stream descending from several hundred feet, filling the glade with mist. There we spread out a lunch of crackers and cut vegetables on a bed of green ti leaves—and, of course, succumbed to the irresistible dip.

Things I'd Never Heard Before

● The *chuck-chuck-chuck* of the little translucent lizards called geckos, clinging to the screens at night.

● The clattering crunch of footsteps on broken lava, a sound like shattering dinner plates.

● The sound of a finger drawn across the underside of a taro leaf—a rasping sound, like torn canvas.

● Wind stirring a bamboo forest, an atonal, clattering sound like nothing so much as bamboo wind chimes.

● The *ttsingg!* of a machete blade glancing off dense fern brake.

● The Pacific surf booming in sea caves—a fearsome sound, like something out of a child's dream.

Vacation as Change

Any vacation worth the plane fare, especially a fitness-type vacation, should change you in some way. Otherwise, why go?

And when we reached the end of our Hawaiian exploration I couldn't help but notice all of us had begun to change. We were all turning brown as coconuts. To my amazement, my body clock had been completely reset to sun time—wide awake at sunrise, around 6:00 (once I woke up without coercion at 5:30 and went for a walk on the beach), and to bed, exhausted, not long after dark at 9:00 or 9:30. I felt tougher, trimmer, more fully alive. My camera bag and my memory were filling up with exposed film. My daypack smelled like guavas and was tucked full of trinkets —an old pandanus nut, a yellow-speckled mitre shell found on the reef, a piece of dark, lovely mesquite wood.

And I had Hawaii in my hair.

—————————■—

Stefan Bechtel

MAKING YOUR
WORKPLACE WORK

Have you snuck up on your office lately and caught it in an awkward position? When was the last time you took a good hard look at the setup to make sure the design works for you? If it's been a while, there are good reasons to take a look now. Learn the secrets of good design and boost your performance.

Ergonomics is the science of applying what is known about human physiology to the design of work stations, furniture, and equipment. Using this science, you can take proven steps to adapt your workspace so that it supports you, rather than thwarts you. You can literally "design out" the hidden enemies that bring on stress, headaches, eyestrain, or cumulative injuries.

Best of all, when you reshape a clumsy environment into one mindful of the way you work, and respectful of your body, the improvements will pay for themselves through higher productivity. Some employers also find that their workmen's compensation costs decrease.

"It makes a whole lot of sense to pay attention to the physical environment,"

says Tim Springer, founder of an ergonomics consulting firm in St. Charles, Illinois. "There's definitely an impact on the bottom line." Over the lifetime of an office building, an employer will spend 90 percent more on personnel costs than on the physical plant, he explains. So, the argument goes, if you can manipulate a proportionately small part of the budget to stimulate a higher yield on your single biggest outlay—salaries—you've made a wise investment.

"You don't have to spend a lot of money to make things better," adds Springer. Nor do the changes have to be that involved. Paying attention to proper posture alone, for instance, can bring dramatic results.

Curious about how useful adjustable workstations were for VDT operators, Springer studied 140 State Farm Insurance Company employees. Counting keystrokes and errors to assess productivity, he found that workers using good quality, adjustable furniture did 10 percent better at data entry than members of a control group, who sat at nonmovable workstations. At another task that required them to call up information on a screen and interact with it in some way, comfortable workers did 15 percent better. Upgrading just the chair brought performance improvements "in the neighborhood of 4 to 6 percent," he says.

Architect Michael Brill of the Buffalo Organization for Technological and Social Innovation reached similar conclusions following a six-year survey of 6,000 workers in 80 offices, many of them in Fortune 500 companies. Workers were interviewed twice: before they moved to a new office and several months after.

One surprising finding for Brill was that "almost all the factors that really affect job performance and job satisfaction are things workers want, things they ask for themselves." He also found that as satisfaction with the environment increases, so does job performance.

Change Doesn't Have to Start at the Top

Right about now, you're probably thinking about your office and wondering, hmmm . . . Maybe you're in a position to

How to Sit at Your Computer

So you think it's elementary, do you? Maybe no one's let you in on the secret, but there is a right way to position yourself at the computer. The best posture is the one that places the least amount of strain on your neck, back, and wrists.

If your chair seat is height-adjustable, set it so that your feet are squarely on the floor. (Or use a phone book or other foot rest.) If you can get the seat to tilt slightly downward, do so until you feel the pressure behind your knees let up. Raise or lower the backrest until it conforms to the natural curve in your back.

If you're a big guy or gal, you may want to set the springs tighter so you can lean back without feeling that the chair is going to tip.

Your work surface should have two heights, one for your keyboard and one for your disk drive and monitor. You can adapt a low table by putting your keyboard on it

and putting the terminal on a raised platform. You can adjust a higher table by adding a keyboard shelf below it.

Put your keyboard at a height that allows you to keep your lower arms roughly parallel to the floor and your elbows at a right angle. "The key relationship is the hands to elbows," says Paul Cornell, a researcher with Steelcase, a Michigan manufacturer of office furniture. Your wrists should be slightly higher than your elbows.

The top of the VDT screen needs to be about eye level so your neck is straight and relaxed. The screen should probably be about 18 to 26 inches from your eyes, depending upon character size.

Bifocal wearers may want to have the screen well below eye level, says Cornell. "If the screen is set too high, they may actually have to be tilting their head backward to see the screen."

Homing in on the Office

Keeping your work life separate from your personal life is a bit trickier when your office is in your home. But if you don't find ways to shut the door behind you, you'll have a hard time turning work off.

That's not to say you need a separate room for an office. An office in a closet can work beautifully. Lots of space isn't as important as smart use of the space you have. You also can segregate work areas with attractive folding screens and area rugs, or by using platforms.

If you're just planning your home office, or about to remodel, think before you buy. Try keeping a journal on an hourly basis for a week or two on how you spend your work time, so you can decide what you really need. After the computer, your big splurge probably will be a comfortable chair suited to your work.

The beauty of a home office is the degree of freedom you have to make it suit you. If you've always hated the plastic, steel, and particleboard environment you were in when you were working for someone else, now's your chance to be creative. Browse in second-hand shops, and furniture and housewares departments to find softer-looking items you can adapt to your use. Beware of highly polished work surfaces. They can bounce light back at you, causing glare.

How do you make a small space seem larger?

During years of research, James A. Wise, a professor at Grand Valley State College, has developed a number of tricks. He has been working with NASA since 1985 to help design space stations that feel larger than they are.

Here are Wise's tips.

• The more regular the space is, whether it's square, circular, or rectangular, the smaller it seems. Irregularly shaped rooms appear larger. Wise found that when he took a rectangular room and angled out one wall by 13 percent, people perceived the room as 22 to 26 percent larger.

• If your space is rectangular, try positioning your furniture on a diagonal in the corner to make the room look larger.

• Don't light from overhead but from the periphery, with fixtures that wash light over the wall. If you must stick with an overhead light, ask a lighting store salesperson for something to help diffuse the light, so it spreads out horizontally.

• Mix fluorescent and incandescent lighting. The subtle differences in color rendering will "break the space apart" and make it appear larger.

• The color you choose is not as important as the shade. The more white in the color, the more it opens up a room.

make some changes. Even if you're not, don't underestimate your power to influence change. Your boss may be more receptive than you think, particularly if you can make a strong case about productivity gains.

Springer remembers a job that came his way after some data entry operators in a firm he'll only identify as a "really conservative" West Coast information services business decided they wanted to feel better at work.

"The employees did their own facilities audit," he says. "They researched available alternatives, got cost information, and presented it to their managers. In essence, they said to management, 'if you reduce this discomfort, we are going to be able to work better.'"

The company asked Springer his opinion of the employee suggestion list. He thought they did "a really fine job. They had a tendency to lowball, so I made some suggestions about spending a little more on items that would be more durable in the long run. Aside from that, the basic concepts were really sound. Once the company followed through, it surpassed their wildest expectations."

"I think one person can make a huge difference," says Susan Dray, manager of the human technology impacts program at Honeywell. "You can build coalitions in positive ways and try to figure out some solutions. When in doubt, network. You can learn a lot talking to other people."

The Changes That Count

To get the most mileage from your office makeover, concentrate on a few key areas. Privacy, Brill's study found, is primary. It has the greatest effect on job performance, job satisfaction, and contentment with the workspace.

"More enclosure almost always seems to work better," says Brill, but he's quick to add that he's not advocating a private office for everyone. "Being out in the open with no protection against noise and visual distraction is really not what you want."

How much enclosure is enough? Well, no one has developed a formula yet and it's not likely anyone will. That's because the right answer for each worker is as individual as the worker. Some people thrive on frequent, spur-of-the-moment interactions with colleagues. Others lose their momentum after a few distractions.

Acoustic privacy—the ability to speak without being overheard and freedom from distracting noise—is even more valued than visual privacy, Brill found. If noise is a problem in your office, consider acoustical dividers to absorb noise and make work areas more private. Noisy printers can be subdued with sound hoods or placed on racks instead of solid surfaces. Segregate the noisiest equipment, such as copiers and postage stamp meters, in a room of their own. And think fabric. Carpets, draperies, and fabric wall treatments, including textile wall-hangings, will help.

Second on Brill's list of how to make the workplace work is layout. If you were starting from scratch, could you come up with a more logical place to put things? Can you arrange your furniture and equipment to give yourself added privacy? Above all, Brill suggests, avoid the cookie cutter approach to layout. "A single layout is crazy. A firm may have six to eight accountants, and they have six to eight approaches to the job."

Whenever possible, arrange furniture

453

so that you can occasionally look out beyond your workspace, into the larger office, through a window or at a painting. Building in this "psychological escape hatch" is important, because it keeps you from feeling penned in, says James A. Wise, professor of facilities management at Grand Valley State College in Allendale, Michigan.

Planning for good posture and good vision are the other essentials for a successful workplace. Researchers have discovered that posture and vision are closely linked. As Rochester ergonomist Sue Rodgers explains, "You can have the most perfect chair, but if there's glare and you have to lean forward to see, it defeats the chair."

Proper lighting is particularly important for VDT workers. Glare, even the kind that's not readily noticeable, can cause headaches and eye fatigue. There are two kinds of glare to watch for: direct and indirect. Indirect glare occurs when light is reflected off a polished surface like your computer monitor or a high-sheen desk. Direct glare is caused by looking into a light source, such as a window or a high-intensity light fixture. And that's why it's not a good idea to put a computer terminal in front of a window. Position it at a 90-degree angle to that window instead.

To check for indirect glare, place a mirror on your workspace and then sit as you normally do. If you see a bright light in the mirror, there's the problem. Eliminate the source of glare if you can. If you can't, control it. A blotter will help curb glare from a shiny work surface. A micromesh filter will do the same for a computer screen. Sometimes a backdrop placed behind the computer terminal, or behind you, can be a big help.

Rodgers has a friend whose office was directly across the street from a "striking English tudor house. The light hit the screen in such a way that there was an exquisitely sharp image of that house on that screen. It created such a sharp contrast that the eye was drawn to the image.

"The eye is always looking for something to focus on," Rodgers adds. "If text is fuzzy around the edges, as it tends to be, the eye tends to be pulled away to what it wants to look at." The competition between the image and the text, she says, tires the eyes. She suggested her friend use a backdrop. The house disappeared from the screen, and the eye fatigue left with it.

Another source of eye fatigue for computer users is glasses that don't match the task. If you wear glasses at work, have your ophthalmologist adjust your prescription for the proper distance to the terminal. "This is especially important for people over 40," says Dr. Martin Mainster, of the Department of Ophthalmology of the University of Kansas Medical Center. "Younger people can zoom in better, but older people have more of a fixed focus system."

The Office Chair as Throne

The lowly office chair has earned new status, as more becomes known about the relationship between good posture and good performance, and poor posture and back problems.

While there is no gold standard among chairs, experts do agree on the characteristics common to ergonomically sound chairs.

THE INNER OFFICE

The most important part of your work environment is what you carry between your ears. Maybe you've got a morning ritual to help you ease into the workday.

The writers of *Positive Living and Health* surveyed a few achievers to ask them about their morning rituals. Here's what they had to say.

Max Rosey.   Rosey, who is among the last of the country's old-time press agents, engineered such stunts as a "wedding at the bottom of the Atlantic Ocean" for the opening of Atlantic City's Steel Pier in 1953, and the "old-shoe" campaign of presidential candidate Adlai Stevenson. "I get up at 5:00 A.M. every day, even if I go to bed at 1:00 A.M." says Rosey, agent now for Nathan's Famous, Hess's department stores, and The Amazing Kreskin. "I get into a hot tub and while I'm lying there, I make a mental list of what I have to do for the day. Then I shower and give myself a good scalp massage. That wakes me up. After I towel off, I write down everything I've thought of."

Marilyn Greene.   Greene, a Schenectady, New York, private investigator, is said to be the country's leading finder of missing children. She works at home. "I like to get up at 5:30 or 6:00 A.M.," says Greene. Then it's down to the kitchen for a cup of coffee. She spends some time with her two search dogs before she lets them out. "It's somewhat distressing to me, having a lot of early morning energy, that I have to wait before getting started on phone calls, particularly to the West Coast. On the other hand, that leaves me a good deal of time to think about what I'm going to do, which is good."

Carolyn Peters.   Peters, creative designer on General Motors' Saturn design team, is responsible for fashioning the instrument panels, consoles, steering wheel, pedals, doors, fabric design, and colors of this "1990s car."

Peters says she gives herself a fresh start every morning by taking a "little vacation in my mind" on her way in to work. Instead of thinking about the projects at hand, she'll concentrate on an upcoming vacation or something else totally different. "It helps me clear my mind," she says.

• They are stable. A five-pointed base is best.

• They are adjustable. Height adjustability is particularly important if several people have to use the same chair.

• They offer forward and backward tilt.

• They offer lumbar support, which helps to maintain the natural curve in the lower part of the back.

• The seat cushion has a "waterfall edge," meaning that it curves downward, minimizing the pressure on the back of the knees.

"Get a good chair," advises Marvin Dainoff, a professor of psychology at Ohio's

455

Miami University and director of its Center for Ergonomic Research. "I give talks and people say, 'These chairs are expensive.' That's crazy. I tell them, 'Yes, you can go into the dime store and buy a pair of sneakers for $9.95. But would you go jogging in them?'

"This isn't furniture," he adds. "What I try to use is the word 'tools'. Your chair and an adjustable work surface are tools."

Changing chairs may not be an option for you at this point. But ergonomist Tim Springer is willing to bet that the one you have now probably can be adjusted to suit you better. "It may need someone with some tools, but oftentimes that is sufficient if the adjustment is done correctly," he says. If the chair doesn't have lumbar support, a back cushion can work wonders.

It's possible that your chair has some adjustment levers you've never noticed. Springer remembers being consulted by a telecommunications company that spent a fortune on very sophisticated chairs, but workers still complained about backaches.

"I couldn't imagine what the problem was, so I had them take me out on the floor. I asked a woman if I could try her chair. She said in her southern accent, 'Darling, you can take this with you. I don't want it.' It turns out these chairs were shipped in the lowest position. Nobody bothered to tell the folks they could adjust them. I found the buttons underneath the seat. They were at a fairly remote spot. When I adjusted the chair, this woman's jaw just dropped."

Springer did a follow-up six months later and found "they were just tickled pink. Not only did complaints from the operators go down, but the company started getting constructive comments from their employees about what else could be done."

Keep That Circulation Going

You've adjusted your lighting and positioned your chair so it's comfortable. That helps, but maybe you still feel stiff and tired at day's end. The problem could be that you're locking yourself into one position for too long. Static postures, held long enough, eventually interfere with blood flow.

"The best way to deal with equipment that isn't perfect," says Rodgers, "is to change positions every so often. Depending upon the job, I'd suggest 1-minute breaks every 45 to 60 minutes to improve posture and the comfort of your visual system. With clerical jobs in the past, a person did more than sit at a desk and type. They had to get up and get the hard copy. With computers, you no longer have the natural breaks you used to have. But people are actually more productive if they can take breaks in the routine."

Get up and move at regular intervals and stretch when you can. Movement is important to your circulatory system. Fixed positions, in which muscles are so contracted the blood stops flowing to them, will cause you to tire quickly. Lack of blood flow allows waste products to build up in the muscles. Over time, numbness and tingling result.

Speaking of circulation, how clean is the air in your office? Do windows open onto the street, or are you in a sealed, energy-efficient environment where the temperature is automatically controlled?

"Sick building syndrome," which has become a major public health issue, results when contaminants build up because ventilation systems recirculate cooled or heated air, instead of bringing in a fresh supply.

MAKING YOUR WORK SPACE "YOU"

Take a good, honest look around your office. How does it really make you feel? Does the place bear your imprint and style or is it about as cheery as the tundra on a sunless day? Could a close friend walking by for the first time pick out where you sit just by the look and feel of the surroundings?

If not, you've got an underachieving office on your hands. The place may look harmless enough, but if it's a poor match for you—your personality, your verve—it might be subtly sabotaging you. Think about the weather on your ride in to work. Did the look and color of the sky, the feel of the air, do anything to your mood? Think of your work atmosphere as a kind of interior weather. What's important is that you can create the climate.

The best way to start is by closing your eyes. Pretend there's nothing there, suggests architect Michael Brill. In your mind's eye, create the ideal workspace. What pieces and parts would it include? How are things arranged? What gives it warmth?

Open your eyes and write down what you saw. Now look at what you have and see how you can approximate your ideal. Can you open up space by getting rid of anything you don't use much? Can you make better use of space by adding some stacked in/out boxes or an under-the-desk file?

Where do things most logically belong? If you're right-handed, chances are you'll want your telephone on the left side of your desk. Then you won't have to switch hands if you need to write down what your caller is saying.

Once you've got the framework, accessorizing can be child's play. Forget about office supply stores for now. Think fun. How about:

• A desk calendar by your favorite cartoonist? Or one with quotes from your favorite author?

• A piece of original pottery or something from the vintage goods antique store that you love to browse in, to hold your pencils and paper clips?

• Bamboo or straw trays or baskets to substitute for the plastic or steel organizers that are too hard-looking for your taste?

• A paperweight that's a real conversation piece; perhaps something you've brought back from your travels?

• A basket or box of morale-boosters: letters of congratulations or praise, that softball you hit clear across the field to make your team league champions, boxes of tea or specialty coffees in your favorite flavors?

• A simple vase to display fresh flowers from your garden?

458

In a sealed building, if the ventilation system is not regularly repaired, adjusted and cleaned, the airborne contaminants could be potent enough to cause allergy problems and respiratory illness. According to the Environmental Protection Agency, the leading causes of poor-quality air are cigarettes, solvent-containing paints and adhesives, and products such as room deodorizers.

If you suspect "sick building syndrome" is at work in your office, you may want to push for installation of an electrostatic precipitator, which will remove airborne particles far better than any desktop air purifier.

Substituting natural materials for synthetic ones will also keep the air fresher. Consider wool or cotton draperies and floor coverings and all-wood furniture. Decorating with lots of plants, particularly philodendrons, spider plants, and aloe vera, will help renew stagnant office air.

MAKE YOUR HOME
A FUN HOUSE

Quick—What color are the sheets on your bed? How many steps are there up to your front door?

Most people wouldn't be able to answer those questions without trotting outside or upstairs to check. Everything is just too familiar—our living rooms look exactly like the ones across the street, down the block, and even the one in that sitcom on TV last night.

When we don't notice our surroundings, they start to blend in with everything else and stop adding their inherent excitement to our lives. Can you imagine eating the same food every day? Cornflakes day in and day out?

Your home doesn't have to be eternal cornflakes. With a pinch of creativity and a dash of scorn for societal norms, you can mold your home into a source of beauty and invigoration. You're the daring type, so take some risks and follow this recipe to change your home from a stiflingly safe snack to the scintillating smorgasbord you've always wanted.

Stir Vigorously

How long has the couch been against the wall opposite the front door with the coffee table right in front of it, arranged just so?

A year? Five years? Longer?

Try moving your furniture around every now and then. A new spot for the breakfront may be hard to find, but most people have the room to shift the easy chair a bit. Just wait until you experience the jolt of awareness a new furniture arrangement will give you each time you walk into the room—you'll wonder why you waited so long to stir things up.

Also, try angling the couch for a change, instead of feeling constrained to place it right against the wall. You could even try the same thing with your bed. "Furniture does not always have to be at right angles with the walls," says New York architect William Breger. "At a different angle, it can create more impact, more excitement, and more joy."

Breathing Beautifully

Do coal miners' canaries die when they enter your parlor? Do important guests wheeze and sneeze all over your damask table linens? The nicest, most attractively decorated home isn't fit for the family dog if the air in it scrapes your throat as it goes down.

Air filters, however, can help. Tips from Dr. Harold S. Nelson, Chairman of the American Academy of Allergy and Immunology's Committee on Environmental Controls, will lead your lungs to a more pristine future.

There are two types of air filters, says Dr. Nelson: HEPA filters, which force air through a fine web that traps the tiny particles, and electronic filters, which either collect airborne particles on electrically charged metal plates or emit negatively charged ions into the air, which attract particles and then deposit them on surfaces.

If you are willing to wash the collection plate in the electrostatic model once a week, Dr. Nelson recommends this type, because it has a long life and maintains consistent levels of air flow. If you are less fastidious, Dr. Nelson suggests you get a HEPA model instead. This type of filter actually becomes more effective as time goes on, since the pollutants it traps make its web even finer. Eventually, however, the openings close over completely and the expensive filter — which can't be cleaned — needs to be replaced.

If you're allergic to cigarette smoke, pets, and pollen and can't or won't get rid of them, Dr. Nelson suggests you only go for the top-of-the-line air filters. They're expensive, he says, but the cheaper ones are a waste of time. Try leasing the machine first, to be sure it will work for you, he says. And once you get it home, allow it to do its best by placing it in the center of the room to be cleaned where it can get at the most room air.

Let It Stand for 1 Hour

Ever spend some time in a sensory deprivation tank? These lightproof, soundproof tanks filled with salty water let you float your way to an inner consciousness that can bring about sometimes extraordinary insights and experiences. The real thing is better of course, but with a little effort, you can transform your bathroom into a sensory deprivation tank and enjoy its benefits at home.

Start off by blacking out the bathroom window — black felt tacked to the frame will do the trick. To block out noise, nail a heavy quilt over the outside of the bathroom door.

Get yourself a thermometer. The water in the tub has to be at skin temperature — 93.5°F — so you won't feel any warmth or coolness (though the water will feel cool at first because we're used to hot water when we take baths).

Professional flotation tanks use 6 pounds of Epsom salts per gallon to make the water salty enough to float on it, but since your head will be out of the water, you won't need that much to be bouyant. Experiment a little to see what works for you—maybe about half that amount.

To make the bathtub comfortable, fill some plastic blow-up pillows with warm water, and let them sit in the tub until they, too, are at skin temperature. You can tuck them under your knees, rest your elbows on them, and lean your head on one.

The air in the bathroom should, like everything else, be 93.5°F, so bring in a portable heater and warm up the room for a while before you start.

Ready to take the plunge? Light a small candle near the tub to light your way in. Turn out the lights, climb into the primordial bath, and blow out the fire.

Bake at 350°F

There's a big difference in climate between Galveston, Texas, the most humid city in the country, and Las Vegas, Nevada, the driest city. But with a humidifier, a dehumidifier, and a thermostat, you can create just about any climate in the world right in your living room.

Suppose you just moved from a dry climate to a humid one. Set up your dehumidifer and voilà—instant cure for homesickness.

Or what if your vacation to Tahiti got cancelled at the last second? It's not quite the same, but you can at least get the flavor of the vacation that never was by turning up the heat, setting the humidifier on high, and putting on a record of tropical rain forest noises.

While you enjoy your imaginary trip around the world, Dr. David Schneider, a New Jersey internist, recommends you remember a few facts.

● Damp air feels warmer than dry air at the same temperature.

● Excessive humidity can aggravate arthritis and rheumatism.

● Cold, humid air can be harmful to people with heart disease.

● Bacteria and mold grow best in warm, moist air.

● Excessively dry air can cause a sore throat and nosebleeds.

Don't Forget the Garnish

A home just isn't a home until it's decorated. "It's crucial to personalize a home," says design researcher Jeff Hayward, director of People, Places, and Design Research in Northampton, Massachusetts. "Otherwise, the house or apartment can seem like a shell that you and your furnishings are in. You won't be happy if you feel like you start 2 inches inside the walls and are trapped between them."

One easy way to get maximum impact for minimum cost is to use color—on walls, furniture, cabinets, doors . . . anywhere it strikes your fancy. Which colors should you use? Well, there are about as many theories around on the effects of color as there are colors themselves. Some people say colors should be matched to the type of sunlight coming in through the windows—warm colors (reds, oranges, and yellows) for southern light and cool colors (blues and greens) for northern light.

Other people say that colored light—

PINK MAGIC

You've heard that red excites you and blue calms you down, but have you heard that pink makes weight lifters drop their barbells?

Baker-Miller pink, a special shade of pink discovered by Dr. Alexander G. Schauss, director of the A.I.B.R. Life Sciences at the American Institute for Biosocial Research in Tacoma, Washington, has been shown to lower heart rates, reduce aggression, help relaxation, and even cause weakness.

"I could scarcely believe it myself," says Dr. Schauss about one of his experiments. "I put a weight lifter in the pink room, and, after just a few minutes, he couldn't lift weights that were normally easy for him."

In another trial, Dr. Schauss painted an admissions cell in the Naval Correctional Center in Seattle all pink—pretty soon, those nasty scuffles that used to happen every day during check-in came to an end.

Since then, the color has been shown to alleviate anxiety and even to help people lose weight.

Thirty-two percent of nervous snackers who used Baker-Miller pink as a relaxation tool and ate a balanced diet of 1,200 calories a day lost weight, reports Dr. Maria Simonsen, director of the Health, Weight, and Stress Clinic at Johns Hopkins Medical Institutions. Only 27 percent of those who used diet and relaxation without Baker-Miller had equal results.

Dr. Schauss thinks the color affects the endocrine system in some way—possibly through neuroendocrine mechanisms linked to the visual system. He also conjectures that the effect may be related to learned sex-role stereotypes about the color pink.

If you want to try Baker-Miller pink yourself, you'll need 1 pint of outdoor semigloss "red trim" paint and 1 gallon of pure white indoor latex paint.

Pour half of the white paint into a separate bucket. Add about one-quarter of the red paint, mixing thoroughly. Once that's blended, add another quarter of the white paint and another quarter of the red paint. Blend them. Keep going like this until all the paint is blended. After mixing, paint the small room you've chosen as soon as possible to prevent the paint from separating. The floor can be painted pink, too, or left a neutral gray or dark brown. Light up with 150-watt incandescent bulbs, and be sure not to stay in for more than 15 minutes at a time.

that is, the light that reflects off a colored object or wall onto your skin and into your eye and brain—vibrates in your body and fills certain health needs. This theory is based on the idea that specific colors correspond with parts of the body. According to Antonio Torrice, an interior decorator and director of Living and Learning Environments in San Francisco, violet is the color associated with the top of the head; the eyes and ears match up with blue; the throat with green; the heart and lungs, yellow; the spleen, orange; and the base of the spine's color is red. So, if you have a problem with your spleen, says Torrice, you'll be naturally attracted to the color orange.

We're not saying that any of these theories are right—or wrong, for that matter. Give them a try, and wait for the vibes.

Don't Eat Alone

Living alone can be tough. But even if you don't know anyone to invite over, your home itself can double as company. "Plants, mirrors, art work, even poster-size photographs of people—there are many things that can act as a surrogate roommate," says psychologist Robert Sommer, author of *Creating Buildings with People in Mind.* Anything you can talk to will make your home seem less lonely.

Half of You Need to Light Up Your Lives

When the snow starts to fall, do your thoughts automatically turn to the Bahamas? When you're waiting for the bus on a winter morning and the sun *still* isn't up, does your mind transport you to a sunny summer meadow? Those thoughts may be a reflection of your body's need for more sunlight—one in two people experience depression or listlessness because of this need, says scientist Dr. Michael Turman of the New York State Psychiatric Institute.

The problem is made worse by our low levels of indoor lighting. "We live essentially in a twilight zone," says neuropsychologist Philip C. Hughes of Medic-Light in Lake Hopatcong, New Jersey. "Light levels in our homes are in the area of what is considered twilight outside."

If you think you might be suffering from light deprivation, try to go outdoors more, and think about installing brighter lights in your home. A visiting researcher from Germany, Siegfried Kasper, working at the National Institute of Mental Health in Bethesda, Maryland, has found that sitting in front of 10 to 15 incandescent lights or a light box comprised of full-spectrum fluorescent lights first thing in the morning makes a difference.

"Put it in the breakfast nook or the bedroom," says Dr. Turman. "Don't look directly at the light. You can eat or read, as long as you are in the field of the illumination, facing it, and not wearing tinted lenses or other things that will reduce the amount of light."

Decorating around the world

When you're thinking about how to change your rooms to make them more regenerative, you might find a global view will give you some ideas. What seems like the only right way for furniture to be arranged to you may seem absolutely crazy to a German or a Japanese person. That's because the way we decorate our homes has a lot to do with what culture we're from, explains anthropologist Edward T. Hall.

Japanese people, for instance, say our rooms look bare to them because we arrange most of our furniture along the walls. They put theirs in the middle of the room to stay away from drafty walls during the winter.

And instead of going from room to room to eat, sleep, and talk with friends, the Japanese stay in one place and let their rooms come to them by moving their paper-thin walls around.

How do you get privacy when you're home? Most likely by going into another room and shutting the door. A German visiting you would probably find that insufficient—their doors are much thicker than ours because they prefer not to be able to hear what is going on in the next room at all.

An Arab, on the other hand, would be upset by your going into the other room and would find our homes lonely. Arabs have very few partitions in their homes because they don't like to be separated from their families. At the same time, they tend to need lots more indoor space than we do. Wealthy Arabs find our small rooms tomblike; their rooms have much higher ceilings, larger spaces, and big windows with distant views.

On the other hand, if you've got about six too many roomies, you'll need to come up with ways to shut them out and establish your own territory. Sommer suggests color changes that say, "your turf ends there by the blue wall and mine begins here by the beige carpet."

Clean Up

For your whole home to be a healthy, happy place to live, you've got to make sure it doesn't have any serious problems. Not enough light is a typical one—the average house has only 11 lighting fixtures—as are faulty electrical outlets or bad locks. Since studies show that household air is often up to ten times as dirty as outside air, indoor pollution could also be lowering the health quotient on your home, says Dr. Bill Wolverton, senior research scientist for NASA.

"Modern buildings often have almost 100 percent synthetic materials inside them," he says. "Things like particleboard, plywood, foam, synthetic rugs, and household cleaners give off formaldehyde and other toxic chemicals. In well-insulated homes, these chemicals can cause unhealthy reactions."

Short of rebuilding your home with only natural products—an expensive affair to say the least—Wolverton says you can counteract the chemicals by bringing houseplants into your home. "We have recently found that houseplants, especially the many types of philodendrons, can absorb indoor pollutants from the environment," he says.

Besides, people like plants: "We know that most people feel better in a room with plants," says Wolverton. "They just make us feel good." And what better place to feel good than at home?

THE OUTER DIMENSIONS OF THE INNER YOU

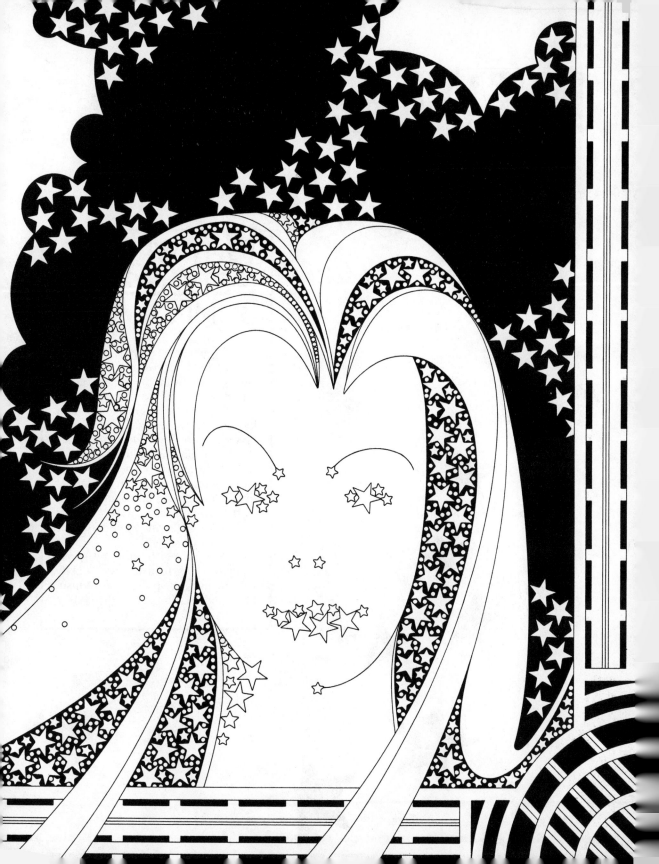

INSTANT INSIGHTS

WHY WE GET GOOSE BUMPS

You might be scared; you might be cold. In either case it's the same — chills creep down your spine and goose bumps pop up all over your body.

Those little bumps could be a leftover survival mechanism from our less-civilized days. Dermatologists speculate that this evolutionary function of our autonomic nerves served two different purposes. In the animal kingdom, it makes hair stand on end so that while under attack, the animal looks bigger and more ferocious than it actually is.

Dermatologists also say goose bumps could be there to preserve body heat by fluffing up the layer of insulating hair.

Dream Potion Now On Tap

Researchers at the University of California at San Diego have discovered an experimental compound called RS-86 that can significantly increase the amount of dream-generating sleep a person can have during the night. (The technical term for this sleep state is REM, or rapid-eye-movement, sleep.)

RS-86 works by prodding acetylcholine, a neurotransmitter believed by Harvard scientists Robert McCarley and J. Allan Hobson to be the "on" switch for REM sleep.

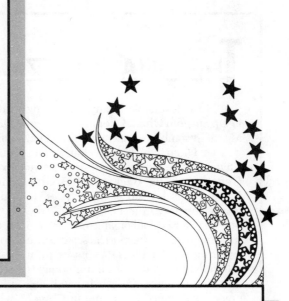

Scratching On A Blackboard Is Monkey Business

A fingernail screeching across a blackboard does more than send chills down your spine—it literally brings out the animal in you. The monkey, to be exact.

So says psychologist Richard Blake of Northwestern University, who's found that 90 percent of the population shivers at the sound. He thought this statistic too high to be a mere coincidence and decided to investigate further. In an acoustic analysis of the scraping sound, Blake discovered it to be amazingly similar to the warning cries of macaque monkeys. The sound efficiently signals danger by grabbing the attention of irritated ear drums, he says.

Blake says his findings "suggest our reaction is an instinct we inherited from our primate ancestors. The human brain obviously still registers a strong vestigial response to this chilling sound."

THE DNA WALTZ

Music lovers, get ready. According to Dr. Susumu Ohno, Chopin's "Funeral March" resembles a cancer-causing gene.

Dr. Ohno, who holds a chair as Distinguished Scientist in Reproductive Genetics at the Beckman Research Institute, has devised a simple system to transcribe the four DNA bases (the building blocks of all organic matter) into the eight notes of the musical scale. Since arrangements of the DNA bases form the individual code for all amino acids of which proteins are constructed, any organic substance has a unique "tune" that represents its makeup.

While this might seem like a laboratory game for dull Friday afternoons, Dr. Ohno is convinced that there is a connection between the genetic information and the resultant melodies. For example, oncogenes, which are cancer-causing genes, sound morbid and slightly out of control when translated into music.

Dr. Ohno's theory was put to the test in Japan when an enzyme that breaks down simple milk sugar translated into a lullaby. The tune was subsequently recorded by a violinist and has been played in several Tokyo kindergartens where it has always helped children fall asleep at nap time — much like a glass of warm milk would.

CLAIRVOYANT CALCULATIONS

Clairvoyance, the ability to mentally see objects not in the immediate environment, is one of the many ESP abilities that has eluded scientific credibility for decades. But recently, two neuroscientists have shown that there may be a direct and traceable link between true clairvoyant functions and changes in the electrical waves the brain produces.

Researchers Norman Don and Charles Warren were able to predict the hits and misses of a subject performing clairvoyant tasks with a 72.7 percent accuracy by using a computerized analysis of the subject's EEG (electroencephalogram), a device used to measure brain wave changes. Don and Warren paid particular attention to activity in the occipital region (the back of the head) when they made their predictions.

Since there was a measurable change in the brain wave pattern of the subject when a correct guess was made, the two researchers now want to see if biofeedback training can allow anyone to achieve that change and perhaps become clairvoyant themselves.

IT'S A GOOD BET THAT COMPULSIVE GAMBLING IS A BRAIN DISORDER

An urge to gamble until every last dollar is gone is more than a lack of self control. It is a disease of the brain, says neurobiologist Leonide Goldstein of the New Jersey Medical School.

Pathological gambling, Goldstein says, is similar to alcoholism—both are the results of lack of impulse control thought to be related to attention deficit disorders (ADD). In his test of 16 men—8 pathological gamblers and 8 nongamblers—Goldstein used an (EEG) electroencephalogram to record brain activity during completion of verbal and nonverbal tasks. Nongamblers, he found, alternated between using right and left hemispheres of the brain while completing the tests. Gamblers' brains alternated less and actually showed reverse stimulation of the hemispheres. That is, gamblers' left hemispheres were activated during the nonverbal procedures, which are usually handled by the right hemisphere.

Goldstein attributes this brain behavior to the connection with ADD symptoms. He says children with ADD often are found to become adult alcoholics, linking ADD with problems in impulse control. The symptoms are the same found in pathologic gamblers, he suggests.

CRACK THE SHELL OF SHYNESS

Shy people may be able to crack out of their shells with a little biochemical prodding, claims Stanford University researcher Roy King.

"Creating a drug to change personality is doable," King says. He says the drug would trigger the release of dopamine, a neurotransmitter in the brain. Dopamine has been found in higher levels in the brains of extroverts and lower than normal levels in the brains of shy people. This future drug, King claims, would increase dopamine production and turn a shy person into an extrovert.

Other tests done with animals show higher dopamine levels correlate with heightened social activity. King says he also found social withdrawal to be a result of low dopamine levels.

THE CASE FOR EXECUTIVE ESP

Maybe every business school ought to teach "Gut Hunches 101." A decade of research has convinced engineer John Mihalasky, an industrial management professor at the New Jersey Institute of Technology, and parapsychologist Douglas Dean, of the link between a chief executive's "precognitive powers" and the profitability of the company.

Dean and Mihalasky, authors of *Executive ESP*, found that more than 80 percent of the CEO's who doubled their companies' profits within a five-year-period had above-average intuitive powers. The high-scorers were also found to be dynamic, "get-it-done-today" types.

And a study of 2,000 public and private sector managers by Weston H. Agor, director of the Master in Public Administration Program at the University of Texas at El Paso, found that top managers used intuition significantly more often than middle- or low-level managers to make decisions.

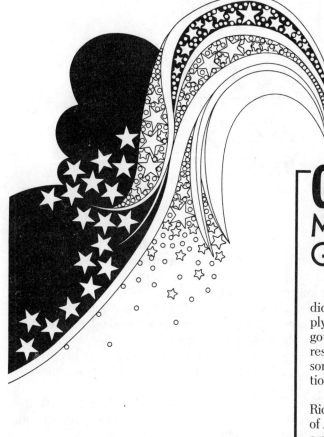

GOUT: THE MAKINGS OF GREATNESS?

Okay, maybe Alexander the Great didn't conquer the known world simply because he had a bad case of gout, but uric acid, the chemical responsible for gout, may have had something to do with Alex's ambitious drive.

According to research chemist Richard Cutler of the National Institue of Aging, many historical high achievers were gout sufferers, Ben Franklin being among the most famous. The connection comes from the fact that uric acid is an antioxidant that shares a molecular structure with many neurostimulants, including caffeine. "It just might turn out to be an important mental stimulant," speculates Cutler.

INTUITION: THE MIND'S COMPASS

The manuscript, masquerading as a children's novel, was rejected by two dozen publishers before it passed into the hands of Eleanor Friede, then an editor at Macmillan. She was entranced. She knew she had an adult book on her hands, a potential blockbuster. In a flash, she saw the slim volume in bookstore windows all across the country.

So Friede pushed Macmillan to publish it. And when the first 75,000 copies sold out, she pressed for a second printing immediately, though the company wasn't keen on the idea. The book? *Jonathan Livingston Seagull.* Friede was on the money. Her find has since sold 3.2 million copies in hardcover and 7 million in paperback.

Mike and Diane were at an art show opening, attended by 20 people Diane knew. She introduced Mike to everyone. In her mind, she was no more ruffled when she introduced him to Tom, who had come with the most striking woman in the room.

But as soon as they left the gallery,

Mike said to Diane, with his characteristic assurance, "Tom's the guy who was after you when I was in California, wasn't he? That city official you mentioned?"

Diane was stunned—and impressed. She had made vague mention, five months ago, of a man who worked for the city, who was interested in her. But she refrained from naming Tom, specifying his title, or describing him. "How'd you put that together?"

"I just know," Mike said. "Just the way he looked at you, and how uncomfortable he seemed around me."

Eleanor's visionary flash, Mike's deft and instantaneous processing of nonverbal cues—such is the awareness we call intuition. "Intuition is what we know for sure without knowing for certain," says Weston H. Agor, director of the Masters of Public Administration Program at the University of Texas at El Paso and president of a consulting firm that teaches intuition skills.

Intuition is what gave the legendary quarterback Fran Tarkenton his edge,

Wanted: Intuitive for Hire

If you're good at leaping to accurate conclusions, if you like finding your own way and exploring the unknown, you're going to go batty in a job that requires you to work logically, sequentially, and within an unalterable set of parameters.

So seek out a job and work environment in which your working style is valued. That's not to say that intuition isn't an asset in every field; it's just that in some it's absolutely crucial. These include research and development, advertising, public relations, crisis management, and trend industries like economic forecasting, fashion/cosmetics, publishing, and entertainment.

Outside of these fields, jobs suited to the intuitive include:

- Buyer.
- Counselor, psychologist.
- Detective.
- Entrepreneur.
- Intelligence operative.
- Inventor.
- Investor, stockbroker.
- Mathematician, physicist.
- Nutritionist.
- Personnel, organizational resource planner.
- Philosopher.
- Scientist.
- Venture capitalist.
- Writer.

broadcasting magnate Ted Turner his nearly flawless sense of timing and Debbi Fields the confidence to begin Mrs. Fields Cookies, a one-store operation that has mushroomed into a three-continent, 200-store empire. And it is what can give you the uncanny knack for making the right choice among the opportunities that come your way in your personal and professional life.

The trick is to learn to harness it. Those who have studied it are convinced we can.

Still skeptical? Do you think intuition is something only other people have? How many times have you said to yourself, "I knew I should have done that?" How many times have you flubbed an answer to a Trivial Pursuit question because you threw away your first guess for one you reasoned out? And how often have you had that "something tells me..." feeling, only to discover later you were right? Imagine how useful it would be if you could amplify that sense of knowingness.

A Natural Talent

During his life, Carl Jung, the celebrated Swiss psychiatrist, promoted the idea that intuition is inborn, a natural human faculty. He saw it as one of four basic psychological functions, along with thinking, feeling, and sensation. Intuition, he said, is what allows us "to explore the unknown and sense possibilities and implications which may not be readily apparent."

Assuming Jung was right—and there is mounting evidence to support his view—we have at our disposal a powerful navigational tool that, like a compass in a cardboard box, waits for us to liberate it and become adept at using it.

Why should intuition concern us? As Jung implied, there are times when intuition really is the best tool the mind has to offer. When the only way to advance is to venture into the unknown, when the facts are few and there's no time to gather more, or when success depends upon factors that have not yet materialized, that's the time to give intuition a heartfelt invitation.

"Hard data deal with the past," observes Philip Goldberg, author of *The Intuitive Edge.* "Anything that can be measured or quantified has to have already happened."

Intuition, on the other hand, looks ahead. "When you are in an intuitive state, you are the future you're envisioning," says Dr. Helen Palmer, a psychologist who heads the California-based Center for the Investigation and Training of Intuition. "Essentially, anything that can be imagined can be known. In a way, intuition relies on the channel of the imagination. It is the next faculty beyond."

Goldberg likens rational thinking and intuition to two pipes that feed into the same faucet. To carry the analogy further, both pipes must be maintained if their particular brand of wisdom is to flow freely. In classes such as logic, geometry, and statistical analysis, we hone our intellect and linear thinking skills. And when we go to the tap for some cold, hard logic, we turn it on, expect it to flow, and it does. But it's the rare mainstream school that offers Intuition 101. So we don't have much experience with that tap.

That may change. Techniques to identify, sharpen, and verify intuition are being taught in places like Dr. Palmer's school, which enrolls 400 to 700 students a quarter; Professor Michael Ray's class in the Stanford University Graduate School of Business and in seminars Agor runs for clients such as Tenneco, Walt Disney Enterprises, and New Jersey Bell. It has become common knowledge in business circles that intuition is a critical component of corporate success. Nowhere is this more true than in the entertainment industry, where the ability to pick the money-making hits depends on tuning in to the changing tastes of a nation.

In a survey of over 2,000 executives and public sector leaders, Agor found that intuition becomes more prevalent as one moves up the management ladder. He found that "top managers differed significantly from middle and lower managers in their ability to use intuition effectively in decision making."

Studies like that one have contributed to our understanding of this elusive skill. Yet, much remains unknown. Intuition scholars usually do a better job defining what it isn't, than what it is.

Consider Goldberg's definition: "Intuition works with the raw materials of information, but it can work with information that is not consciously available, that may have been stored in the past or acquired through subliminal or other sensory means. Rational thinking has to work with whatever the mind is aware of at the time."

If the information isn't consciously available, where is it stored? In what realm of the mind does intuition coalesce?

One theory is that intuition surfaces only after the unconscious mind completes a process very much like conscious reasoning. The difference is that the conscious mind is not aware of the work going on down below.

Dr. Frances E. Vaughan, author of *Awakening Intuition,* takes a different view. She believes intuition originates just below the surface of consciousness and is a form of "direct knowing," a tapping into some core of truth.

"Intuition," she says, "is a sense of certainty. Awakening intuition is equated with following the heart. Truth is recognized in the heart."

For Agor, intuition is a "highly efficient form of knowing. Good education, training, and experience, all enhance it, but insecurity and fear weaken it."

The Intuition Stiflers

Insecurity—the fear of looking stupid, of coming across like a real flake, of being wrong—can lock your intuition in a vise. So can fear of change, intolerance of uncertainty, and an inability to see a problem from more than one angle.

Students of intuition have even made a case for the presence of *anti*-intuitive behavior in people who lack self-esteem. "A need to fail," writes Goldberg, "can program the mind for mistakes and turn us away from correct intuitions."

FEMALE INTUITION: MYTH OR FACT?

Are women naturally intuitive? Do they tend to have more and better hunches than men, or is that just a sexual stereotype? And if it is true, is it biologically based, or a result of social conditioning?

No one knows for sure, but there are some interesting theories. What is known is that the back of the corpus callosum is bigger in women than in men, and that the difference is noticeable even during fetal development.

The corpus callosum is the thick,

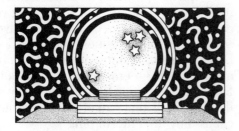

C-shaped bundle of nerve fibers that forms a bridge between the left and right brain hemispheres, allowing communication between them. It transmits memory and learning from one side to the other.

The corpus callosum is also *busier* in women than it is in men, according to Dr. Eran Zaidel, professor of psychology and member of the Brain Research Institute at UCLA. When women are presented with a particular task, he says, the two hemispheres talk to each other more. "I think the female brain may have an ability to integrate complex material in a way the male brain simply doesn't."

And Weston H. Agor, of the University of Texas at El Paso, found in his study of over 2,000 executives and government leaders, that women scored slightly higher than men on a scale designed to measure their ability to use intuition.

478

Yet, intuition is resourceful. Rejected once, it comes knocking at the back door. Eventually it may holler to us from our dreams.

"Intuition gives cues," says Agor, "but we may shove them into the subconscious because we're not willing to deal with what we know to be true. It comes back in dreams. Often, we don't know how to assess that which doesn't fit into what we know to be the existing reality."

And often, we don't know how to separate intuition from other voices: wishful thinking, self-censure, rebelliousness, or impulsiveness. But learning to make that separation is crucial. Dr. Vaughan subscribes to the view that intuition is always right. Screw-ups occur when we confuse intuition with something else or misinterpret the message.

"Beware of how your own fears and desires can get in the way," says Dr. Vaughan. "If I want someone to call me on the phone, for example, I may think that every time it rings, it's that person. That's not intuition."

Using intuition effectively, then, means understanding yourself. The more clearly you see your strengths, weaknesses, tendencies, and vulnerabilities, the easier it will be for you to discern that "this feeling is intuition, but this one over here comes from my fear, belief, or desire that . . ." Don't hesitate to question the source of the mind-chatter you hear.

Reclaim Your Intuitive Power

The surest way to reclaim your intuitive power is to acknowledge that you have it. Still unconvinced? Think back over your experiences and remember the times when some internal prompter pointed you in the right direction—or would have, had you listened to its voice.

Now, "make up your mind to consciously value it," suggests Agor. "Start to get in touch with it and pay attention."

Exactly how do you make contact? Any method that helps you become more attuned to your inner self will help clear the pipeline. Dr. Palmer requires her students to take a class in spiritual discipline along with her class on intuition development. Dr. Vaughan advocates meditation or self-reflection. Other intuitives find rhythmic exercises, like running, bicycling, or swimming, work exceedingly well.

For Dr. Vaughan, the three keys are learning to quiet the mind, focus attention, and remain open.

"By focusing, I mean learning to hold your mind on whatever object you want to pay attention to," she says. "If you're working on a relationship issue, for example, keep that relationship in focus. Most of us have a very short attention span of about 3 minutes. We are very easily distracted. We have to learn to clear the mind and focus to allow that subtle awareness to become more noticeable.

"Like inspiration, intuition comes by itself," she adds. "It's not something you can seize. All you can do is be receptive."

A sense of playfulness helps. As Goldberg observes, an appreciation of whimsy and absurdity seems to favor intuition." Humor and intuition have in common wild, illogical leaps that can often be as practical as they are entertaining."

Intuition's Many Flavors

How you experience intuition is intensely personal. If you're visually oriented, you may see the answer in a pictorial flash, as Friede did. Or maybe the message brings with it a sensation of warmth in your gut, a jolt of electricity, or a rush of awe at the rightness and beauty of it. Maybe yours is a gentle voice that grows more insistent the longer you put it off.

If you can keep track of the sensations that accompany your insights, particularly what you felt when the cue was right on, you'll soon see a pattern you can use to weed out imposters.

Intuition is experienced in different ways and at different levels. Some intuitives are most attuned to their bodies: Specific physical sensations tell them what they need to know. Others are quick to pick up on feelings and relationships. Still others excel at what Dr. Vaughan calls mental intuition, the ability to formulate workable theories, strategies, ideas, and products. The fourth level, according to Dr. Vaughan, is spiritual inspiration, which provides "insights and understandings into the nature of reality."

Intuition Calisthenics

To sharpen your intuitive ability, exercise it. These techniques will help you do just that.

● Next time you enter a bank or toll plaza with long lines, challenge yourself to make a snap decision about which line will move fastest.

● Get purposely lost when you're driving and "feel your way" back home.

● Keep an intuition journal that describes when and how each intuition occurred and what sensations accompanied it.

● Broaden your knowledge by talking to people with whom you have little in common. Explore new places and activities. Read books and periodicals outside your usual fields of interest.

● Set aside some time to venture into a new part of your city or region. Go without a definite plan in mind and let the impulse be your guide.

● Share techniques and knowledge with other intuitives.

● Practice switching your mind into a play mode, whenever you feel yourself locking into one perspective on a problem.

● Brainstorm for the fun of it.

Verify, Verify, Verify

To improve your accuracy, get into the habit of verifying your intuition. But beware of squashing it too early. Give your feelings a chance to fully develop. Then, and only then, should you play scientist. Test your theory. See if you can construct a set of proofs.

First, question the source. Are your emotions in the way? Is it really a hunch, or just a hope? Next, gather whatever facts you can to evaluate your hunch. What's the worst that could happen if you heed your intuition? What might happen if you

INTUITION AND INSIGHT: FRATERNAL TWINS

Milk and cream. A kiss and a hug. Intuition and insight.

The items in each pair are sometimes thought to be interchangeable, but there are times when one partner is definitely more appropriate for the occasion.

Insight, according to *Webster's New Collegiate Dictionary*, means "the act or result of apprehending the inner nature of things."

Intuition, according to the same source, means the faculty of attaining direct knowledge "without evident rational thought and inference."

Insight provides deep understanding of what is or what has been. Maybe all of a sudden you realize what was really going on in a past relationship. Or why something happened in a particular way. Or why an approach isn't working.

Insight is an understanding that usually arises after you focus on a situation and give it much careful thought. Pieces knit together and suddenly the essence of it can be seen for what it is. That's when you get that "Aha!" feeling.

Intuition is more akin to precognition. It is a sensing of relationships and possibilities that have yet to surface. Intuition warns or points or prods. It boasts, "Test me, try me. You'll see I'm right."

don't? Can someone with a different perspective point out pitfalls you don't see?

Sometimes, questioning a gut feeling will give rise to an even fuller understanding of the situation. If your hunch still feels solid after you view it from a number of different angles, chances are it's a good one.

Mastering intuition "is just a matter of education," says Dr. Vaughan. "We've been very preoccupied and concerned with developing mastery in the outer world and ignoring the inner one. When we neglect the intuitive experience, it means people need to do remedial work later on."

So remedy the situation. Become the Columbus of your own inner voyage. It's time to take that compass we call intuition out of its cardboard box.

LUCID DREAMING

You're snug in your own bed, those familiar sheets and blankets secure around you. Except for some rapid eye movements, you're hardly stirring. But as far as you're concerned, you're positively flying beneath the covers. Powered solely by your own will, you glide effortlessly in the sky and only have to think "let's go higher" to do it. The colors swirling around you are so intense, you can feel them as well as see them. They seem to pulse.

Or maybe you're playing tennis on a "dream court," remembering with your body the grace and power of the pro you observed the other day. The racket and ball grow to feel like natural extensions of you. You play effortlessly, beautifully, gliding from one movement to the next.

Yes, you're dreaming. But what's amazing is you *know* you're dreaming. And knowing, you shape the outcome.

This state—the ability to be simultaneously aware of being asleep and experiencing a dream—is what dream researchers dub lucid dreaming. Dr. Stephen LaBerge of Stanford University estimates that one in ten people are naturals at lucid dreaming. If you're not part of that crowd, you can pick up the skill with a little practice and perseverance. Experienced lucid dreamers say it's well worth the effort. There's growing evidence that the benefits you experience in lucid dreams carry over into waking life.

"The dreams are more intense, more beautiful," says psychotherapist Ken Kelzer, who taught himself to lucid dream in 1980. When he first succeeded he says he felt "like I was entering a new land, like the Pilgrims must have felt when they first came to these shores. So many new and marvelous things waiting to be discovered. It's a beautiful paradise."

Sounds great. But is it for real? How is it possible to remain conscious during sleep?

Sleep Consciousness

Although German researcher Paul Tholey has been studying lucid dreams since 1959, Dr. LaBerge was the first to prove physiologically that it is possible to remain conscious during sleep. He'd been

481

482

having lucid dreams for years when he came up with a way to test whether they were actual dreams or just hallucinations.

It had been known since 1952 that dreaming sleep was accompanied by rapid eye movement (REM), which could be measured by electrodes taped near the sleeper's eyes. If the dreamer really was conscious, would it be possible, Dr. LaBerge mused, to indicate that to some outside observer using eye movements in a prearranged sequence? For several nights running in 1978, he hooked himself up to a polysomnograph, a machine that automatically monitors eye movements and other physiological signals. His plan? To move his eyes left-right, left-right, to indicate the start of a lucid dream.

Sure enough, when Dr. LaBerge scanned the polysomnograph records of his sleep, there, embedded among the slow electroencephalogram rhythms of deep sleep and the familiar REM ripples, were four large sweeping zigzags on the eye muscle channel. He was later able to train other lucid dreamers to signal with their eyes.

If lucid dreamers are able to control the eye movements that normally signal the dream state, does that mean that lucid dreams affect the body differently? Preliminary findings suggest that lucid dreaming is more like ordinary dreaming than waking, yet it's a more aroused state of sleep. Perhaps the most significant differences concern nightmares.

"If you're not aware you're dreaming, the whole body reacts to the fright," says Dr. Norbert Sattler, a German clinical psychologist who has been using lucid dreaming in his practice since the early 1970s. "With lucid dreams, you can observe the fright but not experience it with your body."

PRIVATE DREAMS, GROUP VISIONS

If you really want to mine your dreams for wisdom, there's nothing quite like a dream group to keep you on track. How to locate one? Check your local college or night school course listings, or the bulletin boards at area health food and inspirational bookstores.

If you can't find an ongoing group, start your own. A good book to consult for some no-nonsense guidelines to group work is *Working With Dreams,* coauthored by Dr. Montague Ullman and Nan Zimmerman.

Dr. Ullman, a psychiatrist, is convinced that people with no professional dream experience can be great dream coaches, provided they take the right approach. For him, that means the dreamer has complete control over the discussion and shares as little or as much as is comfortable. Group members are not allowed to analyze the dreamer or the dream. They can only comment on what feelings the dream creates for them, and what associations the dream images bring to mind. When the dynamics are right, the results can be dynamite.

What produces the images that you see in your dreams, researchers now think, are bursts of neural activity originating in the brain stem. Named PGO spikes for the areas of the brain they pass through—the pons, the lateral geniculate nucleus, and the occipital lobe of the cerebral cortex—the spikes travel along the same path as the light signals that the retina transmits to the cortex. The PGO spikes affect the cortex almost as if they came from the eyes, producing the images in our dreams.

What's fascinating, but not known, is where the images come from or why any particular image flashes on the dream screen at any given time. Even lucid dreamers don't maintain total control over the images they see; the element of surprise is always there. So is the emotional content. In fact, images alone don't create a nightmare. How you feel about those images determines whether you're uncomfortably frightened or just the star of your own, mildly amusing horror show. Your PGO spikes give you the pictures but something deeper determines your emotional response.

The PGO spikes are an integral part of the REM stage of sleep, which occurs as part of a fairly regular 80- to 90-minute sleep cycle. Most lucid dreams tend to occur during the last dream cycle of the morning, yet experienced lucid dreamers have been known to have several such dreams a night.

"As I get closer to the early morning, I find it's prime time for lucid dreaming," says Kelzer. "As we go deeper into the sleep phase, we are probably able to relax more physically and mentally, and the more we relax, the more we are able to create and maintain."

The Joys of Lucidity

Plenty of us do perfectly well without ever having a lucid dream. Are they really worth the effort it takes to create them?

That depends. Are you after what Kelzer terms a natural state of emotional pleasure and ecstasy? Or what Dr. Jane

Garfield, psychologist and dream expert, calls a heightened awareness, a sense of a greater reality....what one would imagine paradise to be like, glowing from within? Would you like a dream that showers you with sensations, other than merely visual ones, a dream where you can roll in silk or smell the forest after a spring rain? Or climax with a dream lover?

You can have all this and more, depending upon the degree of lucidity you develop.

What more can you accomplish? Greater mental and emotional health, as a result of better integrating the separate —and sometimes conflicting—aspects of your personality. More direct access to your personal power. Dr. Jayne Gackenbach, a psychologist at the University of Northern Iowa, found that the lucid dreamers among the Iowa population she studied even had higher self-esteem and superior physical balance, as measured on a Bongo Board, than nonlucid dreamers.

As Dr. Sattler explains: "Dreams tell us about some aspect of our being. What is it I want to take part in? What is happening in my life? The way we do this in dreams is in a more passive way. We're not aware of what's going on. But we can become a more active part of it.

"Lucid dreams can help us come to all the power that is in us," he continues. "You can overpower a nightmare. You can work in the moment, as dreams develop. It gives you a better understanding of what belongs to me, all of the dark sides."

Lucid dreams do "offer special opportunities for self-development," agrees Dr. Garfield. "The whole concept of having a kind of practice ground in which to test out behavior can be very useful to the

THE SENOI SECRET

The Senoi Indians, who have long fascinated dream researchers, seem to have perfected a way to shape their dreams to serve them.

Anthropologist Kilton Stewart studied these peace-loving and creative Malaysian aborigines in the 1930s and found that although Senoi children have nightmares just like other children, they learn to eliminate bad dreams by the time they reach adolescence. In their place, they substitute pleasurable life-affirming ones. Maybe the sleeper has a wonderful adventure with a friend. Maybe the dream generates solutions to problems or personal insight or offers some art object the dreamer can recreate—an original song, poem, dance, or design.

How do they do it? As soon as they're old enough to share their dreams, Senoi children are taught how to pattern them.

They learn to confront and conquer danger, advance toward maximum pleasure, and achieve a positive outcome.

Here's how to put their secret to work for you. Next time you wake up from a nightmare, tell yourself that the attacker is an aspect of you that you want to confront and conquer. If time permits, you can close your eyes and see yourself fighting back. Once you win, ask your attacker for a gift. If there's no time to redream the scene, remind yourself periodically of your intention to confront and conquer your dream enemy.

Similarly, if you have a pleasant dream, ask yourself how you could make it even better. Resolve to have that dream again, only next time, take it one better. You can practice this by intensifying the pleasurable parts of the dream in a daydream.

---

dreamer. Many of the people who work with me report changes in their tennis-playing ability if they practice those skills within a lucid dream. The trick is to think about the feeling. If you can recapture the sensation of freedom and sureness you had in a lucid dream, you can carry it over into your waking state."

In other words, what you can do with creative visualization, you can do even more effectively within lucid dreams, because things seem that much more real. "When you have a lucid dream, the nervous system is registering it very close to reality," says Dr. Garfield.

Author Your Dreams

Can anyone learn to lucid dream? If you're receptive to the idea and you truly want to have a lucid dream, chances are you're half way there. By all means, give yourself nightly pre-sleep suggestions that you *intend* to have a lucid dream.

Sometimes just learning that it's possible is enough to get you started. Dr. Garfield remembers a phone call she got the day after she did a radio show in the San Francisco Bay area:

"One of the people who called in said 'I heard what you said yesterday. I've been having this nightmare for years about driving off a cliff with my family and falling and getting killed. I told myself that if I have that dream again, I'd change the ending. Well, in the middle of my dream last night, I was getting close to the edge when I realized, oh . . . Dr. Garfield says I don't have to be afraid.' Sometimes," says Dr. Garfield, "it can happen that quickly."

But there are more systematic ways to cultivate lucid dreams. Lay the foundation by paying attention to ordinary dreams. Tell yourself you're going to remember them, and when you do, record them on paper or on tape. Milk them for meaning and appreciate what they yield. If some image keeps reoccurring, maybe a certain person or a specific animal, train yourself to ask, every time you see that object, whether or not you're dreaming.

Once your dreams get the idea you're paying attention, they'll start yielding even more. You'll know when this happens. This is the time to introduce specific techniques to induce lucidity.

One you might try is this Carlos Castaneda method Ken Kelzer used with success:

Relax deeply and clear your mind. Hold up both of your hands in front of you at arms length, focus on them in a detached kind of way, and repeat over and over to yourself: 'I see my hands in my dream, I know I am dreaming.' Then neutralize your gaze by focusing on a clear wall. Repeat the process five or six times at a stretch, several times a day.

If that doesn't feel right, try Dr. Sattler's technique. He advises his clients to question whether they're dreaming or awake. Check yourself a minimum of ten times a day, and be sure to do it at night just before you fall asleep.

"The main thing," he says, "is to adopt a critical view of your normal surroundings. Say, 'I want to find out if this is a dream or not. How did I come to this place?' If you train this way for a long time, the question surfaces in your dream."

You can also try to retain consciousness as you're falling asleep. Watch the pictures floating in front of your eyes and try to remember what that feels like, to be awake as you dream. Similarly, if you have time in the morning, try to redream the dream in a more pleasant way, as you drift back to sleep.

Above all, be patient. Dr. Sattler finds that clients who use his technique faithfully may take anywhere from two to four weeks to have their first lucid dreams. Until yours occurs, use your ordinary dreams to help you.

"Begin looking at the dream," says Dr. Garfield, "and say to yourself 'Now where in here could I have become lucid? What might I have noticed that's incongruous and could indicate it's a dream?' The most peculiar and unusual things are accepted as a matter of course in our dreams. The trick is to be attentive to the unusual."

Some of us seem to have our own internal prompters on this. Dr. Garfield still remembers a scriptwriter who took her lucid dreaming class years back. The dream was about a woman who had been in a well, but was coming out of it. Across the bottom of the dream script was an asterisk, with the words "we can assume she can breathe out of water!"

Zeroing In

"Prelucid" is the word dream researchers use to describe the dream state that hovers just at the edge of lucidity. If you've ever dreamed that you've awakened, or if you're dreaming that you're having a dream, or talking about your dreams, then you're almost there, says Dr. Gackenbach. "These are the experiences you tend to have first. When the lucid dream comes through, it will be quite clear you're having one. They're like nothing else."

You'll find that your lucid dreams differ from ordinary ones in several distinct ways, she says. Most obvious is that you know you're dreaming and you have waking recall. Beyond that, lucid dreams are realistic. You probably won't find yourself deep in conversation with a cow. There are likely to be only a few characters involved. And you'll find your senses are heightened. You may even experience what one writer calls synesthesia, the blending of sensory impressions. Meaning, you may be able to see sound waves as well as hear the sound. Or smell colors.

The characteristics build, as you become more and more aware in your dreams, says Dr. Gackenbach. "Do you have waking recall? Do you remember who you are, where you live? Can you successfully complete a task? You have control. Go and see somebody.

"With lucid dreams, there is a cognitive component. The rational, left hemisphere gets involved. You have auditory and kinesthetic experiences."

Getting Good

You've succeeded a couple of times to have just a snippet of a lucid dream. But the minute you realized you were dreaming, you lost it. Maybe you bolted

awake, from the excitement, or you slipped into a nonlucid state.

How do you control that, so you can give yourself enough time in the lucid dream to create the outcome you want?

"You have to control your emotions," says Dr. Gackenbach. "Say to yourself, 'I am dreaming. I am keeping my emotions subdued.' It's a real balancing act. Any excess and you seem to lose it."

"You need to maintain a slightly detached feeling and hold on to this awareness so you don't slip back into regular dreaming," adds Dr. Garfield. "Balancing yourself between these two states is very much like the focusing requirement in meditation."

Take It to the Limit

The neat thing about lucid dreams is that there's always a new threshold to cross. Have you learned to have them? Then learn to maintain the lucid state in your dreams for as long as you want it. Once you can hold on to the state, you can begin to experiment with its many possibilities and really have fun. Fly. Enjoy intimate encounters in a rain forest. Hike the Himalayan ranges.

Psychologist Judy Malamud believes that lucid dreamers advance through a certain progression as they get better at their skills.

"If you know you are dreaming, you know you are the creative source," she says. Then you realize that what you see is a self-reflective environment: that it actually reflects some aspect of your perception. You are experiencing an alternate reality that is not the same as the so-called objective world.

MILLION-DOLLAR DREAMS

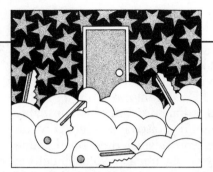

You never know. You can tell some people to "dream their way to success" and they'll take you literally.

Here are five people who did exactly that.

Conrad Hilton. When Hilton decided to buy the Stevens House, now the Chicago Hilton, he originally bid $165,000. But that morning he woke up with the number $180,000 firmly in mind. So he changed his bid. The next highest bid was $179,800.

Elias Howe. Elias Howe spent several years working out the invention of a lockstitch sewing machine. Originally, he put the thread hole in the middle of the needle, but he couldn't get the machine to work to his satisfaction. One night, he dreamed he was captured by a tribe of savages who took him prisoner before their king. The king commanded him "on the pain of death to finish the machine at once." But he couldn't. He was shaking with fear.

In the dream, dark-skinned and painted warriors surrounded Howe and led him to the place of execution. He looked at them and it struck him that the spears they carried had eye-shaped holes near the tip. He awoke in a fright, only to realize that if he threaded the needle through an eye-shaped hole near the tip, he'd get that lockstitch machine to work.

Otto Loewi. This winner of the 1936 Nobel prize in physiology or medicine discovered in a dream a way to prove his theory about the chemical transmission of nerve impulses. Seventeen years earlier, he had a hunch that nerve impulses had a chemical as well as electrical component. But he let the idea slide because he couldn't think of an experiment to prove it. One night in 1920, the hunch, and the design of an experiment to prove it, came to him in a dream. Loewi woke, scrawled something on a piece of paper, and fell back asleep. The next morning he couldn't decipher the scrawl.

The following night, the dream returned. Jarred awake, Loewi went immediately to the lab and did the experiment on a frog's heart. His results laid the foundation for future work in that area.

Robert Louis Stevenson. Plagued by nightmares into his early adulthood, Stevenson helped put himself to sleep by imaging pleasant stories. His dreams grew less frightening, and he began using them as the basis for stories, which he later sold. One story Stevenson created this way was "The Strange Case of Dr. Jekyll and Mr. Hyde." He had been trying in vain for two days to come up with a plot to illustrate an idea of his, and on the second night, he dreamed that Hyde, "pursued for some crime, took the powder and underwent the change in the presence of his pursuers."

Guiseppe Tartini. This composer, who is credited with the invention of the modern violin bow, had a dream as a 21-year-old that the devil had become his slave. In his dream, Tartini handed the devil his violin to see what he could do with it. He heard a sonata "of such exquisite beauty as surpassed the boldest flights of my imagination." Tartini awoke and tried to recapture what he could remember. The result? *The Devil's Sonata,* his best-known work.

488

Let's say that you dream about a Doberman pinscher who is straining against his leash in an effort to break free from it and sink his teeth into you. If you saw the dog in an ordinary dream, you'd probably run from it. If you see it in a lucid dream, in which you haven't developed much control, you may imagine yourself getting hold of a weapon you can use to defend yourself against the dog. Or getting into a car and speeding away.

As you become even more aware in your dreams, you may see that Doberman and realize you're only dreaming. The dog can bark and rattle his leash all he wants, but he can't hurt you. And if you're *really* lucid, you'll realize that Doberman represents something in you and you can ask the animal what it wants to tell you about yourself. Do you have a fear? A fear of whom or what? How can you resolve it?

"What I am ultimately aiming for is to get in touch with the part of the mind that creates life scripts, whether that's in the dream or waking life," says Malamud. "A part of you is creating the whole waking world of experience in your dreams.

You may begin to carry that over into your waking life as well.

"People can have mastery over the forces that threaten them in the imagination. It's a developmental process."

When Malamud lectures on lucid dreaming, or gives workshops, she always reminds her listeners to get in touch with the emotional content of their dreams. How did you like what you created? How did it make you feel? Is there another way to create what you created?

Eventually, say the people who study lucid dreams, the skill of making things happen, of looking for the most pleasing alternative, will help you feel freer to create positive situations for yourself during your waking hours.

"The state is so powerful it has an impact," says Kelzer, who speaks from experience. "There's an automatic carryover to the waking state."

"It goes both ways," adds Dr. Garfield. "What you're thinking about in the waking state affects dreams. Experiences in your dream state carries over into waking life."

TAPPING THE "WISE MAN" WITHIN

Channeling—allegedly, the practice of using the body as a conduit to transmit the wisdom of spiritual beings—is a source of rapidly rising interest. Substantial proof for this phenomenon is nonexistent. But one current theory suggests that when channelers go into a trance, they may connect, not with a supernatural being, but with a higher part of their own minds—sort of a wise companion within. What this means is that the "channeled" voice may be none other than the channeler's own subconscious talking. This part of the mind, psychologists say, has greater cognitive and creative powers than the conscious personality.

"There are many names for this other part of the mind," says Dr. Willis Harman, president of the Institute of Noetic Sciences in California. "Some call it the supraconscious, while others label it the true self or the hidden observer. We all have it and occasionally hear from it. But for the most part, it lies suppressed deep within the subconscious."

Observing the Hidden Observer

Professor Ernest Hilgard of Stanford University discovered signs of this hidden observer during his famous ice-bucket experiment, Dr. Harman explains. Hilgard hypnotized a subject, then made a hypnotic suggestion that the man's left hand was perfectly comfortable when in fact the hand was immersed in a bucket of crushed ice and cold water. When asked how his hand felt, the subject replied that it was fine. Then, Hilgard put a pencil into the subject's right hand and asked him to write something. The subject protested, "Ouch, it hurts."

"Hilgard deduced from this that there is a hidden observer in the mind that isn't fooled by hypnotic suggestion and is available to make its observations known if you want to tease them out," says Dr. Harman.

In his book *Higher Creativity*, Dr. Harman provides us with a hidden observer

490

scenario we can all relate to. It happens at night when we're asleep. "Cars zoom by outside. A siren wails in the distance, and the person sleeping next to you is snoring like a chain saw. Nothing seems to wake you. Suddenly, a door creaks open downstairs and you're out of bed like a shot. That noise was four times softer than anything else going on, but that part of your mind that watches over you picked it out as possible trouble and woke you."

This observer is only one manifestation of your true self. "The true self is in fact your real creative center," says Dr. Harman. "When an executive follows a hunch or when an artist creates a truly great work, he or she is reaching into that hidden territory."

But why does the true self remain hidden? "Psychotherapy holds that the ordinary self fears being thrown out of the driver's seat by the real self," says Dr. Harman. Or it may be that your ordinary self fears your true potential. Realizing our greater potential means change and more responsibility. So we keep the true self locked up in the unconscious.

Why the true or higher self seems to have much greater cognitive and creative abilities than the ordinary self is a matter for speculation. Perhaps the ordinary self acts as a buffer, allowing information to pass through while shielding the true self from the distractions and emotional stomachaches of daily life. The true self then comes to its conclusions unfettered by ego-based prejudices.

Whatever the workings, being on speaking terms with your inner self has many benefits. Rather than passively waiting for that flash of intuition or insight,

wouldn't it be nice to call on your inner self whenever you need to?

A Direct Line

"Two possible routes to take are active relaxation and guided imagery," suggests Dr. Harman. "Both help to quiet the outer static of the ordinary self and the world around you so that you can hear what your inner self has to say."

To evoke the relaxation response, four things are necessary: a quiet environment, a comfortable position to eliminate distractions, a mental device to calm the storm of stray thoughts whirling inside your head, and a passive attitude to allow interesting things to happen.

The mental device, called a mantra in Eastern religions, can be secularized by choosing any one-syllable sound. "You can even use the word 'one' as your chosen sound," suggests Dr. Harman. Allow your mind to work through any thoughts at hand, then, as it begins to quiet, introduce the mantra. Repeat the word over and over to yourself. If other thoughts drift into your consciousness, don't fight them. Allow them to happen, then gradually refocus your mind on your chosen one-syllable word.

As you relax and your conscious self quiets down, your inner self can come forward and may share some valuable insight with you. If your inner voice is a little timid at first, don't despair. Just try again.

When *Prevention* editor Mark Bricklin wants to gain a little insight into a particular problem, he uses guided imagery to meet up with the wise old man. "Take 10 minutes to get into a relaxed state. Then close your eyes and picture yourself on a dirt path winding through a thick, green forest," suggests Bricklin. "Walk the path until just up ahead you see an old man standing there."

Imagine that this is the wisest man in the world. Walk up to him and ask him a question concerning any problem you have. You may be surprised at the answer. "Interestingly enough, I find that sometimes he'll answer my question with another question," says Bricklin. "That gets me thinking in a whole new direction. I start seeing my problem in a different light."

Both techniques take practice to achieve results. Once you master the process, however, try consulting your inner wise man regularly. You may begin to notice that you like the decisions you're making. In fact, don't be surprised when they seem to fit so well with your true desires, plans, and needs. After all, who knows what you want better than your true self.

M. G.

HOW TO HAVE
A MYSTICAL EXPERIENCE

Mystical experiences are not necessarily extraordinary events that happen only to extraordinary people such as dedicated meditators or peyote eaters. You may deliberately induce a mystical state by paying attention to subtle feelings and ideas lying just beneath the layers of everyday awareness. That is what mystics and gurus have been telling people for thousands of years. Quite simply, begin to notice — in a nonjudgmental way — how you talk about your life, rationalize your behavior, explain the world around you. By shifting your awareness from mundane concerns and temporarily suspending your "belief systems," you may be more ready to experience life from the vantage point of the sage. You may even feel connected to something greater than yourself. Your rigid concept of time will probably dissolve into a sense of timelessness, blurring the distinctions between past, present, and future.

To achieve a subtle shift in perspective and induce a mystical experience without dramatically altering your way of life, you may find it helpful to practice the following exercises. Proceed at your own pace; practice when you're sober, you feel emotionally relaxed, and when you won't be interrupted. *Warning:* Because these exercises are designed to challenge the sense you have of yourself and of reality, we recommend that you check with your doctor if you feel uncertain about your ability to handle them. If you have a history of psychiatric problems, consult your therapist or psychiatrist. You may terminate any exercise whenever you like and complete it later. Even though these exercises are intended to be practiced alone, you may adapt them for small groups. Some exercises are designed to be practiced during the holiday season, a time when you usually feel more open to other people and more willing to look at your life from a new point of view.

■ Exercise 1: Imagine

■ Objective

To understand who you've become (your identity) by pretending your memo-

492

ries are merely a product of your imagination; to ask yourself, "Is there a more basic and immutable part of my identity beneath the superficial roles I assume? Is there some aspect of my life—a particular experience or another person—that is impossible to imagine as an illusion?

Setting

Choose a place where you're completely alone for a couple of hours. (You also may practice this exercise if you're alone among a group of strangers—on an airplane or in a movie theater.)

Instructions

1. Sit in a comfortable chair, close your eyes, and take a deep breath. As you continue to breathe slowly, let your life pass before you: childhood events, adolescent experiences, major life accomplishments or mistakes, memories of family members and friends. Don't become analytical about past relationships or get stuck on particular experiences. Just let your impressions come and go. How does it feel to be the person you've become?

2. Take another deep breath. As you exhale, concentrate on how alone you are at this moment. Pay attention to your physical environment and your body's sensations. Continue to breathe slowly.

3. Now imagine that your present situation and immediate surroundings represent the whole of reality. Everything you remember about the world and your life, the people and events in it, is imaginary. In fact, you've just come into existence in the past few moments.

If you are surrounded by strangers, imagine that they are also experiencing their lives as an illusion.

Benefits

With regular practice you may begin to experience everyday reality in a different way—not as boring, habitual, or conflicted. You may feel freer to consider more satisfying careers, start creative projects, or ask potentially threatening questions like, "What do I want out of life?" Ask yourself, "Who might I be if all I remember about my life is an illusion?"

Exercise 2: The Ghost of Christmas Past

Objective

To transcend the restrictions imposed by our limited concept of time and to communicate with the child you once were.

Setting

Choose a spot that was important to you as a child during the holiday season—a church, an attic room, or possibly the home of a favorite relative.

Instructions

1. Take a few moments to remember how you felt when you first visited this place as a child. Let go of your adult perspective. Concentrate on your worldview as a child. What questions were important to you at that time? Maybe you felt misunderstood and secretly wished for a wise grown-up friend to answer your questions.

2. Focus on your childhood feelings until you identify feelings you had as a child that you've continued to experience as a adult.

3. Now imagine that time does not exist and that you can communicate directly with your childhood self. Exchange viewpoints with each other: As the adult, share with the child what the adult now knows about life; as the child, tell the adult about the child's aspirations, desires, and goals — things the adult may have forgotten.

4. Complete this exercise by giving a present to the child. Ask the child what he or she would like — a toy or a trip to the zoo or an amusement park.

Benefits

The child's insights may help soften the hardened or jaded parts of your adult personality. The adult point of view may help resolve conflicted childhood feelings. You also may experience sensations of timelessness, as though you somehow exist simultaneously as a child and an adult. Some of the distinction between past and present may begin dissolving.

Exercise 3: Back to the Future

Objective

To transcend the restrictions imposed by our limited concept of time and connect with whom you'll become in the future.

Setting

Return to the location you chose to practice Exercise 2. For this exercise,

however, you must contract with yourself to go back to this place at some point in the future. The exact date may be left open, or you may want to specify a particular time, say, on New Year's Eve in five years. You may use this spot anytime as psychologically sacred ground, a place to reflect on your present life from the vantage point of the future.

Instructions

1. Take a few moments to think about your current problems. Are you dissatisfied with your job? Unhappy in a relationship? Afraid to try something new? Don't analyze your problems — just let them float by you.

2. Now imagine you're at this spot in the future, reviewing your present concerns with the experience you've gained in the intervening years. Ask your future self to talk to you about your current problems.

Benefits

If you feel frustrated about your present situation, the insights you receive from your future self may help alleviate some of your tension or unhappiness; you will be less likely to feel stuck because you're willing to look at your life from a future perspective. You also may experience sensations of timelessness, which may begin to loosen your rigid concept of time.

Exercise 4: Silent Nights

Objective

To spend a weekend in silence.

Setting

Stay at home, go camping, or rent a cabin near a lake or forest—far away from civilization. If you choose to remain at home, don't watch television or listen to the radio. Unplug the phone.

Instructions

1. Set aside an entire weekend, preferably during the holiday season, to be silent. Don't talk to anyone.

2. To avoid embarrassing situations, explain your plans to a friend and ask your confidant to be your interpreter.

3. If you remain at home and need to go out, don't cross the street to avoid meeting a friend. If necessary, your interpreter will explain what is happening. Don't use a pen and paper to write messages.

Benefits

Self-imposed silence will allow you to feel both the joys and restrictions of verbal communication. You'll probably experience a flood of emotions varying from frustration to euphoria because you will be completely alone with your thoughts and feelings. Notice the way people respond to you when they realize you "cannot" talk.

Exercise 5:
Perchance to Dream

Objective

To induce a mystical experience by depriving yourself of sleep. (*Warning:* You must be stable both physically and psy-

chologically to practice this exercise. If you have any reservations, check with your doctor.)

Setting

Home.

Instructions

1. Remain awake for at least 24 hours. To conserve your energy, don't engage in strenuous physical activity.

2. Use the time when you would be asleep to write letters or Christmas cards or to prepare new dishes for holiday meals. If you choose activities you enjoy, your attentions will be diverted from thinking about the sleep you are missing.

3. After a couple of hours, find a comfortable place to sit and look directly at an illuminated watch or clock that has a second hand. Dim the lights and then watch the clock for a while.

4. Take a deep breath and think of a significant event that you're really looking forward to. Estimate the number of days before the event happens. Then count the hours, minutes, and seconds before this event occurs. Take another deep breath. Watch the second hand sweep around the clock—seconds quickly add up to minutes, and the minutes add up to hours.

Benefits

Sleep deprivation often induces a sense of intense objectivity, as though you were observing your experiences from a distance. When you see yourself in such a way, you may feel free to question your identity or the roles you play in a non-threatening manner.

Sleep deprivation also may induce déjà vu experiences in which unfamiliar situations seem oddly familiar. But there's no rational explanation for your feelings. If you experience déjà vu during sleep deprivation, don't try to figure out why the experience seems familiar. Imagine that you've really been "here" at another time. Indulge yourself in the fantasy and see what happens.

When you watch time in the way you have done in this exercise, you may begin to appreciate its subjective quality and realize that our perception of time is largely based on cultural traditions. As the hours pass, your sense of time may begin to change. Your internal focus of attention affects your subjective experience of time.

Exercise 6: Grand Central

Objective

To understand the ways in which you are simultaneously radically different from and very similar to other people.

Setting

Pick a crowded location such as a busy airport, bus terminal, or train station. Spend a day sitting in one place observing people come and go during the holiday season. If you don't have the time or patience to sit for a day, try to spend a couple of hours watching the crowds pass by.

Instructions

1. Notice the stationary objects in your environment—benches, vending machines, newsstands, restaurants, coffeehouses.

2. Watch the moving crowd and the coming and going of buses, trains, airplanes, taxicabs. After an hour you'll probably begin to notice patterns of motion and activity that at first seemed to move in a random way.

3. As you watch the people, consider the possibility that no one around you perceives reality in the exact same way. Pick out a stranger, and compare your reality to his reality. Don't dwell on the superficial differences between you, such as physical appearance, racial identity, and cultural background, but consider how differently the two of you perceive the world. Your belief—I share the same reality with this stranger—may be an illusion. Ask yourself, for example, if you have any way of knowing if the two of you perceive the color red the same way.

4. Relax, take a deep breath, and turn your attention back to your general surroundings. Now consider what you have in common with the people you're watching: You're all alive during this moment in human history; your lives have crossed paths even if at a comfortable distance.

Benefits

It takes only an unexpected shift in circumstances—a terrorist attack, an earthquake, a fire—to tighten the loose connections that bind you to the people around you. In such circumstances many individual differences can quickly disappear, and people see what they have in common with one another. But you do not have to share a traumatic experience to induce a sense of camaraderie. Picture yourself and the strangers you're watching as a single group, one entity moving without individual perceptions. You probably will feel closer to the people around you. At the same time, when you consider the possibility that your perception of reality is unique, you may get a dramatic clue to your own identity. Ask yourself: If I'm alone in the way I perceive reality, what do my perceptions tell me about who I am? Repeat this question to yourself until its meaning sinks in.

Exercise 7:
Singular Sensation

Objective

To experience all of reality as unified and not as a collection of disparate objects.

Setting

Choose any ordinary surrounding— your favorite chair at home, a park bench, a beach. Make sure you feel relaxed.

Instructions

1. Focus on some common object in your immediate environment such as a candy dish, a seashell, a leaf. Make certain that the object is close to you.

2. Take a deep breath and concentrate on the object until it's all you see or think about. As you exhale, consider the fact that a candy dish, for example, is just a receptacle. Depending on its function, it could be an incense burner or an ashtray.

3. Imagine what its structure might be like on the molecular or quantum

level. If you and the object are composed of the same basic particles, perhaps you are not as different from the object as you imagined.

Benefits

Mystics claim that all reality is unified. It might be helpful to experience reality, if only for a few fleeting moments, from this alternate perspective.

Exercise 8:
The Daily News

Objective

To achieve a sense of identity with the rest of humanity.

Setting

Living room.

Instructions

1. Spend at least two weeks avoiding contact with television news, newspapers, or magazines. Even though you will hear bits of news or see an occasional headline, you probably will begin to feel disconnected from events in the world.

2. After two weeks, choose an evening to watch the 11 o'clock news. Turn off all the lights. Sit far enough away from the TV so you maintain a sense of distance and objectivity. Turn off the sound on the television. Your goal: to concentrate on the images, not on the commentators' interpretations.

3. Watch the facial expressions of the male and female anchors who report

497

the day's events. Are their facial expressions appropriate in light of the images they present? Do they smile as they introduce stories accompanied by violent images or tragic scenes? How much of the news is upbeat? How much is an accounting of the day's misfortunes around the world? Pay particular attention to the sequence of news stories and to the commercials that are interspersed between the various reports.

4. Continue this exercise on a nightly basis for about ten days sitting in the dark, watching the news with the sound turned off. You may interrupt your periods of silent observation with additional news blackouts to help you maintain objectivity and a sense of distance.

Benefits

Ask yourself how your view of the world and your understanding of human nature are influenced by regular exposure to these images. Don't judge the motives of the reporters, but imagine you're an alien from another planet observing human behavior for the first time. What are you learning?

Exercise 9: Trading Places

Objective

To trade places mentally with a dog, cat, canary, or animal in the zoo.

Setting

Home or the zoo.

Instructions

1. Relax and sit in front of the animal so that you can easily look into each other's eyes. Make sure the animal feels secure with you.

2. Take a deep breath. As you slowly exhale, look into the animal's eyes, and imagine that a part of your awareness is being transmitted through your breath into the animal's mind. Watch the animal breathe, and imagine that a part of its awareness is being transmitted into your mind.

3. Continue looking directly into the animal's eyes until you can feel your consciousness merge with the animal's consciousness.

4. If you feel comfortable merging with a domestic animal, then try to merge with an animal at the zoo.

Benefits

As the boundaries between you and the animal dissolve, you may feel as if you've really traded places with a member of another species, as though a part of you has become the animal—this is the height of subjective merging. You may begin to feel more compassion for other species. You'll also probably recognize some of the artificial difference between the human and animal worlds.

Exercise 10: Big Sky

Objective

To help you reflect on the past year and prepare for the year to come.

Setting

Find a comfortable spot where you can see the sky on New Year's Eve.

Instructions

1. At midnight, relax and look up at the constellations. Remember that people have viewed these same constellations for millions of years and that these same constellations will be visible long after you have died. Consider that people around the world can watch the same star patterns.

2. As you watch the sky, review your past year, and imagine what the new year will be like.

3. Continue to watch the constellations and think about some distant place you would like to visit. Ask yourself how these same constellations would look above that location. Imagine that you're already there in that place, looking up at the same pattern of stars. Continue drifting back and forth between locales until you're in both locations at the same time.

Benefits

The grandeur and immensity of the night sky will probably induce a sense of wonder at the world and a serene acceptance of your place in it, a prerequisite for any positive changes you may want to make in your life. As you travel back and forth between locales, the limitations of space and time seem less important. You may look ahead ten years without worrying about whether you'll be satisfied with

your life—you've already begun to accept your past and what that makes you. You're now open to influencing your future in a positive way.

Exercise 11: A Room with a View

Objective

To induce a sense of objectivity about your life and a feeling of connectedness to the rest of the cosmos.

Setting

A quiet, dark, and secluded spot from which you can clearly observe the constellations.

Instructions

1. Stand with your head turned slightly upward, your legs slightly apart, and your hands at your sides. Take a deep breath and concentrate on a particular star in your favorite constellation.

2. Imagine the star as a point of consciousness in space, as though the center of your forehead and the star were connected by invisible lines of force.

3. When you feel connected to the star, imagine that you are a constellation composed of individual stars located at different points all over your body.

4. Take another deep breath, and as you exhale, imagine that your body is dissolving. Only the stars marking your overall shape remain.

5. As you continue slowly inhaling and exhaling, imagine that the stars marking out your shape mirror the positions of the stars in the constellation you are viewing—as if the constellation is a reflection of yourself. With a little more imagination, you may become a reflection of the constellation. Alternately, imagine that you're on Earth looking up at the constellation and that you're in space looking back at Earth.

Benefits

By developing the ability to let go of your physical form and look back at your life on Earth, you may begin to look at your life from an objective distance, reducing stress and gaining insights into your place in the universe. Seen from space, your life may seem insignificant in relation to the rest of the cosmos, but remember: You're connected to some larger reality represented by the constellation. Everyday experience then may seem to take on much greater significance to you.

Exercise 12: Urban Renewal

Objective

To experience the relationship between your personal life and the lives of people in the past and the future.

Setting

The demolition site of a condemned building, followed by the site of a building under construction.

Instructions

1. Position yourself at a safe distance from the demolition site, and observe the building as it is being slowly torn down.

2. Imagine how permanent the building must have seemed to the people who once lived there. Pay attention to the relationship between the different floors and rooms. Don't they seem close to one another once the outer walls are gone? Think about all the people who have lived in the building, their worldviews, occupations, even the activities and conversations carried on in the building.

3. Go immediately to visit the site of a building that is currently under construction. Consider that the workers are not merely constructing another structure but are creating a reality for those who will live or work in the new building. Who will live here? What will they say to one another?

4. Make an agreement with yourself to explore the interior of the new building once it is completed. When you explore the finished building, imagine that you really are leaving a mental trace of your own experiences there for future generations to think about.

Benefits

By experiencing some of the ways in which even the most seemingly constant aspects of your environment may be only a temporary part of a particular time in history, you may feel less confined by your assumptions about everyday reality or the immediate worldviews of those around you. By realizing that nothing is permanent, you may also be more willing to risk making positive changes in your life.

Road to Somewhere

These exercises are like seeds you plant and eagerly wait to sprout. Some of these exercises may not affect you; others probably will. There is no guarantee you will have a mystical experience. But if you practice them, you probably will become aware of feelings, thoughts, and questions about your place in the universe —the subtle stuff we ignore daily or are not even conscious of. You cannot change what you will not accept or even look at about yourself—and that willingness to scrutinize yourself is the peephole to an altered state of consciousness, a mystical view of life.

FIVE DAYS
OF SERENITY FOR $575

Flying into Monterey Airport, my mind was filled with doubts even as my eyes enjoyed the natural splendor of the California coastline from a 3,000-foot vantage point. Here I was, a somewhat uptight, East-Coast homeboy about to be dropped for a five-day course at what has come to be known as the granddaddy of the whole West Coast, hot tubbin', New Age scene: the Esalen Institute.

My flight from Pennsylvania was just long enough for me to work up a healthy dose of both respect and uneasiness concerning this assignment. On the one hand, since its birth in 1961, the Esalen Institute has played host to some of the most respected names in psychology and the human potential movement. Abraham Maslow, B. F. Skinner, Fritz Perls, Buckminster Fuller, and Aldous Huxley are just a few of the heavyweights who have come to Esalen to teach, write, or to simply enjoy the ambience. On the other hand, magazine articles that covered Esalen during the 1960s and 1970s hinted at a cosmic factor that made me wonder just how many times I'd have to use the words "life force," "karma," and "self-actualization" before I hit my native turf again.

Esalen is situated about an hour south of Monterey. By the time I got there, not only had my doubts evaporated, but I was fairly sure that if Heaven had a highway, it must look a lot like the one I had just driven down. On my right was the ocean, heaving itself against the solitary cliffs and washing up along unpeopled beaches that have never seen a T-shirt shop or Tastee-Freez stand. Sea lions played in the surf. To the left were mountains, mysterious mountains that gradually disappeared into the morning mist like a whisper. No matter what your state of mind is as you leave the airport, you'll show up at the gates of Esalen as I did: wide-eyed with wonder.

At the main office, I picked up a room key and found out where my group was meeting that evening. I was signed up for Big Sur Wilderness Experience, one of four programs being offered that particular week. All I knew about it was that it had something to do with hiking and was being run by a Steven Harper.

Having dispensed with the formalities, I checked out my room. To be honest, I had been prepared for something less than a Hilton suite and more like a Boy Scout camp cabin. But in fact the room was very comfortable, and the wooden walls and skylight made for a mellow, contemplative space. A thoughtful hand had laid some wildflowers on the bed and stocked a small dish on the dresser with incense. A bowl of ripe apples gave a final touch to the gently welcoming atmosphere.

Strolling around the grounds, the first thing I noticed was a sense of leisurely freedom. Here and there, people dotted the thick, spongy lawn eating their lunches and gazing out over the ocean. Beneath a tree, a woman sat cross-legged playing a flute while, up near the dining room, two young men were running at each other, furiously butting chests and laughing as they fell to the ground. Nowhere did I see that vacationer's desperate need to have fun or die trying. There was no rush here.

That first night, I met my group, and as we spent the evening getting acquainted, I began to realize that these people were not the flower-children-grown-up refugees of the 1960s I had so fondly imagined they would be. Our international contingent consisted of Anna from Spain, Sebastian from the Canary Islands, and Sylvan from Quebec. Among the rest of the group, there were three fun-loving and boisterous women from the Baltimore area; a psychoanalyst from Virginia Beach; a public relations exec from Woodstock, New York; and an actor from Santa Monica. Including myself and Steve, the leader, we made a comfortable group of 13. And the diversity of the group was mirrored in each person's reason for being there. Some just liked to hike, others had heard about Esalen and were curious. On the whole, a friendly, likable, and well-grounded bunch. And yet, as we went around the room, our spoken expectations seemed to secretly hint at just a little more than a hike in the woods. I think we had all come to see a bit of Esalen magic, to have an *experience*.

The Cosmos in Small Bites

The experience started almost immediately as Steve began guiding us through a few little exercises. "Focus on your breathing," he directed. "What is the quality of attention you are willing to give to your breath?" To be honest, I give more attention to old "Star Trek" reruns than to my breathing, and even in the short few minutes we practiced, I found my mind wandering.

"If your mind wanders, it's okay," said Steve reassuringly. "Each time it happens, gently encourage it back to the business of breathing. There's no need for force." He also suggested thinking the word "in" on the intake and "out" as we exhaled. Believe it or not, this simple technique worked better for me than the most exotic mantra or visual imagery. The multitude of distracting little worries, details, and thoughts usually floating around in my head seemed to evaporate as I matched my breathing to the words "in" and "out."

Simplicity seemed to be the byword in all the techniques Steve offered. We were neither expected nor encouraged to swallow the cosmos in one bite. I found that the more I immersed myself in the simple, the richer and more multi-hued it

503

504

became. Little rituals we performed became magical. My favorite was the way we began our hikes in the morning. All of us would gather at the entrance to a wilderness area and enjoy a moment of silence that ended with a deep bow to the woods. As we acknowledged the woods and made a respectful gesture toward them, I found myself, for the first time, recognizing the woods as alive, as having a personality. Through the entire hike, that feeling never left me, and the forest became slightly enchanted. At the end of each hike, we bowed once more in thanks for the experience. Maybe this ritual sounds just a little precious, but try it for yourself the next time you go hiking and see if it doesn't make a difference.

As for the hikes themselves, each was a perfect little 4- to 5-mile package, well within the capabilities of our group, which ranged in age from the midtwenties to the midfifties. But the mountainous terrain did ensure a sensible aerobic workout. Each morning, we'd assemble after breakfast, divvy up the food to stash in our daypacks, and drive to one of the many state parks that comprise almost all of the Big Sur area. On the trail, Steve was a treasure trove of nature information as he pointed out various miniecosystems, unusual plant life, and even sites that marked previous habitation by the Essalen Indians, a tribe now extinct. Steve's love for the wilderness was reflected in his careful instructions on how to leave the woods as we found them.

The trails we took led us through the most diverse landscape I'd ever seen. One day we climbed a mountain and emerged into sunlight above a low-lying fog. The next, we strolled along a deserted beach.

In between were redwood forests, grassy glens, amazing views of rolling hillsides, and a waterfall or two. There were moments when I was amazed at how silently a group of 13 could pass through the woods.

Back by late afternoon, our time was our own to enjoy the pool or the famous natural hot springs and then have dinner and a glass of wine in the dining hall. After dinner, our group would meet for a couple of hours to try new exercises, talk, or make up ridiculous (incredibly ridiculous!) stories concerning the ghost of Esalen. We also learned about something Steve called the hara. It's the center of a person's energy, as well as the body's center of gravity, and it lies deep within the belly. By letting awareness sink into your belly and then performing physical action from this center, Steve showed us how our movements become more stable, fluid, and, in general, more effective. To focus awareness, we might need to give ourselves a few pats on the stomach and emit the same low grunts one hears from sumo wrestlers as they take their stance. Many times there was as much laughter as grunting, which was fine by me. I tend to change the channel when things get too dogmatic.

Afloat in a Circle of Trust

The last night at Esalen was something special. Steve had gotten an herbalist to prepare a large hot tub with many and varying plants. When we arrived, the tub was surrounded by candles with flowers floating on the water. Believe it or not, we then proceeded to rub each other down with baking soda, rock salt, and cornmeal, taking quick showers between applications. If you've never tried this, be advised it turns your skin into silk.

Then it was into the hot tub where we formed a circle. In the center of our circle, we all took turns being floated on our backs, supported by 12 sets of hands while everyone else chanted and hummed to beat the band. It was one of the best experiences of my life. As I came up out of the circle, I couldn't help laughing out loud and thinking about how much I actually trusted this group of strangers I hadn't known a week ago. I felt that with these people I could do or say anything I wanted without feeling foolish. What really suprised me was that try as I would, I couldn't remember the last time I had felt this way.

Driving back up Route 1 toward the airport and reality the next day, I tried to figure out exactly what Esalen was. A retreat? A classroom? A New Age playground for adults? Then something Steve said came back to me. He'd called it a laboratory, and I think I was just beginning to understand what he had meant. Esalen is a place where you can research and make discoveries about yourself in an environment that acts as a catalyst to the process. Inherent abilities we all possess to enjoy ourselves, the people around us, and our world are just a few experiments away from being released in a place like this.

■

M. G.

(*Editor's Note:* Five-day programs at Esalen cost approximately $575 and include room and board. For more information concerning the Esalen Institute or for a catalog of upcoming courses and seminars, write to Esalen Institute, Big Sur, CA 93920.)

INDEX

Page references in *italic* indicate tables.

A

Absorbing Power (of nutrients), *72*
Acetylcholine, 469
Acting, *392-93*
Activities, determining form of, 397-99
Activity, sleep and, 198
Activity and rest cycle, 230
Acupressure, 243-44, 257. *See also* Shiatsu
    Jin Shin Do Bodymind, 281-83
Acupuncture, 243
Adenosine, 81
Adolescents, 178, 299
Adventure, high-risk, *392-93*
Advice, giving, *392-93*
Aerobics, 15
Affairs, extramarital, 346
Aging. *See also* Elderly
    meditation to slow, 221
    memory loss and, 30, 31, 32
    mental abilities and, 408-10
    reaction time and, 413
Air filters, 460
Air pollution
    in cities, 434-35
    in home, 464-65
    in workplace, 456, 458
Alcohol, 63-64, 84-87
Alcoholism, imagery and, 276-77
Alertness, sleep and, 241
Alexander, F. M., 189, 245-46, 257

Alexander Technique, 189, 245-46, 257
Allergies, 47
Altruism, 111-20, 179-82
Alzheimer's disease, treatment of, 31
Ambitions, fulfilled late in life, 407-8, 409
Anger, 178, 362-63
Angina pectoris, 159
Animals, trading places with, exercise to
    experience, 498
Antibodies, 166
Anxiety. *See also* Stress
    anticipatory, 176-77
    coping with, 176-77
    memory affected by, 33
    muscle relaxation and, 201
    music to reduce, 284
    therapeutic poems to reduce, 308
Aptitude tests, 398
Architecture, physical reaction to, 423
Arguments, how to stop, 348
Aromatherapy, 247-48
Art, physical reaction to, 423
Arthritis, rheumatoid, 237
Association, memory improved by, 36-37
Associations, 399-400
Attention, memory aided by, 31, 32
Attention deficit disorders (ADD), 471
Attitude, 216-17, 226-27
Attractiveness, perception of personality based
    on, 110

Rodale Press, Inc., publishes PREVENTION, America's leading health magazine.
For information on how to order your subscription,
write to PREVENTION, Emmaus, PA 18098.